# The End of an Antibiotic Era

Rinke van den Brink

# The End of an Antibiotic Era

## Bacteria's Triumph over a Universal Remedy

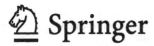 Springer

Rinke van den Brink
Dutch Broadcasting Foundation (NOS)
Hilversum, The Netherlands

ISBN 978-3-030-70722-4          ISBN 978-3-030-70723-1    (eBook)
https://doi.org/10.1007/978-3-030-70723-1

Based on a translation from the Dutch language edition: *Het einde van de antibiotica* by Rinke van den Brink, © De Geus 2013. All Rights Reserved.

Illustration by Stephen Sewell

This Springer imprint is published by the registered company Springer Nature Switzerland AG.
The registered company address is: Gewerbestrasse 11, 6330 Cham, Switzerland

# Preface

**"Imagine there is a fire in your house"**

*Imagine that there is a fire in your house, a fire that started in the roof-top apartment. Who would not start helping to stop the fire, knowing that it could reach your apartment too. Nobody would ever think that closing all doors and windows and ignoring the apartment on fire would be helpful. Nobody would ever think that reducing the amount of water and resources for the top floor apartment would be helpful.*

However, it seems that nowadays we do have the latter behavior in Europe with respect to infectious diseases.

The ongoing COVID-19 pandemic shows that in Europe a coordinated action to control SARS-CoV-2 is lacking. The common goal to stop this pandemic would mean to control the fire in one region or country before it reaches another. Each country is solely responsible for its own prevention, but we see that this is not enough to protect all Europeans. European regions where hotspots are starting need massive financial and infrastructural support from the European Union (EU). Furthermore, the strategy needs to be the same, but at different time points during the pandemic, different measures need to be taken by different European regions within the member states. The COVID-19 pandemic shows in a rapid crisis what has been visible for more than two decades with respect to the very topic in this book, antimicrobial resistance (AMR).

We can also imagine that the fire in the house stands for multidrug-resistant organisms (MDRO), such as methicillin-resistant *Staphylococcus aureus* (MRSA), vancomycin-resistant *Enterococcus faecium* (VRE), carbapenem-resistant *Enterobacteriaceae* (CRE), and many others, and that the above-described house is the EU. All those MDROs have reached the hospitals within our EU and are spreading within and between those hospitals. While we mainly continue to describe the problem, compare countries with each other, and wonder about the extreme differences in prevalence, others believe that the sole production of new antimicrobial agents will extinguish the fire.

Instead, we should start implementing a plethora of different prevention activities at all levels of healthcare within all European countries to successfully combat the fire. We should begin with mutual and multidisciplinary collaboration following the real-life transmission routes. But this would require an increased European awareness to those measures.

With regard to the prevention of AMR and the prevalence of MDRO, some countries are considered to be a very good example for other countries, at least in Europe. The Netherlands and Scandinavian countries for example are at the forefront of low MDRO prevalence for centuries. However, since 2010, also the Netherlands registers large outbreaks of VRE (mainly VRE-*vanB*). The problem is that introduction of VRE is often across the border from neighboring countries. A few years ago, Germany decided not to isolate any patients solely colonized with VRE anymore. This is mainly due to the fact that the German healthcare system does not easily facilitate infection control measures such as isolations, due to the simple fact that the remuneration of hospitals is based upon the use of the hospital beds and the few single-bed rooms. The more beds are used, the higher the income. The Dutch system is based on the principle that you do not get automatically more when admitting and treating more patients. Moreover, and most importantly, Dutch hospitals only need to use 50–60% of their bed capacity in order to get their full funding. This means that isolation measures are facilitated in one and jeopardized in the other system, two systems that are present in two countries sharing a border with each other.

This means that we need to take a closer look at the real and underlying factors, for example, the factors of a healthcare system that drive citizens to become patients more frequently, the number of doctors, and the risk of exposure to healthcare, doctors, pharmaceuticals, and in consequence antibiotics. Interestingly, the use of antibiotics is often not presented independently from the use of other pharmaceuticals or with regard to the workforce; usual statistics only show how many nurses per inhabitants work in a country, whereas it would be preferable to see how many nurses per admitted patients work per country or healthcare institution.

Recent data showed that in most European countries inter-regional transmission of MDRO is already ongoing, and in several Southern and Eastern European countries an endemic level has been reached for certain MDROs. At the same time, countries such as Germany let VRE spread within and between hospitals in the whole of the country, leading to major outbreaks and to an increase in prevalence. Allowing VRE to spread will open the door for other microorganisms that take similar transmission routes, such as CRE. Next to being an MDRO on its own, especially with the increased risk for immunocompromised patients, VRE could be seen as an indicator for the level of prevention maturity of a given healthcare system. In countries with a low level of prevention maturity, even experts will argue that it is not worth to prevent VRE, especially the less resistant *vanB* variant, because the burden of prevention is much higher than the burden of disease. Nevertheless, this is a very short-term thought, especially in countries with high economic power such as Germany or the Netherlands, where resources to enable prevention should be available. The problem is thus not the resources but the system itself. The doctors and even infection control experts who are part of this system might start accepting the given limitations, relativizing the necessity of protecting people from infections. The fact that there are not enough beds for isolation within a healthcare system does not mean that there is no possibility to create and finance them.

It seems to be a systemic and therefore a health-political decision whether to fully support prevention or not, in any given European country. We believe that we need to transform our healthcare systems from today's use of a more or less production-economic model into a prevention-economic model, wherein remuneration is not bound to a higher number of cases, but to higher quality of care. But this is only possible if at the same time hospitals are not any more forced to compete with neighboring hospitals within the same healthcare region. In times of chronic diseases and long-term care with iterative re-admissions, competition in healthcare is starting to become a possible risk for quality of care and public health. Today a patient in a tertiary care hospital will tomorrow be transferred to the long-term care facility and a month later admitted again to another regional hospital. Asking hospitals in a given healthcare region to compete with each other is to ask your left hand to compete with your right hand instead of both focusing on extinguishing the fire that has started in the roof-top apartment in your house.

Those healthcare regions are organically grown collective systems and composed by all healthcare institutions and practices in a given geographic region. They can be mathematically defined by analyzing the usage pattern of the citizens for those institutions and practices. All healthcare institutions and doctors are therefore together responsible for the optimal and efficient care and cure of the citizens of their own region. The costs are made together and regions that work together in an optimized way will do it in the most cost-efficient way. The responsible economic unit will then not be any more the single hospital, nursing home or doctor, but the healthcare region. Some people start worrying here, but the positive aspects of competition remain, but now between the different healthcare regions, on the basis of national or even better international quality indicators that make a comparison between regions possible.

This is a feasible way to go, and will allow us to organize regional care and cure, but especially also integrated diagnostic and infection prevention and control. We can do this by creating diagnostic and preventive coherence of data, and knowledge on resistance circulating in the region that is most often missing and the major reason for a rapid spread of MDROs in many countries. But how to organize an integrative approach, where next to antibiotic stewardship, diagnostic and infection prevention stewardship is combined in a single hospital, but also in a coherent way in the whole healthcare region, where different stakeholders take different responsibilities helping each other to prevent the transmission and spread of MDROs? This is crucial, as we see now during the COVID-19 pandemic. AMR can be thus taken as a preventive challenge that fosters structures and expertise every day in order to be prepared for an infectious disease crisis you probably would think you could never be prepared for.

Another difficulty lies in the fact that over the past decades, we have trained our healthcare workers to be competent, but unfortunately also very competitive and exclusive. Today, young doctors start their specialist career as general doctors, but when they reach their specialist competence, they feel different to other fields. However, with more and more complex and chronic diseases, there is no specialist field that is able to treat a patient on its own; multidisciplinarity will be normal and required for optimal patient cure and care. Our medical professionals have to learn that knowing solely everything in your own field is just not enough; you need to become a mosaic stone in the whole mosaic of multidisciplinary cure and care of patients. We need to become not only more competent but also meta-competent.

The same is true for European competence. Especially in infection prevention and control, many different local, national, and international recommendations exist to tackle MDRO within the different levels of the healthcare system. The differences are often based upon difference in national evidence, most often due to difference in socioeconomic status and structure. What sense makes a national guideline in a future European Union of Health. Our doctors and experts discuss with colleagues across borders and they are all allowed to work across the borders. Thus, we need to teach them European competence in order to be able to adapt their knowledge gained in one healthcare system within another system.

This is exactly the outcome of our euregional projects: where we took, e.g., the Dutch search and destroy policy for the prevention of MRSA and transformed it into an MRSA search and follow strategy on the German side of the border. This transformation allowed the implementation of the essential components of the successful Dutch strategy of identifying carriers and free them from MRSA, whenever possible alongside the much more complex patient path through the specific German healthcare system. A copy and paste approach across the border would not have worked out successfully, as the healthcare systems are different. This example shows how we could further develop European competence, but it also shows how border regions can be used as transformation spots for good practice. Border regions can serve as "living labs" where a given guideline or recommendation of the country from one side of the border can be transformed and translated to be feasible and successfully implemented on the other side of the border. This will ultimately result in the adaptation of a good practice example that can spread further into the remaining country.

We would then see the strength of Europe's diversity and could be enthusiastic about the particularities of the different people, systems, and approaches, comparable with a healthy ecosystem, where we mutually take or leave the lead to the most successful way to go. In strengthening Europe by cooperation, we will be able to protect the European people from health threats, and in order to extinguish the fire in our house, we can repel MDRO from our continent again. As a challenge, let us try to get Europe CRE free again by 2030. Who is committing himself with us?

## This Book

On our way to reach this goal together this book is a great direction sign. The author Rinke van den Brink is since 2005 the editor for healthcare at NOS, the Dutch Broadcast Foundation, and since 1982 active as a journalist who has worked for weekly magazines, radio, and television. Next to his journalistic activities, Rinke van den Brink has also always had a talent for writing books. He has published four books about extreme right-wing politics in West Europe, among which are *De Internationale van de Haat* (1994) and *In de greep van de angst* (2005). In 1993, he received the ADO Media Prize from the "Anti Discriminatie Overleg" for his way of systematically following the extreme right wing since years. The jury highlighted that his writing is fascinating and very readable, so that his stories, no matter how somber the content may be, read like a novel. During his years as NOS editor for healthcare, he was responsible for a number of major scoops in the Netherlands, such as stories about Q fever, ESBL-producing bacteria on (chicken) meat, and the outbreak of the multiresistant Klebsiella at the Maasstad Hospital in 2010.

So, it came as no surprise that he published a book dealing with the tenuous topic of AMR, first published in Dutch in 2013 with the title *Het einde van de antibiotica*, which was then updated, translated, and published in German in 2015 and now the present English version.

Antibiotics and antibiotic resistance have been a headline topic around the world for many years, but definitely have received more attention since the reports and notifications from the World Health Organization in 2014. News stories about fatal bacterial outbreaks are no rarity anymore. Highlighting that antibiotics, which were for a very long time the magic bullet that drastically reduced the risk of dying from various infectious diseases, have lost their magic now in the twenty-first century. This is the result of one major disadvantage of antibiotics: bacteria have become insensitive to their effect.

In *The End of the Antibiotics*, Rinke van den Brink describes what antibiotic resistance and subsequently outbreaks of antibiotic-resistant bacteria mean for the individual patient, the physician, director, policymaker, and many more stakeholders. Extensive consideration is given to the use of antibiotics in animal husbandry and the important role of different stakeholders. He describes the successful measures in Sweden and Denmark but also mentions the risks of illegal use of antibiotics and globalization in livestock farming that remain a big problem. When reading this book, it becomes clear, by all the different examples that Rinke van den Brink illustrates, that antibiotic resistance is not a national problem, which can only be solved by collaboration and by dealing with it in an international fashion. He speaks to a variety of international specialists and asks them about possible solutions to this urgent global problem, such as other reward systems for the development of new antibiotics, the use of older antibiotics, prevention through improved hygiene, changes in antibiotic use in livestock farming, and antibiotic stewardship for hospitals.

Altogether, the book *The End of Antibiotics* presents a nice comprehensive overview of the hot topic of antibiotics and antibiotic resistance to the reader and will hopefully pave the way for extinguishing the fire together in our house.

Groningen, 03.01.2021

Corinna Glasner and Alex W. Friedrich

Hilversum, The Netherlands                                          Rinke van den Brink

# Acknowledgments

There is no greater pleasure than writing a book. When I was busy with this book every evening at the end of the summer of 2012, I dreamt one day of saying that. Now I am setting it down here, in black and white. Television, radio, writing texts for websites, newspapers, weekly or monthly magazines – those are all very fine, but nothing in comparison to writing a book. Researching thoroughly, conducting countless interviews with often highly motivated experts – it was a fascinating activity, and gave me an enormous amount of joy. Just like writing the book itself. I hope that the reader will sense this joy, and share my fascination for this topic. If I can also succeed in making it clear how urgent this topic is, then *The End of Antibiotics* will have been a success.

I had a lot of support during the writing of this book. The management at NOS and my superiors in the inland editorial team gave me the freedom to immerse myself thoroughly in the subject of antibiotic resistance so that I could write a book about it. A long procession of scientists and other individuals, both at home and abroad, often took a great deal of time to answer my questions. With several of these, an e-mail correspondence developed, which was at times very intensive. They all took the trouble to explain factual issues I could not understand and answer further questions. There was a whole crowd of fellow readers who commented on all or some of the texts. That helped me enormously. But of course, only I am responsible for the content of this book.

Without wishing to relegate others to the background, at this point I would like to mention the names of four people to whom I am quite particularly grateful for their support as readers, sources of information, and guides through the strange world of antibiotic resistance: Christina Vandenbroucke-Grauls, Jan Kluijtmans, Inge Gyssens, and Alex Friedrich. Without you, this book would never have come into being! The same applies to my family, my wife, and my children, who once again had to get by with a part-time partner/father for a while.

Rinke van den Brink, Amsterdam, February 2013

The German version of this book is a considerably revised and expanded version of the original Dutch edition. The German edition would never have come about without the unremitting efforts of Prof. Dr Alex W. Friedrich to publish the book in German. Nor without the support of, and great deal of work carried out by, Annette Dwars and, above all, Antje Wunderlich.

Rinke van den Brink, Amsterdam, May 2015

For the English version of this book, I rewrote considerable parts of the German edition. I updated it where necessary and added a great deal of new information to the manuscript. Once again, Prof. Alex W. Friedrich was the driving force behind the publication of this English version of my book. Corinna Glasner, Annette Dwars, and Antje Wunderlich were important sources of support during this project. Alastair Jamieson-Lane corrected the English manuscript. The author remains of course entirely responsible of the content of this book.

Rinke van den Brink, Amsterdam, April 2021

The author received grants for the research and writing of the original Dutch edition of this book from the *Fonds voor Bijzondere Journalistieke Projecten* (https://fondsbjp.nl/dutch-fund-for-journalism/) and from the *Fonds Pascal Decroos* (www.fondspascaldecroos.org).

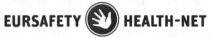

For both the German and the English edition the author received grants of the non-profit EurSafety Fund.

**EURSAFETY**  **HEALTH-NET**

# Contents

# About the Author

**Rinke van den Brink** (1955) is journalist and writer. Since 2005, he is health editor at NOS News in the Netherlands, working in a multimedia editorial staff. He published his first articles in 1977 and is since 1982 a professional journalist. He worked for different radio stations in the Netherlands and was correspondent in Amsterdam for different foreign, French-language newspapers and radio and TV stations. He worked for a long time for the Dutch weekly *Vrij Nederland* and wrote through the years four books on extreme-right political movements in Western Europe. In March 2013, he published after years of research *Het einde van de antibiotica* (*The End of Antibiotics*) a book on antimicrobial resistance and infectious diseases. In 2015, a strongly revised and enlarged German edition of this book was published. It has been revised again for the actual English edition. In 2020, the author published an autobiographical book on how he became victim of an abdominal sepsis after a medical error and how this sepsis triggered a severe psychosis. The author describes in detail the enormous impact of what happened to him and his family and how he succeeded in overcoming this black period in his life thanks to exemplary psychiatric care.

# Introduction

**1**

The elderly lady, let us call her Lucy, in the Gastroenterology Department of the University Medical Centre Utrecht was incurably sick, there was not much more the doctors could for her. They wanted to transfer her to a nursing home, but no nursing home was willing to accept her; she had fallen critically ill right in the middle of an outbreak of VRE at the UMC Utrecht and, unfortunately, had been infected. Vancomycin-resistant Enterococci (VRE) is one of the nastiest forms of antibiotic-resistant bacteria a hospital can have. It is extremely contagious, and very difficult to remove from a hospital once it has moved in there. And so, no nursing home was willing to admit her. The protocol for dealing with such cases was strictly observed. For months, Lucy lay lonely and isolated in a small room. Finally, she became severely psychotic, and died in the clinic. This drama unfolded in 2000. 'In such cases I find myself wondering: What's worse, the illness or the treatment?' says Professor of molecular epidemiology of infectious diseases Marc Bonten, up until April 1 2021 Head of the Department of Medical Microbiology at the UMC Utrecht. 'We have to constantly keep an eye on what we're doing to people, what effect our infection prevention measures and treatments are having on patients. In my opinion, far too often departments are simply closed. This very quickly gives rise to bottlenecks in patient care. If you close an intensive care unit you can't perform operations, and then as a result critically ill people have to be transferred to other hospitals. That's a real problem'.

The individual well-being of Lucy had collided with the collective interests of public health. This tension forms one of the key topics when discussing the rapid increase in antibiotic resistance worldwide. 'All doctors wants to do everything possible for their patients', says Jan Kluytmans, Professor at the University Medical Centre Utrecht and Head of the Department of Medical Microbiology at the Amphia Hospital in Breda. 'They want to help them, they want them to get better. But it's very difficult to keep an eye on collective interests at the same time. In principle you should always ask yourself what effects the treatment of an individual patient will have on public health. With most medicines such considerations only play a subordinate role, if any at all. But when you use antibiotics, then you have to confront this issue. A doctor's education doesn't give you any extra help here. When you've finished your studies you take the Hippocratic Oath, and that too is all about the individual patient'. In Chap. 2 of this book, *In the beginning there was antibiotic resistance*, I will investigate this problem in detail.

The inflexible rules and strict protocols at the UMC Utrecht may have had a disastrous impact on the well-being of Lucy early this century, but they were drawn up for good reasons. In any institution, a multiresistant bacterium is a nightmare for every doctor, nurse and manager. For any healthcare institution, dealing with multiresistant bacteria means dealing with patients who can only be treated with great difficulty or in some cases, not at all. It means isolating patients at great expense, and subjecting doctors and nurses to exceptionally strict hygienic regulations. It means temporarily closing entire departments so that they may be thoroughly cleaned with disinfectants. Chapter 3 deals with the human and economic costs caused by antibiotic resistance.

## Outbreaks

If a hospital or other healthcare institution does not follow the guidelines or carry out the required measures, there is a high risk that a disaster scenario will develop like the one that occurred at the Maasstad Hospital in Rotterdam in 2010 and 2011. The hospital was plagued by an outbreak of a multiresistant *Klebsiella* bacteria strain for 2 years. The hospital delayed carrying out the necessary measures, and the bacteria spread like wildfire. Similar events occurred during two outbreaks in Germany: the outbreak of an ESBL-producing *Klebsiella pneumoniae* bacterium in the neonatal department of the Bremen-Mitte Clinic, and the KPC-outbreak[1] at the University of Leipzig Medical Centre, which lasted almost 3 years. In the end, three people died as a direct result of the bacterium in Rotterdam; it may also have played a role in ten other deaths as well. In nine more infected patients that passed away, it was not possible to establish whether there was a link with the multiresistant *Klebsiella* strain or not. Finally, the bacterium played no part in the death of 14 other patients infected with the *Klebsiella* strain. Patients began to avoid the Maasstad Hospital *en masse*. The events in the Maasstad Hospital prove once and for all the crucial importance of a good functioning infection prevention system. During outbreaks like the one that hit the Maasstad Hospital so hard, it is essential that microbiology experts and hygiene specialists work closely together. Where they fail to do so, incidents of this kind will repeatedly occur. At the Maasstad Hospital there was, unfortunately, no cooperation between these two professional groups. In Chap. 4, *Major outbreak at Maasstad Hospital*, I describe in detail the decisions, the circumstances and all other elements that lead to the outbreak, along with its long-term consequences.

---

[1]KPC = *Klebsiella pneumoniae* carbapenemase. Carbapenemase is an enzyme that makes bacteria resistant to the important carbapenem class of antibiotics. Carbapenems are high-performance antibiotics with relatively few side effects.

It is pure bad luck when some nasty bacterium arrives in a hospital. This happens much more often than people generally assume and it is unavoidable, as is illustrated in Chap. 5, *A thin layer of faeces on everything you touch*. To prevent that an isolated case of a patient carrying a resistant bug becomes an outbreak, good infection prevention is decisive. In its size and severity the outbreak in Rotterdam was extraordinary—as were the outbreaks in Leipzig and, to a lesser extent, Bremen. Without question, the cause for this was the inadequate management of each outbreak.

Large-scale use of antibiotics in intensive livestock farming is not without its consequences for human beings. In recent years a number of studies have been published that reveal its far-reaching effects. For example, most chicken meat that is commercially available in the Netherlands contains antibiotic-resistant ESBL-producing bacteria. The same also applies, to a lesser extent, to meat from other animals (Overdevest et al. 2011). ESBL (extended spectrum beta-lactamases) are a group of enzymes that make two important groups of antibiotics ineffective—penicillins and cephalosporins. The latter are antibiotics that are administered to hospital patients by infusion therapy if their GP cannot bring infection under control with oral antibiotics. The main producers of ESBL are commonly occurring intestinal bacteria such as *E. coli*[2] and *Klebsiella pneumoniae*. However, the resistant bacteria are also found in the soil (Knapp et al. 2010), in water (Blaak et al. 2010, 2011), and often on vegetables as well (Reuland et al. 2014).

According to the data over 2015 of the European Centre for Disease Prevention and Control (ECDC), every year an estimated 33,000 people die in Europe as a consequence of infections caused by multiresistant bacteria (Cassini et al. 2019). In 2010, at a conference in Uppsala, the Pakistani professor Zulfiqar A. Bhutta presented a study showing that, in only five southeast Asian countries, roughly 100,000 children die every year from infections caused by multiresistant bacteria (Bhutta 2010).

An ECDC report from 2009 estimates that the costs arising from antibiotic resistance in the EU amount to around 1.5 billion euros per year, while the number of annual deaths due to infections caused by multiresistant microbes was estimated at 25,000 (ECDC/EMEA 2009). The figure in the United States is at least 35 billion dollars per year, according to a 2009 study (Roberts et al. 2009) and according to the CDC at least 20 billion dollars in direct healthcare costs and 35 billion dollars in societal costs caused by lost productivity (CDC 2013). ESBL and the conflict between economic interests and those of public health are the principal topic of Chap. 6, *The beginning of the end*.

---

[2]*Escherichia coli* or, for brevity's sake, *E. coli* were named after their discoverer, Theodor Escherich.

## Resistance To Carbapenems

At the end of 2011, the Health Council of Belgium published a statement regarding the management of the greatly increased number of bacteria that were resistant to carbapenem antibiotics, which are regarded as last-resort reserve medicines (Glupczynski and Gordts 2011a, b). In such cases the only recourse left to doctors is experimental treatments, such as the antibiotic colistin that is more than 60 years old, whose use was discontinued as a result of side effects including kidney damage. Alternatively, they might use tigecycline, a newer medicine with fewer side effects—which, however, is at best mildly effective against the infection.

The *Klebsiella* bacterium that caused the major outbreak at the Maasstad Hospital in Rotterdam is one of these bacteria that are resistant to carbapenem antibiotics. These were rarely found in the Netherlands before the outbreak in Maasstad and they are still scarce; but the situation is quite different in hospitals in many other countries among which Greece, Poland, Romania and Spain. In these countries—and, for example in India (Singh et al. 2019) and the United States—the use of antibiotics, and of these last-resort carbapenems, is high in hospitals and other healthcare facilities, but also in the community.

In 2009, over three and a half times as many antibiotics were consumed outside healthcare facilities in Greece as in the Netherlands. In the same year, the Cypriots took three times as many antibiotics as the Dutch, the French and Belgians two and a half times as many. The Germans consumed around a third more antibiotics than the Dutch. And things had basically not changed by 2019 either. And the higher the use of antibiotics, the higher the antibiotic resistance rates. Chapter 7, *The end in sight?* revolves around this topic of resistance to carbapenems.

## Animals Full of Resistant Bacteria

In the veterinary sector the picture has long been quite different. Until 2011, the Netherlands was one of the leading antibiotics users in this sector. Dutch veterinary surgeons, in particular, used antibiotics extravagantly. And note: these antibiotics are often the same as those used in human medicine. Veterinarians are at the same time pharmacists. They sell livestock farmers the antibiotics—and all other medicines— that they themselves prescribe. Around five per cent of veterinarians are responsible for 85 per cent of the turnover in antibiotics. They earn vast amounts of money from this.

Only in the veterinary sector in Greece and the United States were even more antibiotics used than in Netherlands (CDC 2019a, b; CDC 2017). The high rate of antibiotics used in the Netherlands can partially be explained by the prescription of preventive antibiotics, which are mixed in with the feed, and by herd treatment; if a few animals in a livestock pen become sick, then all the animals are given antibiotics. It was only in 2010, and mostly from 2011 onwards, that a start was made to control the use of antibiotics in the veterinary sector. According to the official wholesale sales figures, in 2019 livestock farmers were already using 70 per cent less antibiotics as in 2009 (Heederik et al. 2020). The use of antibiotics in livestock farming is the main topic of Chap. 8, 'Looking behind the figures'.

## The Role of Medical Microbiology

Since I reported on the *Klebsiella* outbreak at the Maasstad Hospital and its inadequate management on 31 May 2011, there have been dozens more reported outbreaks of multiresistant bacteria in the Netherlands. It is not yet fully clear what conclusions can be drawn from this knowledge. There was no mandatory obligation to report bacterial outbreaks. So until then, no-one knew whether these were all the outbreaks of resistant bacteria that occurred within the relevant timeframe, or whether perhaps only half of them. The fact is that for several years, more and more resistant bacteria have been found in hospital patients, nursing home residents, and even among the general public. And this does not just apply to the Netherlands. More than half the outbreaks that I counted in the records for the Netherlands involved MRSA (methicillin-resistant *Staphylococcus aureus*), the classic hospital bacterium. Besides the hospital variant there are two other MRSA types in circulation: a livestock variant that appears most frequently in pigs, and a third kind that can infect people who have neither been in hospital nor had contact with animals. The MRSA management in Dutch hospitals, which is based on the 'search and destroy' principle, is very strict, but it is successful. According to a 2011 study carried out in Utrecht, the costs of this programme are considerably lower than the costs arising from the outbreaks they avoid (Wassenberg et al. 2012). Generally speaking, outbreaks are identified at an early stage.

In October 2011, in a response to parliamentary questioning, Dutch health minister Edith Schippers reported that every year an estimated seven people die of an infection caused by MRSA in the Netherlands (Tweede Kamer 2011–2012, 286). By comparison, in the United States, almost 19,000 patients died from the consequences of an infection caused by MRSA in 2005 (Klevens et al. 2007), and in 2011, after major efforts to decrease that number, the figure was still an estimated 10,600 in 2017 (CDC 2019a, b). In the United Kingdom, the number of deaths resulting from sepsis (blood poisoning) caused by MRSA fell from a peak value of 1652 in 2006 to 364 cases in 2011 (ONS 2012). The decreasing trend in the number of deaths due to a MRSA-bacteraemia continued. In the fiscal year 2018/2019, England reported 191 deaths within 30 days after a MRSA-bacteraemia (PHE 2019). According to ECDC data for 2019, in the United Kingdom the MRSA rate—the percentage of invasive *Staphylococcus aureus* resistant to methicillin—was 6.0%, a sharp decrease compared to the 10.8% in 2015 (ECDC 2020).

In Germany, the trend in the rate of MRSA in blood cultures was similar. In 2015 the prevalence of MRSA in these cultures was 11.3%. In 2019 it had decreased to 6.7% (ECDC 2020). In the German state of North Rhine-Westphalia, with 17 million inhabitants comparable to the Netherlands in population, MRSA occurred 32 times more frequently in 2010 than in the Netherlands. If MRSA management similar to that used in the Netherlands were introduced in North Rhine-Westphalia, it was estimated that the number of deaths per year could be reduced by 150 (Van Cleef et al. 2012). In North Rhine-Westphalia the evolution of the MRSA-rate did not differ from the trend in Germany as a whole: the number of MRSA-infections decreased In Germany from 3612 in 2015 to 1784 in 2019. In North Rhine-Westphalia, it decreased over the same 5 years from 1146 to 575 cases of MRSA-infections, almost without exception bacteraemia. In 2019 in Germany a total of 129 deaths was attributed directly to the MRSA-bacteraemia, a death rate of 7.3%. Applied to North Rhine-Westphalia this would mean that 42 deaths occurred in 2019 due to a MRSA-bacteraemia (RKI 2020). That is still much more than the roughly five deaths due to a MRSA-bacteraemia that occur yearly in the Netherlands (Bonten 2018).

It will not be easy to bring the MRSA-rate and the death rate due to MRSA-bacteraemia in North Rhine-Westphalia further down to the Dutch level. According to statements by Professor Alex Friedrich of the University Medical Centre Groningen, by the end of 2012 only ten per cent of German hospitals had microbiologists, as a result of budget cuts. In the other hospitals their posts had been abolished, and the in-house microbiological laboratories—if indeed there were any—had been closed. Big commercial laboratories have taken over this work for the German hospitals, which number around 2000. Generally speaking, these laboratories fulfil their responsibilities well—the only problem is that the hospitals which request the tests often lack the expertise to decide which tests should be carried out and how to react appropriately to the results. The German Bundestag recognised this problem. In summer 2011, the 400 biggest German hospitals—those with more than 400 beds each—were legally required to re-employ microbiologists or other medical experts for hospital hygiene. All the other hospitals have to collaborate with external experts on issues of hospital hygiene (Bundesamt für Justiz 2011). But progress has been made over the last years. Chapter 9 is mainly focused on the role and importance of medical microbiology. During the ongoing SARS-CoV-2 pandemic of 2020 the big microbiological laboratories proved the usefulness of their large scale: they were able to perform huge numbers of PCR tests to establish whether a person is carrying the coronavirus or not.

## Travel as a Source of Infection

Until about 10 years ago, it was mostly patients in hospitals who became infected with multiresistant bacteria. More recently, however, they are often colonised by resistant bacteria already when they arrive at the hospital. Besides the food chain, people's travel habits also play a major role in spreading antibiotic resistance. The first Dutch patient with an OXA-48[3] producing *Klebsiella* bacterium was admitted to a hospital in Amsterdam after a lung operation in New Delhi. The big KPC outbreak that kept the University of Leipzig Medical Centre in its thrall for almost 3 years

---

[3]OXA-48 is an enzyme that makes bacteria resistant to the highly effective carbapenem antibiotics.

began with the admission of a patient who had become infected with KPC at a hospital in Rhodes.

In 2010, microbiologists at Linköping University in Sweden succeeded in confirming a link between travel and antibiotic resistance (Östholm-Balkhed et al. 2013). The scientists tested people who were getting vaccinated before a long-haul trip to see whether they were carriers of ESBL-producing bacteria. Before they left, ESBL was confirmed in four per cent of the people tested. After they returned, the figure was 32 per cent.

In many countries around the world antibiotic resistance is a much bigger problem than in Germany, the Netherlands or other European countries. In December 2011 the scientific journal *Clinical Infectious Diseases* published a horror story regarding antibiotic resistance (Udwadia et al. 2012). A group of Indian scientists had found a variant of a tuberculosis bacterium—which had first been confirmed in Iran in 2009—that was completely resistant to all antibiotics commonly in use against the disease. As described in the article, twelve cases of this form of tuberculosis had already appeared at the Hinduja Hospital in Mumbai. The 'Totally Drug-Resistant TB' (TDR-TB) that surfaced in India also goes travelling: along with backpackers, or the numerous medical tourists who have operations in India. In October 2012, during a broadcast of the science programme *Labyrint,* Dutch TB experts warned that it was only a matter of time before patients with untreatable tuberculosis surfaced in the Netherlands or other countries as well (Labyrint TV 2012). Patients would then actually have to be placed in isolation for the rest of their lives to protect public health. The scenario outlined by the Dutch TB experts had already become reality in South Africa. In the medical journal *The Lancet* a group of scientists headed by Professor Keertan Dheda of the medical faculty of the Groote Schuur Hospital in Cape Town described precisely this problem (Pietersen et al. 2014). South Africans with extremely drug-resistant TB (XDR-TB) who can no longer be treated are sent home, because there are no longer any beds for them to be treated under isolation conditions. These patients are often poor people who live together with many others in small dwellings. The danger of infection is colossal. The experts call for new medicines to be developed against tuberculosis, but at the same time also demand that sanatoria once again be opened for tuberculosis patients where they can be housed and treated appropriately.

## Medical Tourism

Every year many patients—from Pakistan, the Middle East, the United States and, above all, the United Kingdom—travel to India for operations. A considerable number of patients return home with multiresistant bacteria, and they often bring these into their local healthcare facilities. It is in this way, for example, that NDM-producing bacteria[4] find their way to Europe. In the United Kingdom, medical

---

[4]The enzyme that makes the bacteria resistant was named after the place where it was first identified: New Delhi metallo beta lactamase.

tourism by the large Pakistani and Indian communities is giving rise to serious concern.

'We need a new Alexander Fleming', says Professor Patrice Nordmann, Professor for Microbiology at the Faculty of Sciences and Medicine of the University of Fribourg, Switzerland. 'As a result of migration from Africa and Asia to Europe, but also because of own travel habits, resistant bacteria are spreading faster and faster all over the world. The Klebsiella bacterium that led to the outbreak at the Maasstad Hospital in Rotterdam is identical to a Klebsiella strain I had to deal with at a hospital I used to work in. And this strain comes from Morocco'.

Edwin Boel was President of the Dutch Society for Medical Microbiology (NVMM) until the end of November 2013. Since its founding in 2018 he is President of the Association of Laboratories for Medical Microbiology and as such he became in 2020 coordinator of the Health Ministry's Taskforce on Testing for SARS-CoV-2. He works at the University Medical Centre in Utrecht and sees grounds for serious concern. 'The spread of resistance is proceeding so fast. A few years ago the issue was still ESBL, and we could still treat it with carbapenems. But now, resistance even to these is cropping up more and more frequently. We can hardly keep pace with these developments'.

Professor Herman Goossens, Head of the Department for Medical Microbiology at Antwerp University Hospital in Wilrijk, also sees a bright spot in all this gloom. 'We are slowly becoming aware that a major problem is heading our way. We are dealing with one of the biggest threats to public health here. It is very important to make ourselves aware of this. It's even an essential requirement for being able to master the problem. We need to be clear about this'.

Professor Roel Coutinho, Director of the Centre for Infectious Disease Control (CIb) at the RIVM[5] until August 2013, supports this view. 'In Greek hospitals, *Klebsiella pneumoniae* bacteria are already widespread. These are resistant to carbapenems—the last effective antibiotics we have. The same also applies to India and other far eastern countries. We cannot close our borders to bacteria. They're coming towards us, and quickly. That's a big problem for public health'.

This problem can only be tackled by collaboration across borders. International collaboration in the field of infection prevention, and the campaign against increasing antibiotic resistance, are described in detail in Chap. 10, which is devoted to cross-border projects.

## New Antibiotics

Antibiotics are not just administered in hospitals in order to fight infections, but also to prevent them—for example, during major medical interventions such as hip replacements and open-heart surgery. Or for patients who have to undergo intensive

---

[5]Rijksinstituut voor Volksgezondheid en Milieu (Dutch National Institute for Public Health and the Environment).

chemotherapy. Without effective antibiotics, treatments such as these are scarcely possible due to the risk of infection. Antibiotics are also given to premature babies.

Dr. Alexander Mellmann works as Medical Specialist for Hygiene and Environmental Medicine at the University Hospital Münster—one of the few bastions of medical microbiology and hospital hygiene remaining in Germany, after their responsibilities in many German hospitals were outsourced to external providers in the early decades of this century. 'There are only very few new antibiotics', he says, 'and we are seeing more and more patients for whom not a single medicine works any more. Antibiotics are very powerful and keen-edged weapons, but if used improperly or too frequently they can very quickly become blunted'.

'Antibiotic resistance is unavoidable', says Professor Christina Vandenbroucke-Grauls, former Head of the Department of Medical Microbiology at the VU University Medical Centre Amsterdam (VUmc). 'The antibiotic resistance problem is increasing, and it seems to be coming at us from all angles. There are resistant bacteria and resistance genes in the ground, in the major rivers, in animals, on vegetables and in human beings. It has long since ceased to be problem confined to hospitals. And, thanks to our travel habits, we're spreading it all over the world. The only thing we can do is slow down the increase of the problem by means of good infection prevention and correct use of antibiotics. But what we really need are new antibiotics'.

And there is the rub: hardly any new antibiotics are being developed. 'There are some interesting medicines that might come on the market in the not-too-distant future', said Professor Christian Giske to me back in 2012. He works as a microbiologist at the renowned Karolinska Institute in Stockholm and the university hospital of the same name. 'But in fact these are more like variations of already existing drugs. With them, we can gain a little more time. All our efforts should be targeted towards containing the problem. Because after these few medicines arrive, there's nothing more. The pipeline is empty'.

Many large pharmaceutical companies have stopped investing in the research and development of new antibiotics. The latest was the biggest pharmaceutical company in the world Johnson & Johnson in September 2019 (NDR 2019a, b). In 2018 two other major companies Novartis (Bloomberg 2018) and Sanofi (ReAct 2018) pulled out of developing antibacterials and antivirals. AstraZeneca did so in 2016 (Antibiotic Research 2016). All four companies were in 2016 founding members of the AMR Industry Alliance and pledged to invest in research and development of antibiotics (AMR Industry Alliance 2016).

The reasons for this can be found in the specific nature of these medicines. Antibiotics must kill bacteria without harming the people being treated. Just like cancer medicines, for example. If a company develops a good new antibiotic and launches it on the market, then health authorities worldwide ask all doctors to use the drug only in extreme emergencies, in order to postpone the formation of resistance for as long as possible. And if they prescribe it all the same, it is almost always only for a short period of 1 or 2 weeks. For the pharmaceutical industry, this is not a very interesting business model. From an economic viewpoint, it is far more promising to develop medicines for a chronic illness, which patients must take for several years.

However, if no new antibiotics should appear on the market, then many doctors and scientists believe that there is a threat of regressing to the time before the discovery of penicillin.

'Of course we need new antibiotics', said Mats Ulfendahl, General Secretary of the Department of Health and Pharmacy of the Swedish Research Council almost 10 years ago to me. 'Because resistances are repeatedly being formed. But that's not enough. In India, 600 million people don't have a toilet. This promotes the spread of drug-resistant and other forms of bacteria, as well as infectious diseases. The same applies to other poor countries. We must also solve these problems'. At the beginning of 2020, the World Health Organisation (WHO) issued two reports on this problem underlining the limited number of new antibiotics in development and stressing the fact that most of them do not target the (multi)resistant Gram-negative bacteria, who form the main threat (WHO 2020a, b). In July 2020 the AMR Action Fund was launched, an initiative of more than 20 pharmaceutical companies, the WHO, the European Investment Bank and the Wellcome Trust (AMR Action Fund 2020). Remarkably there are some companies among the founders who announced earlier their retreat from the research and development of new antibiotics. The eleventh and final chapter discusses the dearth of new antibiotics, and other solutions for the pressing problems of antibiotic resistance.

## International Awareness

'Antibiotics losing the fight against deadly bacteria' ran the headline in the *Independent on Sunday* already on 18 September 2011 (Independent 2011). And the *New York Times* of 29 December 2013 published seven opinion pieces under the headline: 'Avoiding a Time When Bacteria Can No Longer Be Stopped' (The New York Times 2013). The nightmare scenario described by both newspapers sums up the opinion of many experts very well. Yet it still does not trigger sufficient anxiety to radically restrict the misuse of antibiotics: misuse in human medicine, and also in mass livestock farming, with far-reaching consequences for public health, food safety and the economy. According to statements by Dame Sally Davies, at the time the British Chief Medical Officer and, therefore, the highest-ranking health official in the United Kingdom, antibiotic resistance is 'a catastrophic threat for the population' (The Guardian 2013), which 'should be ranked along with terrorism on a list of threats to the nation' (BBC 2013). Davies made these remarks on 11 March 2013 at the occasion of the presentation of the second part of her annual report for 2011 (Davies et al. 2013).

In autumn 2013, the British medical journal *The Lancet* referred to the situation under the title *Antibiotic resistance: a final warning* (The Lancet 2013). And Jim O'Neill, chair of the Review on Antimicrobial Resistance, an expert committee founded at the request of the former British prime minister David Cameron in 2014, put it this way in his final report of June 2016: 'It is now clear to me, as it has been to scientific experts for a long time, that tackling AMR is absolutely essential. It needs to be seen as the economic and security threat that it is, and be at the forefront of the minds of heads of state, finance ministers, agriculture ministers, and of course health ministers, for years to come' (O'Neill 2016).

The regional conference of the Food and Agriculture Organisation of the United Nations (FAO) for Asia and the Pacific launched a clear warning in a document (FAO 2020) adopted in February 2020 in Bhutan. 'The greatest burden from AMR is projected to occur in Africa and Asia where weak health systems, weak infrastructure, limited technical capacity, and higher prevalence of infectious diseases exist and where legislation, regulatory surveillance and monitoring systems on the use of antimicrobials are inadequate'.

Antibiotic resistance is a global health problem closely linked to economic development, globalization, lack of innovative new antibiotics and overuse of the existing antimicrobial drugs. That is what this book is all about.

# References

AMR Action Fund. (2020). *Bridging the gap between science and patients*. Accessed March 27, 2021, from https://www.amractionfund.com/

AMR Industry Alliance. (2016). *Our members*. Accessed March 27, 2021, from https://www.amrindustryalliance.org/our-members/

Antibiotic Research. (2016). *AstraZeneca pulls out of antibiotic drug development*. Accessed March 27, 2021, from https://bit.ly/39mePHH

BBC. (2013). *Antibiotic resistance 'as big a risk as terrorism'- medical chief*. Accessed March 27, 2021, from https://www.bbc.co.uk/news/health-21737844

Bhutta, Z. A. (2010). *Millennium development goals and child survival: Does antimicrobial resistance matter?* In Presented at the conference global need for effective antibiotics – Moving towards concerted action, Uppsala, 6–8 September 2010. Accessed October 18, 2020, from https://bit.ly/393MJ32

Blaak, H., Schets, F. M., & Italiaander, R., et al. (2010). *Antibioticaresistente bacteriën in Nederlands oppervlaktewater in veeteeltrijk gebied*. Accessed 18 Oct 2020, see page 5 for an English abstract from https://bit.ly/3q9Nsqv

Blaak, H., Van Rooijen, S. R., & Schuijt, M. S. (2011). *Prevalence of antibiotic resistant bacteria in the rivers Meuse, Rhine, and New Meuse*. Accessed October 18, 2020, from https://bit.ly/2L03RyN

Bloomberg. (2018). *Novartis exits antibiotic research, cuts 140 jobs in bay area*. Accessed March 27, 2021, from https://bloom.bg/3w4XywA

Bonten, M. (2018). *AMR deaths in Europe*. Reflections on infection prevention and control. Accessed from https://reflectionsipc.com/2018/11/07/amr-deaths-in-europe/#more-4078

Bundesamt für Justiz. (2011). *Gesetz zur Verhütung und Bekämpfung von Infektionskrankheiten beim Menschen*. In German. (see sections 3, 8 and 23). Accessed March 27, 2021, from http://www.gesetze-im-internet.de/ifsg/index.html

Cassini, A., Högberg, L. D., Plachouras, D., et al. (2019). Attributable deaths and disability-adjusted life-years caused by infections with antibiotic-resistant bacteria in the EU and the European Economic Area in 2015: A population-level modelling analysis. *The Lancet Infectious Diseases, 19*, 56–66. https://doi.org/10.1016/S1473-3099(18)30605-4.

CDC (Centers for Disease Control and Prevention). (2013). *Antibiotic resistance threats in the United States, 2013*. Accessed October 18, 2020, from https://www.cdc.gov/drugresistance/pdf/ar-threats-2013-508.pdf

CDC (Centers for Disease Control and Prevention). (2017). *Antibiotic use in the United States, 2017 progress and opportunities*. Accessed October 18, 2020, from https://bit.ly/2L7p5KU

CDC (Centers for Disease Control and Prevention). (2019a). *Antibiotic resistance threats in the United States, 2019*. Accessed October 18, 2020, from www.cdc.gov/DrugResistance/Biggest-Threats.html

CDC (Centers for Disease Control and Prevention). (2019b). *Antibiotic use in the United States, 2018 update: Progress and opportunities*. Accessed October 18, 2020, from https://bit.ly/3hOgGYX

Davies, S., et al. (2013). *Annual report of the Chief Medical Officer Volume Two, 2011 infections and the rise of antimicrobial resistance*. Accessed October 18, 2020, from https://bit.ly/2Xkfi6M

ECDC. (2020). *Antimicrobial resistance in the EU/EEA (EARS-Net) – Annual Epidemiological Report for 2019*. Accessed January 7, 2021, from https://bit.ly/3ntksIw

ECDC/EMEA (European Centre for Disease Prevention and Control/European Medicines Agency). (2009). *Joint technical report. The bacterial challenge: Time to react A call to narrow the gap between multidrug-resistant bacteria in the EU and the development of new antibacterial agents*. https://doi.org/10.2900/2518. Accessed October 18, 2020, from https://bit.ly/38k3GXS

FAO Regional Conference for Asia and the Pacific. (2020, 17–20 February). *Thirty-fifth session, Thimphu, Bhutan*. Report on Antimicrobial Resistance (AMR). Accessed March 27, 2021, from http://www.fao.org/3/nb741en/nb741en.pdf

Glupczynski, Y., & Gordts, B. (2011a). *Maatregelen te nemen naar aanleiding van de toename van carbapenemase producerende enterobacteriën (CPE) in België. Advies van de Hoge Gezondheidsraad nr. 8791*. In Dutch. Accessed October 18, 2020, from http://bit.do/fHkQ5

Glupczynski, Y., & Gordts, B. (2011b). *Mesures à prendre suite à l'émergence des entérobactéries productrices de carbapénémases (CPE) en Belgique*. Avis du Conseil Supérieur de la Santé N° 8791. Accessed October 18, 2020, from http://bit.do/fHkRg

Heederik, D. J. J., Bonten, M. J. M., Van Geijlswijk, I. M., et al. (2020). *Usage of antibiotics in agricultural livestock in the Netherlands in 2019 trends and benchmarking of livestock farms and veterinarians SDa/1153/2020*. Accessed October 18, 2020, from https://www.autoriteitdiergeneesmiddelen.nl/en/available-now

Independent. (2011). *Antibiotics losing the fight against deadly bacteria*. Accessed March 27, 2021, from https://bit.ly/31qOxQm

Klevens, R. M., Morrison, M. A., Nadle, J., et al. (2007). Invasive methicillin-resistant Staphylococcus aureus infections in the United States. *JAMA, 298*(15), 1763–1771. https://www.cdc.gov/mrsa/pdf/InvasiveMRSA_JAMA2007.pdf

Knapp, C. W., Dolfing, J., Ehlert, P. A. I., et al. (2010). Evidence of increasing antibiotic resistance gene abundances in archived soils since 1940. *Environmental Science & Technology, 44*(2), 580–587. https://doi.org/10.1021/es901221x. https://pubs.acs.org/doi/abs/10.1021/es901221x

Labyrint, T. V. (2012). *Uitgewerkte antibiotica*. In Dutch. Accessed March 27, 2021, from https://www.npostart.nl/labyrint/17-10-2012/VPWON_1179058

NDR. (2019a). *Antibiotika-Forschung: warum Unternehmen aussteigen*. In German. Accessed March 27, 2021, from https://bit.ly/3sv9oh5

NDR. (2019b). *The end of antibiotics?* Accessed March 27, 2021, from https://bit.ly/3szs9Ag

O'Neill, J. (2016). *Review on antimicrobial resistance. Tackling drug-resistant infections globally: Final report and recommendations*. Accessed October 18, 2020, from https://bit.ly/2Xmade4

ONS. (2012). *Office for National Statistics. Statistical Bulletin. Deaths involving MRSA: England and Wales, 2007 to 2011*. Accessed from https://bit.ly/2Xfa3Fs

Östholm-Balkhed, A., Tärnberg, M., Nilsson, M., et al. (2013). Travel-associated faecal colonization with ESBL-producing Enterobacteriaceae: Incidence and risk factors. *Journal of Antimicrobial Chemotherapy, 68*(9), 2144–2153. https://doi.org/10.1093/jac/dkt167.

Overdevest, I., Willemsen, I., Rijnsburger, M., et al. (2011). Extended-spectrum β-lactamase genes of Escherichia coli in chicken meat and humans, the Netherlands. *Emerging Infectious Diseases, 17*(7), 1216–1222. https://doi.org/10.3201/eid1707.110209. https://wwwnc.cdc.gov/eid/article/17/7/11-0209_article.

PHE. (2019). *Public Health England. Thirty-day all-cause mortality following MRSA, MSSA and Gram-negative bacteraemia and C. difficile infections 2018/19.* Accessed January 7, 2021, from https://bit.ly/397bhIl

Pietersen, E., Ignatius, E., Streicher, E., et al. (2014). Long-term outcomes of patients with extensively drug-resistant tuberculosis in South-Africa: A cohort study. *The Lancet, 383* (9924), 1230–1239. https://doi.org/10.1016/S0140-6736(13)62675-6.

ReAct. (2018). *Despite industry declaration AMR commitments Sanofi quits R&D on anti-infectives.* Accessed March 27, 2021, from https://bit.ly/39kO9aj

Reuland, E. A., al Naiemi, N., Raadsen, S. A., et al. (2014). Prevalence of ESBL-producing Enterobacteriaceae in raw vegetables. *European Journal of Clinical Microbiology & Infectious Diseases, 33*, 1843–1846. https://doi.org/10.1007/s10096-014-2142-7.

RKI. (2020). *Robert Koch Institut. Infektionsepidemiologisches Jahrbuch meldepflichtiger Krankheiten für 2019.* In German. Accessed January 7, 2021, from https://bit.ly/35iZllN

Roberts, R. R., Hota, B., Ahmad, I., et al. (2009). Hospital and societal costs of antimicrobial-resistant infections in a Chicago Teaching Hospital: Implications for antibiotic stewardship. *Clinical Infectious Diseases, 49*(8), 1175–1184. https://doi.org/10.1086/605630.

Singh, S. K., Sengupta, S., Antony, R., et al. (2019). Variations in antibiotic use across India: Multi-centre study through Global Point Prevalence survey. *Journal of Hospital Infection, 103*(3), 280–283. https://doi.org/10.1016/j.jhin.2019.05.014.

The Guardian. (2013). *Antibiotics catastrophe warning from chief-medical officer – video.* Accessed March 27, 2021, from https://bit.ly/3w3VxRc

The Lancet. (2013). Antibiotic resistance: A final warning. *The Lancet, 382*(9898), 1072. https://doi.org/10.1016/S0140-6736(13)62008-5.

The New York Times. (2013). *Avoiding a time when bacteria can no longer be stopped.* Accessed March 27, 2021, from https://nyti.ms/39hM672

Udwadia, Z. F., Amale, R. A., Ajbani, K. K., et al. (2012). Totally drug-resistant tuberculosis in India. *Clinical Infectious Diseases, 54*(4), 579–581. https://doi.org/10.1093/cid/cir889.

Van Cleef, A. G. L., Kluytmans, J. A. J. W., Van Benthem, B. H. B., et al. (2012). Cross border comparison of MRSA bacteraemia between The Netherlands and North Rhine-Westphalia (Germany): A cross-sectional study. *PLoS One.* https://doi.org/10.1371/journal.pone.0042787.

Wassenberg, M., Kluytmans, J., Erdkamp, S., et al. (2012). Costs and benefits of rapid screening of methicillin-resistant *Staphylococcus aureus* carriage in intensive care units: A prospective multicenter study. *Critical Care, 16*, R22. https://doi.org/10.1186/cc11184.

WHO. (2020a). *2019 Antibacterial agents in clinical development: an analysis of the antibacterial clinical development pipeline.* Accessed March 27, 2021, from https://bit.ly/2QLRcBZ

WHO. (2020b). *Antibacterial agents in preclinical development: an open access database.* Accessed March 27, 2021, from https://bit.ly/3fh7Qn5

# In the Beginning There Was Antibiotic Resistance

2

With most problems, we can identify the beginning more or less clearly—but this is not the case with antibiotic resistance. It sounds like a modern concept, a term that postdates the discovery of penicillin and the subsequent development of other antibiotics. But the reality is quite the opposite. Antibiotic resistance is older than humanity—far older, in fact.

Millions of years ago, an extensive network of caves appeared in what is today the US state of New Mexico. The Lechuguilla Cave is situated in the Carlsbad Caverns National Park in the extreme south of New Mexico, near the border with Texas. A listed UNESCO World Heritage Site, the cave is more than 200 km long and over 500 m deep. The deepest parts were cut off from the outside world between 7 and 4 million years ago. They form a primordial ecosystem, unaffected by external factors of any kind. The Lechuguilla Cave, therefore, affords a unique opportunity to study the existence of antibiotic resistance in a natural environment. The bacteria in the cave have never come into contact with antibiotics made by humans. Scientists from the McMaster University in Hamilton, Canada and the University of Akron in Ohio descended into the cave to collect samples at three different positions. They describe their extraordinary discoveries in a study published by the open access journal *Plos One* (Bhullar et al. 2012). The three locations were chosen because practically no other human being had ever been there.

There were no footprints or other traces of human presence. The archives of the Carlsbad Cavern National Park reveal that until then only a handful of scientists, at most, had even been anywhere near the place where the samples were taken. The scientists who, now and again, had previously obtained permission to visit the cave had been restricted to an official path, from which the present sampling sites were some way distant. Moreover, no water entered the site where the samples were taken, either directly or by condensation. The scientists from Hamilton and Akron were able to remove almost 100 different bacteria strains from the Lechuguilla Cave. The Canadian and American scientists tested these strains for resistance to 26 different antibiotics. Some of these antibiotics also occur in nature; of the rest, some consisted partly of natural ingredients and some were developed entirely in the laboratory.

© The Author(s), under exclusive license to Springer Nature Switzerland AG 2021
R. van den Brink, *The End of an Antibiotic Era*,
https://doi.org/10.1007/978-3-030-70723-1_2

Roughly two-thirds of all the bacteria strains were resistant to three or four different classes of antibiotics. Three strains were even resistant to 14 different antibiotics. Generally speaking, the resistance pattern of the Lechuguilla Cave bacteria did not differ significantly from that of the bacteria in our own environment. As already mentioned, the ecosystem of the Lechuguilla Cave was cut off from the outside world millions of years ago, long before the excessive use of antibiotics for human beings and in intensive livestock farming. Yet, nevertheless, the scientists were able to establish multiple resistances against antibiotics there, and to a considerable extent. The scientists even found two resistance mechanisms that had been unknown up to that time. They came to the conclusion that resistance is a natural phenomenon.

However, this deduction was nothing new. In September 2011, other scientists at the same institution, McMaster University in Hamilton, Ontario, had already published a study in *Nature* that came to the same conclusion (D'Costa et al. 2011). They had investigated soil samples from permafrost regions in the Canadian north-west for the presence of genes resistant to modern beta-lactam antibiotics[1] and vancomycin.[2] They found genes resistant to these modern antibiotics in samples that were at least 30,000 years old. 'Resistance to antibiotics is as old as the world', says Christina Vandenbroucke-Grauls, Professor for Medical Microbiology at the VU Medical Centre in Amsterdam until her retirement in October 2017.

## Genetic Pressure Cooker

Let us suppose that a patient goes to the doctor with, say, a bladder infection, and is given an antibiotic. It kills the bacteria that cause the infection, but it may also kill all sorts of other bacteria which the patient actually needs. After treatment, a readjustment of the bacterial balance takes place. Other bacteria that happen to be situated in the urinary tract, and which possess the resistance gene that makes them immune to the antibiotic used, will survive the treatment. If these resistant bacteria are the same as those that caused the infection, they will not be destroyed.

After treatment, with no further competition from other bacteria, these resistant bacteria can multiply unchecked. And that happens at a dizzying pace. 'Bacteria undergo a much faster evolution than animals or humans', explains Professor Alex Friedrich. Born in Nuremberg, he worked as Senior Physician at the Institute of

---

[1]Beta-lactam antibiotics kill bacteria by upsetting the synthesis of the bacterial cell wall, which then dissolves. The group of beta-lactam antibiotics includes penicillins, cephalosporins, carbapenems and monobactams. Because of their low toxicity and outstanding efficacy against bacteria that react to them, they are frequently used. Resistances against beta-lactam antibiotics are often found together with resistances against other antibiotics. In such cases there are few other effective agents to choose from, but these are preferably not used since they are either toxic, less effective or both.

[2]Vancomycin, a member of the class of glycopeptides, is a natural antibiotic which works by destabilising the bacterial cell wall. Vancomycin is administered for infections that have been caused by methicillin-resistant staphylococcus aureus (MRSA), methicillin-resistant *staphylococcus epidermidis* (MRSE) and *Clostridium difficile*.

Hygiene of the University Hospital Münster before becoming Professor for Medical Microbiology and, in 2011, Head of the Department for Medical Microbiology and Hospital Hygiene at the University Medical Centre Groningen. 'With human beings, we get a new generation roughly every 25 years. If you look back to the time of the Neanderthals—in other words, roughly 30,000 years—we've had around 1200 generations since then. Bacteria have a generation time of 20 min. This means that they produce 72 generations per day. For those 30,000 years of our evolution since the time of the Neanderthals, bacteria don't even need 17 days. Each generation can adapt to its environment. And antibiotics give an additional boost to the tempo of bacterial development'.

Humans and animals have only one way to pass on their genetic information, which is through their direct descendants. Bacteria can do it in two ways. As Friedrich explains, 'bacteria can not only pass on genetic information to their descendants, but also to members of the same generation. This is rather like people with blond hair going to Africa, living there with black-haired people, and then developing black hair themselves as protection against the sun. Bacteria are actually able to transfer characteristics in this way. This is described as *horizontal gene transfer*. Passing on characteristics to one's descendants is called *vertical gene transfer*. Bacteria are able to transfer both resistance genes and virulence genes between one another in both of these ways.[3] This accelerates their evolution even more'.

For horizontal gene transfer, it is not necessary for bacteria to belong to the same species. The genetic information that makes bacteria resistant is often found on plasmids—tiny, ring-shaped DNA strands that are easily transferred from one bacterium to another. This can occur between *E. coli* or *Klebsiella* and campylobacter[4] or bacteria which cause cholera or typhus. But it occurs more easily between bacteria of the same family such as *E. coli* and *Klebsiella,* which both belong to the family of enterobacteria (Enterobacteriaceae). 'Bacteria are masters of adaptation. They react to the use of antibiotics in their environment by developing resistance. They want to survive, and to do it they deploy the available resistance genes'.

---

[3]Virulence genes determine how intensely pathogenic a bacterium is.

[4]Campylobacter is a family of bacteria that cause the most frequently occurring zoonoses, i.e. diseases that can be transmitted from animals to humans. For many animals—including poultry, livestock, birds, cats, young dogs and rodents—the bacterium is a normal intestinal bacterium. The bacteria are also transmitted by flies and they are also present in ground and surface water. The infection can result in acute, aqueous and occasionally bloody diarrhoea, accompanied by severe stomach cramps and, sometimes, fever. Very small children, older people, those infected with HIV and patients with impaired immunity are most at risk of severe complications. In 2017, more than 250,000 laboratory-confirmed cases of campylobacteriosis in EU/EEA countries were reported to the ECDC. This is equivalent to 64.9 cases per 100,000 members of the population, an increase compared to the 60.8 cases per 100.000 in 2013. Children below the age of 5 years are most susceptible to campylobacteriosis (ECDC 2019).

## Selection Pressure

The more antibiotics are used, the faster this process occurs. And this applies not only to the use of antibiotics in human medicine, but also to their application in intensive livestock farming. 'When animals are given antibiotics', says Friedrich, 'these find their way back into the environment through their slurry and droppings, and into plants and water. Admittedly, they are present there in very tiny, subthera-peutic concentrations – but even this gives rise to selection pressure that accelerates the bacteria's adaptive process'. A study by scientists at the universities of Newcastle and Wageningen, published in the January 2010 issue of Environmental Science and Technology (Knapp et al. 2010), demonstrates that the number of resistance genes in Netherlands soil has increased severely in the last 70 years. The scientists investigated soil samples taken from various locations in the Netherlands at regular intervals between 1940 and 2008. They established an exponential rise in resistance genes in the soil samples. Two genes that make bacteria resistant against beta-lactam antibiotics occurred more than 15 times more frequently in 2008 than in 1940. The same picture emerges in the major Dutch rivers. At the end of 2011, the Netherlands National Institute for Public Health and the Environment (RIVM) published a study on the incidence of antibiotic-resistant bacteria in the Maas, Rhine and Nieuwe Maas rivers (Blaak et al. 2011). On average, between a third and a half of the *E. coli* (intestinal enterococci), *Campylobacter*, *Salmonella* and *Staphylococcus aureus* strains they found were resistant to one or more antibiotics. These bacteria find their way into the rivers through dung, slurry or only partially treated wastewater— e.g. from hospitals where many people are treated with antibiotics. A study from the University of York showed similar results for the presence of antibiotics in rivers. In this study, researchers looked for 14 different widely used antibiotics in rivers in 72 countries on six continents. On two-third of the monitored spots antibiotics were found, sometimes in concentrations up to 300 times the concentration considered as safe, meaning resistance is much more likely to develop and spread (York University 2019).

Some clinics in Germany and the Netherlands now use self-disinfecting sink syphons. Syphons are tubes in an upside-down U shape by which liquids like wastewater can be transferred to a lower level over an intermediate elevation. The self-disinfecting syphons are a German invention that ensures that no resistant bacteria find their way into the (waste)water via the washbasin and outflow. These syphons continuously disinfect the water with heat and ultrasound. In Germany, these self-disinfecting syphons have been installed in places such as the intensive care units (bone marrow transplant, neonatal and oncological) at the university clinics of Tübingen (Willmann et al. 2015), Munich and Greifswald, and at the hospital in Bischofswerda. In August 2002, the traditional syphons in the washbasins at the Bischofswerda hospital intensive care unit were replaced with self-disinfecting models. This occurred after an ongoing increase in hospital bacteria. In the 2 years after the new syphons were installed, the number of healthcare-associated infections fell by around 60 per cent. The consumption of antibiotics at the intensive care unit fell by around a third, and the time patients stayed in the unit was reduced by more than 1 day (Sissoko et al. 2004).

Researchers from the University Clinic in Leiden studied the use of these disinfection devices during an ongoing outbreak of multidrug-resistant *Pseudomonas aeruginosa* on the ICU's of the hospital. Both sink drains and patients were colonized at a level of around 50 per cent and more. During the study ICU A was equipped with a disinfection device in the sink drain, ICU B was not. On ICU A there was a dramatic drop in colonisation of syphons and patients by *Pseudomonas aeruginosa*. On the control ICU B the researchers found an increase in colonisation until this ICU was also equipped with the device. The conclusion of their study published in 2019 is clear: 'Colonization with MDR-PA in sink drains in an ICU was effectively managed by installing disinfection devices to the siphons of sinks. Colonization of patients was also significantly reduced, suggesting that sink drains can be a source of clinical outbreaks with *P. aeruginosa* and that disinfecting devices may help to interrupt these outbreaks' (De Jonge et al. 2019).

At the Reinier de Graaf Hospital in Delft, the wastewater is purified before it is released into the sewer system. This medical facility was the first in the Netherlands to purify its own refuse and wastewater in order to produce clean water and biogas. This is achieved by a plant that processes biodegradable chamber pots and urinals and their contents, hospital waste and food residues by means of fermentation, filtration and oxidation (Pharmafilter 2012). By the end of 2019 this same system is used by five other hospitals in the Netherlands, while several others are considering buying it. One of the hospitals using it, the Zaans Medical Center, decided half in September 2019 to replace the system in use than since 2 years. It did so after a study by an independent engineers firm established that the system caused severe blockages by remainders of solid waste such as perspex test tubes in the sewing system of the hospital, a sewing system which construction could have been better. These blockages led to many floodings of the toilets bringing back the content of the sewer in the toilets and the hospital. It also contributed to the continuous spread of a multiresistant *Citrobacter freundii* producing the enzyme NDM5. In 18 months 39 patients were contaminated with that microbe. One of the patients died of an infection by the *Citrobacter freundii*. Other hospitals that use the same plant to process their waste either do not use the processor for the solid waste or only use it to process biodegradable chamber pots and urinals and their contents.

---

## Alexander Fleming's Warning

Resistance to antibiotics has always existed and in all places. It sounds paradoxical, but there was resistance to antibiotics before human beings began producing them. The reason for this is that many antibiotics occur in nature and are based on natural ingredients. Penicillin, the first known antibiotic, was discovered by accident by the Scottish microbiologist Alexander Fleming. He observed that no bacteria were growing in some of his culture trays. A mould fungus, which had spread there, was obviously preventing the growth of the bacteria. Fleming investigated the mould fungus and discovered that it had a lethal effect on several bacteria. The fungus produced a substance to protect itself against them. Bacteria defend themselves against other bacteria in the same way. For example, *Pseudomonas* produces substances that kill *staphylococcus aureus*.

Fleming published his discovery in 1929 and called it 'penicillin'. However, subsequently it took until 1940 before two other scientists—Ernest Boris Chain and Howard Walter Florey—developed a practical procedure for isolating penicillin from the mould fungus, enabling it to be manufactured as a medicine. In 1945, Fleming, Florey and Chain together received the Nobel Prize for medicine for their collective discovery. In the acceptance speech given by Alexander Fleming after the prize had been awarded, he warned against the emergence of resistance to his miracle cure. As he stated in his Nobel Lecture of 11 December 1945: 'It is not difficult to make microbes resistant to penicillin in the laboratory by exposing them to concentrations not sufficient to kill them [. . .] The time may come when penicillin can be bought by anyone in the shops. Then there is the danger that the ignorant man may easily underdose himself and by exposing his microbes to non-lethal quantities of the drug make them resistant' (Nobel Prize Committee 1945).

Since then, in large parts of the world antibiotics have actually become as easily available as Fleming predicted. They are cheap medicines—too cheap, in fact, in the opinion of many doctors, scientists and pharmaceutical industry staff. The price in no way reflects the value of these antibiotics: medicines that cure diseases and save lives and that, additionally only need to be taken for a short time. The low price guarantees that it is far too easy to fall back on antibiotics—certainly in the Western world, but in part also in other countries such as India. Their price has no inhibiting effect. And because of this unnecessary use of antibiotics, selection of bacteria with resistance genes favours the spread of resistance. It is pure Darwinism: bacteria defend themselves against threats.

## Knowledge

Eva Ombaka's problems with antibiotics are different from the excessively low prices quoted by many Western specialists. I met her at the beginning of September 2010, at a conference in Uppsala entitled *The Global Need for Effective Antibiotics— Moving towards Concerted Action* (Cars et al. 2011). She is a pharmacist, and the driving force behind campaigns for cautious use of antibiotics in Tanzania. Such campaigns are urgently needed. This is not because antibiotics are handled so wastefully in her country. Quite the opposite: for large sections of the population in Tanzania, and many other African countries, antibiotics are not even available, because they are too expensive for most people. The 'low price' so often discussed in Uppsala is, therefore, an extremely relative concept. 'In fact,' says Ombaka, 'in Tanzania a doctor can only prescribe antibiotics, which the patient must then pick up at a chemist's. Both doctor and pharmacist are supposed to take the time to explain to the patient how antibiotics work, how they are to be taken—and that he or she must undergo a complete course of antibiotics, since otherwise underdosing will help the bacteria to develop resistances'. In western Europe and the rest of the developed world, the consensual trend is increasingly towards shorter treatments with higher doses of antibiotics, as Christina Vandenbroucke, for example said during her retirement ceremony lecture at the VU University Medical Centre on 6 October 2017 (Vandenbroucke-Grauls 2018).

In Tanzania and several other countries besides, says Eva Ombaka, the reality is quite different. 'Even when there is a doctor who prescribes antibiotics—and this is not the case everywhere in Tanzania and other parts of Africa—unfortunately the explanation for the patient is often skipped. As a result, as soon as patients feel better after taking a couple of tablets, they keep the remainder of the antibiotics course to use if they should start feeling worse again. 'For most patients in Tanzania and other parts of Africa, in fact, antibiotics are expensive. Only very few people can afford to buy a complete course. Most antibiotics in Tanzania are sold without a prescription. As a result, antibiotics are far too readily available: from drugstore-type corner shops, at markets or on the street. Poor people then buy themselves one tablet— "Just give me one of those pink ones"—or two, if they can afford it. And an underdose of antibiotics does not even help against an infection, but only stimulates the growth of resistances. Moreover, antibiotics are of no use against flu or other viral diseases. If a person takes antibiotics all the same, by doing so they are only promoting the development of resistance. But try telling that to a Tanzanian mother with a sick child', says Eva Ombaka. 'Explain to her that it's no good to take only half a course of antibiotics', she continues. 'Or even just one tablet. Antibiotics must, therefore, be affordable'. So affordable that poor people, too, can have access to these lifesaving medicines. And yes—she laughs—if antibiotics were cheaper, then in Africa too people would fall back on them more readily, with all the consequences. For Ombaka, everything revolves around knowledge. This knowledge must be communicated: people must learn what antibiotics involve. And that will take time, a lot of time. According to Ombaka, a comprehensive information campaign is required. 'If necessary we must go from village to village explaining how antibiotics are to be used. We must explain to people that antibiotics are medicines that can save lives, but also that they only preserve their value if they are handled carefully'. She is confident that this can succeed. 'Nowadays, people with HIV also know how they must use their medicines. This has changed their lives. The same can also be achieved with antibiotics. But before this, poor people in Africa and other parts of the world must nevertheless be given access to antibiotics. This is also in the interests of rich countries', says Ombaka. Otherwise, soon there will no longer be any effective antibiotics there either. Because antibiotic resistance can, in fact, travel.

In India, Greece and the Balkans, cases of patients who succumb to infections from (almost) completely resistant bacteria are becoming more and more frequent. In spring 2010, 64-year-old Jos Jonker was on holiday in India. 'When he arrived in New Delhi at the end of February, he actually started to feel unwell immediately', his daughter Liz explained to me at the end of March that year. 'He suffered from breathing difficulties caused by a collapsed lung'. That was on Monday. Her father was admitted to a good hospital. 'His operation went well, but on Saturday complications began to appear. A pulmonary fibrosis was diagnosed, and he had to have another operation'. In the end, Jos Jonker had to be treated for more than 2 weeks in two different Indian hospitals. In addition, he suffered two strokes in succession, which left him paralysed. In these Indian hospitals, Jos Jonker received many antibiotics. 'That was the first thing they gave him', his daughter tells me in the corridor outside her father's room at the Sint Lucas Andreas Hospital in Amsterdam. He is lying in strict isolation in a room with an airlock. At this point in time, her father possessed no more than a quarter of his lung capacity. Liz Jakobs herself was actually afraid of becoming infected with the resistant bacteria her father was carrying. 'I have a little five-year-old daughter', she said, 'yes, sometimes I worry. I hope I'm not infecting myself'. Before his trip to India, her father was an energetic man. 'He lived in a top-floor flat and never had any problems climbing up the stairs. Now he can't do anything anymore. He will never get better again'. Shortly after I spoke to Liz Jakobs her father passed away. In the final analysis (Kalpoe et al. 2011), the cause was pneumonia that had been caused by a *Klebsiella* strain producing OXA-48.

## The American Military

The introduction of penicillin to medicine initiated by Chain and Florey received an enormous boost when the American army became involved in its industrial production. This had already begun at the start of the Second World War, but the Americans first became seriously involved when they intervened in the hostilities. The British and Americans began an intensive collaboration on an Anglo-American penicillin project. Leading British and American scientists, government authorities and major pharmaceutical companies such as Merck, Pfizer and Abbott worked closely together. Already in 1940, the American scientist Mary Hunt succeeded in isolating a significantly improved form of penicillin. The Pentagon invested considerable sums in the manufacture of penicillin. From 1943 onwards it was produced on a large scale in 29 factories so that on D-Day, the start of the invasion on the Normandy beaches, enough penicillin was available for every soldier. When the invasion began, 3 million courses of penicillin were held in storage. Between D-Day on 6 June 1944 and the end of the Second World War on 8 May 1945, hardly any more allied soldiers died of wound infections. In the First World War, 15 per cent of soldiers still died from such infections. During the Second World War, the US Army distributed a propaganda poster depicting a healthcare worker treating a wounded soldier. The poster bore the words 'Thanks to penicillin ... He will come home!' referring back to the First World War when many American—and other—soldiers died as a consequence of wound infections and the sexually transmitted diseases syphilis and gonorrhoea. The latter disease is increasingly becoming difficult to treat due to growing drug resistance (WHO 2012; ECDC 2012a, b).[5]

---

[5]In June 2012, the World Health Organisation (WHO) warned that it would become more difficult to treat gonorrhoea because the bacteria that cause the disease are becoming increasingly resistant to

Jan Kluijtmans, a microbiologist at the Amphia Hospital in Breda and Professor at the University Medical Centre Utrecht, uses every opportunity to show this poster during the presentations and lectures he gives all over the world. The slides he presents afterwards show the rates of mortality caused by infectious diseases in the United States. Around 1900, almost 800 people out of every 100,000 US inhabitants died of infectious diseases. At the time penicillin was discovered, this figure had already been reduced to around 250 per 100,000 inhabitants. After penicillin was introduced, this number fell further, to less than 50 per 100,000 inhabitants. Similar sharp declines in mortality caused by infectious diseases can be observed everywhere penicillin and other antibiotics are used. 'By showing these slides', says Kluijtmans, 'I want to stress that the fall in mortality caused by infectious diseases had already begun decades before penicillin began to be used. Nevertheless, the availability of penicillin has had a very significant impact on the mortality of the population, of a kind never achieved by any other medicine'.

## Water Supply and Sewer Systems

At the time penicillin was introduced in the Western world, infectious diseases had already ceased to be the mass killers they were at the beginning of the twentieth century and during the preceding centuries. Making penicillin available was the third major step in the fight against infectious diseases. The introduction of water supply systems and, later, wastewater sewers had already been able to reduce mortality through infectious diseases considerably. The effects of constructing sewer and water supply systems on the reduction of infectious disease mortality cannot be overestimated. Between 1870 and 1970, the standardised mortality rate[6] in the Netherlands fell by almost 75 per cent (Mackenbach 2007). A similar trend can be demonstrated in Belgium. Between 1880 and 1940, life expectancy increased by 2–3 years every decade (Devos 2006). We see identical developments in Germany, the United Kingdom and other developed countries (Riley 2005). A large proportion of this decline in mortality rate can be attributed to the fact that all possible types of infectious diseases occur less and less often. It was precisely for this reason that, in January 2007, the readers of the prestigious *British Medical Journal* voted sewer and water supply systems the most important milestones (BMJ 2007) in medicine since 1840—ahead of the discovery of antibiotics, anaesthetics and vaccination (Ferriman 2007).

According to the 2006 study *Global burden of disease and risk factors* (Lopez et al. 2006), in 2001 1.8 million people died of diarrhoea in low- to middle-income

---

antibiotics. Cases of gonorrhoea that were resistant to cephalosporins—the last antibiotic available to treat this sexually transmitted disease—have already been reported In Australia, Japan, France, Norway, Sweden and the United Kingdom. Also in June 2012, the European Centre for Disease Prevention and Control (ECDC) published an action plan (ECDC 2012b).

[6]Mortality figures that have been corrected to reflect the composition of the population in terms of age and gender.

countries (World Bank 2020).[7] Polluted water, lack of sanitary facilities and poor hygiene were responsible for 88 per cent of these fatalities (Lopez et al. 2006). In December 2012, the 2010 version of the *Global burden of disease and risk factors* was published (The Lancet 2012). It reported significant advances in the reduction of diarrhoeal deaths—by nearly a half. Nevertheless, according to the scientists' data, every year almost one and a half million children still died of diarrhoea caused by germs for which effective vaccines are available (Lozano et al. 2012). The decrease in deaths due to unsafe sanitation and drinking water continued over the next few years. The 2016 *Global burden of disease* study, published in September 2017, emphasised the fact that both unsafe sanitation and unsafe water became less important as causes of deaths and illness between 1990 and 2016 (The Lancet 2017). These trends were confirmed in the 2017 Global burden of disease study published in October 2018 (Gakidou et al. 2017; IHME 2018). But at the same time, in lower- and middle-income countries, sanitation, safe water and access to hand-washing facilities remain areas where much still needs to be achieved. In the 2020 edition of the Global Burden of Disease the editorialists of *The Lancet* take stock of the developments in this century. I quote this editorial 'Global health: time for radical change?' here in its entirety:

> What strategies should governments adopt to improve the health of their citizens? Amid the COVID-19 syndemic it would be easy to focus attention on global health security—at a minimum, strong public health and health-care systems. WHO has based its global health strategy on three pillars: universal health coverage, health emergencies, and better health and wellbeing. The indispensable elements of robust public health and health care are well known and endlessly rehearsed—a capable health workforce; effective, safe, and high quality service delivery; health information systems; access to essential medicines; sufficient financing; and good governance. But has the gaze of global health been too narrow? Have health leaders and advocates been missing the most important determinants of human health? The latest report of the Global Burden of Diseases, Injuries, and Risk Factors Study (GBD) 2019 raises uncomfortable questions about the direction global health has taken in the 21st century. On the one hand, the news seems good. The health of the world's population is steadily improving. Global life expectancy at birth increased from 67·2 years in 2000 to 73·5 years in 2019. Healthy life expectancy has increased in 202 of 204 countries and territories. In 21 countries, healthy life expectancy at birth increased by more than 10 years between 1990 and 2019, with gains of up to 19·1 years. The estimated number of deaths in children under 5 years decreased from 9·6 million in 2000 to 5 million in 2019. Indeed, the falls in rates of age-standardised disability-adjusted life-years since 1990 have been the largest for communicable, maternal, neonatal, and nutritional diseases—and progress has been fastest in the past decade. But GBD also reveals, once again, that health depends on more than health systems. The strong correlation between health and the sociodemographic index—a summary metric of a country's overall development based on average income per capita, educational attainment, and total fertility rates—suggests that the health sector should consider redefining its scope of concern. GBD 2019 also offers a revised theory of the demographic transition, delineating seven separate stages. A particular

---

[7]These categories are used by the World Bank. According to the World Bank website 'for the current 2021 fiscal year, low-income economies are defined as those with a Gross National Income (GNI) per capita, calculated using the World Bank Atlas Method, of $ 1035 or less in 2019; lower middle-income economies are those with a GNI per capita between $ 1036 and $ 4045.

innovation is the idea of late-transition and post-transition stages, disaggregated for migration status. 35 countries, largely in sub-Saharan Africa and the Middle East, are in mid-transition, with falling birth and death rates (as of 2019, no countries were in the pre-transition stage). Countries such as Brazil, China, and the USA are in the late-transition stage, with death rates plateauing, while birth rates continue to decrease. The final post-transition stage is when the birth rate is lower than the death rate and natural population growth is negative—as seen in Japan, Italy, and Russia. An important and overlooked influence on these demographic stages is migration. 17 countries, including Spain, Greece, and many eastern European countries, are in "a precarious state"—in the post-transition stage, with net emigration. Here, policies are needed to lessen the social and economic effects of an increasingly inverted population pyramid— encouraging immigration could be one way to help. None of these arguments should suggest that universal health coverage and global health security are irrelevant to health. As the GBD 2019 authors argue, some countries have longer life expectancies than their stage of development would predict. These over performing nations—such as Niger, Ethiopia, Portugal, and Spain—probably have superior public health and health-care policies. What GBD 2019 does suggest is that the global health community needs to radically rethink its vision. An exclusive focus on health care is a mistake. Health is created from a broader prospectus that includes the quality of education (primary to tertiary), economic growth, gender equality, and migration policy. This conclusion is immediately relevant to national strategies to address COVID-19. Although attention should be given to controlling community transmission of severe acute respiratory syndrome coronavirus 2 and protecting those most vulnerable to its consequences, success will require a more capacious strategy. COVID-19 is a syndemic of coronavirus infection combined with an epidemic of non-communicable diseases, both interacting on a social substrate of poverty and inequality. The message of GBD is that unless deeply embedded structural inequities in society are tackled and unless a more liberal approach to immigration policies is adopted, communities will not be protected from future infectious outbreaks and population health will not achieve the gains that global health advocates seek. It's time for the global health community to change direction (The Lancet 2020).

A report published in June 2019 by UNICEF and the World Health Organisation (UNICEF and WHO 2019) also underlined that considerable progress was made over the last 10 years in the field of water, sanitation and hygiene. Nevertheless, still roughly 2.2 billion people lack access to safely managed clean drinking water, 2 billion do not have access at all to toilets or only to unsafe toilets and 3 billion lack basic handwashing facilities. The principal culprits in this respect are the open sewers found in the slums of the developing world's megalopolises. They ensure that wastewater contaminated with urine and excrement can find its way into drinking water, producing a lethal cocktail. Since the appearance of the hit film Slumdog Millionaire, awarded eight Oscars, the whole world knows what the sewer system in the slums of Mumbai is like. Six hundred million people in India have no toilets, or still prefer to defecate in the open. Up until 2014 in India's rural regions four out of ten people have a toilet, while more than 80 per cent of people in cities have them. Since the government of Narendra Modi assumed power in India in 2014, the campaign Swachh Bharat Mission (Clean India Mission 2020) has been launched to increase the number of households with toilets. According to the 2018–2019 National Annual Rural Sanitation Survey, more than 93 per cent of rural households had access to toilets (NARSS 2019). The Clean India Mission campaign website even claims that 95 per cent of rural households have access to toilets and 100 per cent of urban households. An official report of the National Statistical Office disputes these figures. The NSO-survey comes to the conclusion that 71 per cent of rural households and 96 per cent of urban households have access to toilets. Having a toilet does not always mean using it. In rural areas, almost 96 per cent of women and 95 per cent of men use the toilet. In urban areas 98 per cent of men and women do. But the availability of many more toilets does not solve all the problems. The sewer system is far from complete, and many wastewater pipes are leaky. As a result, the lakes and rivers are contaminated with germs, and cholera, therefore, is widespread in India (NSO 2019; BBC News 2019).

## Carbapenems by the Dozen

In addition to the lack of wastewater sewers and water supply systems and consequent lack of hygiene, there is still another important cause for the spread of antibiotic resistance: the use of antibiotics itself and, above all, using them improperly and incorrectly. Professor Herman Goossens, Head of the Department for Medical Microbiology at Antwerp University Hospital, saw a whole range of examples of this during a trip to India in October 2011. 'India's 1.2 billion inhabitants not only have a frightening shortage of sanitary facilities and, therefore, a lack of basic hygiene; in this vast country, there is also an infinite multitude of places where there is no medical provision of any sort. All you can do is buy tablets—just like that, across the counter—without any doctor being involved. And this includes antibiotics'. The extensive pharmaceutical industry in the country therefore eagerly exploits the possibilities of this unorganised, unregulated market— 'with all the problems that such behaviour brings', as Goossens puts it. 'In India there are dozens of different meropenems on the market. Meropenem is an important antibiotic belonging to the class of carbapenems. Many of these Indian medicines contain too little active ingredient, or none at all. Medicines with insufficient active ingredients guarantee there will be even more resistances. And the tablets are on sale everywhere'. Alex Friedrich adds: 'If you administer patients antibiotics against a bacterial infection, then usually these should be given for a short time and at a high dosage. In this way, the pathogens are killed and the selection pressure[8] that is responsible for the development of resistances remains as low as possible. If you give too little for too long, the pathogens are not killed, and all you do is support the development of resistances by selection pressure'.

---

[8]When an antibiotic is administered to a patient this drug neutralises or kills microbes that are sensitive to its working, while those resistant stay alive and can procreate without the competition of the neutralised and killed microbes. This mechanism is called selection pressure.

## Bactericidal and Bacteriostatic Agents

Impressed by the success of penicillin, during the 1950s the pharmaceutical industry threw itself enthusiastically into the development of different antibiotics. New products appeared on the market constantly throughout the second half of the twentieth century. They may roughly be divided into two main groups: antibiotics which kill bacteria—bactericidal agents—and antibiotics which inhibit the growth of bacteria—bacteriostatic agents.[9] All these new antibiotics were important, because Alexander Fleming had been more than right when he warned of the development of penicillin resistance. In the United Kingdom, this already became clear in the immediate post-war years (Smith et al. 1969) above all in the case of *Staphylococci aureus* bacteria that cause infections such as furuncle. The majority of people carry these bacteria in their noses, and pass them on to others through hand contact. People with reduced immunity or wounds can therefore easily become infected. This occurs particularly often in hospitals. Within a few years, the percentage of resistant strains of *Staphylococcus aureus* in UK hospitals rose to almost 60 per cent—a fourfold increase. In the United States, exactly the same development occurred in the corresponding period just after the war (Kirby 1945). In some US hospitals at that time, three of the four bacterial strains were already resistant to penicillin. Today, almost all staphylococci strains are penicillin resistant. In the United States, the situation was already on the point of lapsing back to the days before penicillin was discovered in the 1950s.

But then, just in time, the pharmaceutical industry launched in 1960 methicillin on the market, which also helped for a while. It is true that the first case of staphylococci that were resistant to the new medicine was announced after less than a year (Knox 1961), but it took another 10–15 years before methicillin resistance became a major problem. It was then that, above all in European hospitals, outbreaks of the dreaded 'MRSA'—methicillin-resistant *Staphylococcus aureus*—began to increase. By the second half of the 1970s, MRSA was still only responsible for a few problems in Europe, but instead, there were even more in the United States. In the 1980s, Europe again found itself forced to cope with the MRSA problem. On each occasion, new antibiotics were used—for example ciprofloxacin, an antibiotic belonging to the class of fluoroquinolones—and, every time, after a while resistance to the new drug once again developed. On 18 November 2011—European Antibiotic Awareness Day—the European Centre for Disease Prevention and Control (ECDC) presented some figures on the incidence of MRSA in the European Union member states. MRSA remained the leading cause of infections in hospitals and other healthcare institutions. Infections caused by MRSA prolonged the time patients spent in hospital and increased mortality rates (ECDC 2011). At a press conference in Brussels, the ECDC director at that time—Marc Sprenger—said that

---

[9]Beta-lactam antibiotics, aminoglycosides, (fluoro-) quinolones, vancomycin, rifampicin, nitroimidazole derivatives and sulphonamides/trimethoprim are bactericidal medicines. Tetracycline, macrolides, chloramphenicol and thiamphenicol have bacteriostatic effects.

the situation in the EU with regard to the campaign against MRSA had somewhat improved. Nevertheless, in almost a quarter of all EU countries, the percentage of MRSA still remained between 25 and 50. These countries are coloured deep red on the map of Europe. In Portugal and Romania, where the red is even darker, the percentage of MRSA has even risen to more than half of all infections caused by *Staphylococcus aureus*.

The data Marc Sprenger—since summer 2015, and until he became in January 2021 Special Envoy Covid-19 Vaccination for Dutch Caribbean on behalf of Dutch Government, he was director of the WHO's secretariat for antimicrobial resistance— presented were surveillance data. Surveillance of antimicrobial resistance tracks changes in microbial populations. It permits the early detection of resistant strains of public health importance and makes the prompt notification and investigation of outbreaks possible. The ultimate goal of strengthening surveillance is to address with more success the challenge of antibiotic resistance and to improve the outcome for individual patients.

Over the last couple of years, the decline in the total number of invasive MRSA isolates has been lower compared with the period 2009–2012. But the decrease of MRSA did continue in 2019 like it did in previous years, states the ECDC annual report on antimicrobial surveillance in Europe 2019, published in November 2020. 'Despite this positive development, MRSA remains an important pathogen in Europe. S. aureus is one of the most common causes of bloodstream infections, exhibiting a high burden in terms of morbidity and mortality' (ECDC 2020b). The population-weighted mean percentage of MRSA among invasive *Staphylococcus aureus* isolates was 15.5 per cent with large differences between countries ranging from 1.1% in Norway to 46.7% in Romania. Six countries reported MRSA percentages still above 25% (ECDC 2020a).

## New Threats

But when we speak of antibiotic resistance, we are no longer just talking about MRSA. Certainly, MRSA is the best known and most widespread germ, 'but we know a great deal about it and can keep it under control to a certain extent', says Hermann Goossens. He is regarded as one of the trailblazers in the fight against antibiotic resistance—and not just in Belgium, but throughout Europe. 'We've already known about MRSA bacteria for such a long time, and we've learnt to live with them. We don't worry about them so very much, because we've established that they're on the decline in many European countries. Of course, MRSA is very much still with us. But we can still treat MRSA infections. There are still medicines that work.' Our real concern is not with MRSA—a gram-positive bacterium—but with the gram-negative bacteria.'[10]

---

[10]The Danish microbiologist Hans Christian Gram (1853–1938) developed the Gram staining technique, which enables types of bacteria to be distinguished by staining them with crystal violet

The bacterial cell is surrounded by a membrane, and this in turn is surrounded by a cell wall. Gram-negative bacteria are distinguished from Gram-positive types by their much thinner cell wall. But they have an additional membrane around the cell wall. This distinction is important for combatting infections. Many antibiotics are targeted specifically at the cell walls of bacteria, since human and animal cells have no cell walls. In this way, the antibiotics kill off pathogenic bacteria without causing damage to human or animal cells.

'At present, we are seeing an enormous increase in infections caused by gram-negative bacteria, above all in Asia. This continent isn't just developing into a vast economic power: at the same time, it's a huge reservoir of antibiotic resistance and a major danger for global public health. We're therefore watching China and India with great interest – the two biggest global economic powers of the future and, at the same time, the countries which present the greatest threat where antibiotic resistance is concerned'.

These troublesome Gram-negative bacteria include, for example *Klebsiella pneumoniae*. Named after their discoverer, Theodor Klebs, the *Klebsiella* has a huge potential to cause disease. This bacterium is one of the main causes of urinary tract infections, pneumonias and since *Klebsiella* is an intestinal bacterium, it is easily spread from one patient to another through hand contact with hospital staff. In fact, until now multiresistant *Klebsiella* have mostly been found in hospitals. But it is precisely here that one finds the sick and enfeebled people who most easily succumb to infections. And since the average length of a hospital stay is becoming increasingly shorter, the patients in hospitals are, on average, becoming increasingly sicker.

The former Head of the ECDC, Marc Sprenger, came straight to the point on European Antibiotic Awareness Day, 2011. 'Since 2009 we have seen a dramatic increase in resistance to antibiotics of the carbapenem class in the European Union. In 2009 it only occurred in Greece, although *Klebsiella* strains that were resistant to carbapenems were also found in Italy and Cyprus. In 2010, we also established a rising trend in Austria, Cyprus, Hungary and Italy (ECDC 2011). This is all the more alarming because carbapenems are the last available option for treatment of infections caused by multiresistant gram-negative bacteria. 'Antibiotics from the carbapenem class can still be administered for cases of ESBL. But the options for treating patients who are suffering from an infection by carbapenem-resistant bacteria are very limited'. A year later, Sprenger presented the figures for 2011 at the European Antibiotic Awareness Day Symposium 2012. In Italy, more than a quarter of all *Klebsiella* infections had been caused by *Klebsiella* strains that were resistant to carbapenems. In Greece, the figure was actually more than half of *Klebsiella* infections (ECDC 2012a, b).

In 2012, Greece and Italy were still struggling against the high proportion of infections that were caused by carbapenem-resistant *Klebsiella pneumoniae*. *Carbapenemase-producing Enterobacteriaceae* (CPE) bacteria are endemic to

---

iodine complex, decolouring them with alcohol, and counterstaining them with fuchsin. Gram-negative bacteria are coloured red, and Gram-positive bacteria appear bluish-violet.

these countries. Meanwhile in Germany and Belgium, CPE bacteria have been appearing in individual regions. In the Netherlands, there were sporadic outbreaks in hospitals (ECDC 2013). At the European Antibiotic Awareness Day Symposium in 2015, the ECDC presented new figures. The average percentage in the EU, Iceland and Norway, adjusted for population structure, rose from 4.6% in 2010 to 7.3% in 2014. This increase was mainly caused by southern and south-eastern European countries. The same applies to the increase in carbapenem resistance found in *Pseudomonas aeruginosa* and *Acinetobacter* spp. (ECDC 2015).

The ECDC Report Surveillance of antimicrobial resistance in 2019, published in November 2020, shows a limited further increase of the average percentage of carbapenem-resistant *Klebsiella pneumoniae* to an population-weighted average in the EU, Iceland and Norway (EU/EEA) from 6.5 in 2015 to 7.9% in 2019 (ECDC 2020a, b). This was again mainly caused by southern and south-eastern European countries, where the rates of *Klebsiella pneumoniae* resistant to carbapenems remain extremely high in Greece (58.3%) and also very high in Romania (32.3%), Italy (28.5%) and Bulgaria (27%) (ECDC 2020a, b). The population-weighted EU/EEA-average of carbapenem resistance in *Pseudomonas aeruginosa* decreased over 5 years from 19.3 to 16.5% in 2019. For *Acinetobacter* spp. not much changed in the same period of time. ECDC registered an increase from 32.1 in 2015 to 32.6% in 2019 (ECDC 2020a, b).

## Colistin

In countries with high levels of carbapenem resistance, it is inevitable that colistin—one of the very few remaining treatment options—is used relatively often instead.[11] As a result, combined resistance to carbapenems and colistin is observed more frequently there (ECDC 2018). In 2015, between 5% and 10% of all carbapenem-resistant invasive *Klebsiella pneumoniae* isolates in Greece, Italy, Romania, Cyprus and Malta were also resistant to colistin. This trend continued in 2016: of all invasive *K. pneumoniae* isolates reported to the ECDC in that year, between 5 and 10% were resistant to both carbapenems and colistin in Italy, and between 10 and 25% in Greece, Romania and Cyprus. Resistance against colistin is also appearing regularly in *Acinetobacter* spp. in Europe. In 2015, 4% of all invasive *Acinetobacter* isolates possessed resistance to colistin—a percentage that did not change in 2016.

If there is resistance to carbapenems, there are still two other medicines left: colistin, to which reference has already been made, and tigecycline. It is known that tigecycline is more frequently ineffective than other antibiotics, and that mortality rates during treatment can be slightly higher than with other agents (Prasad et al.

---

[11]Colistin belongs to the family of polymixins, a group of polypeptide antibiotics discovered in 1947. They have broad-spectrum activity against Gram-negative bacteria, including most species of the Enterobacteriaceae family. The two polymyxins currently in clinical use are polymyxin B and polymyxin E (colistin), which differ from one another by one amino acid only, and have comparable biological activity.

2012). Jacobien Veenemans, Assistant Physician for Clinical Microbiology at the Amphia Hospital in Breda, presented some data on this at the annual Symposium of the Working Group for Antibiotics Guidelines (SWAB) in 2012. The conclusion drawn from these data was that it would be better to avoid the use of tigecycline, particularly for critically ill patients, if any other medicines were still available. A number of Gram-negative bacteria easily become resistant to this drug. Over half of all enterobacter[12] causing infections are resistant to tigecycline. *E. coli* is often susceptible to tigecycline. The other drug, colistin, is notorious for its side-effects, in particular its damaging effect on the kidneys. Since safer drugs were developed, colistin—a medicine that is over 50 years old—has not been as widely used in human medicine as before.

In many countries, such as Brazil, India, China or Argentina it is given to chicks as a means of boosting growth. In recent years, many doctors and microbiologists have again been voicing concerns about colistin's side-effects. However, sometimes there is no other option.

'Medicines that we would have preferred not to use in the past, because they are poisonous, are suddenly regarded as not that bad at all if the alternative is death', says Australian professor Lindsay Grayson, Head of the Department of Infectious Diseases & Microbiology at the Austin Hospital in Melbourne and editor of the handbook *Kucer's The Use of Antibiotics*. But the side-effects of the medicine seem to have abated as well. 'That has something to do with the old method of manufacturing colistin', explains James Stuart Cohen, a clinical microbiologist at the Alkmaar Medical Centre in the Netherlands. 'The way it used to be produced, it gave rise to renal toxicity in some patients. The production process has now been changed, and since then this problem has occurred much less often. I rarely encounter any kidney problems when I give patients colistin. If I don't have any other options, I am very happy to prescribe it for my patients'. The old antibiotic chloramphenicol is also still effective against Gram-negative bacteria on occasions. 'It penetrates everything', says Stuart Cohen, 'it's actually a broad-spectrum version of tigecycline. But it's also a scary drug to use, because sometimes it can lead to a very severe bone marrow suppression in which the marrow almost—or completely—ceases to function. In this case the bone marrow no longer produces blood platelets or white blood cells any more. And, moreover, this is irreversible. For this reason, chloramphenicol is hardly ever still used in Western countries, but in India and Africa everyone uses it'.

'The same applies to colistin,' says Lindsay Grayson, whom we have already mentioned. 'It's no surprise that colistin is a bestseller in India. This is because of the multiresistant NDM-1 bacteria'. The NDM-1 enzyme makes bacteria resistant against all carbapenem antibiotics. Administering colistin intravenously is then one of the few remaining treatment options. And now that colistin is once again in more frequent use—and not just in India, in the United Kingdom there was a 40%

---

[12]Enterobacteriaceae or enterobacter are a family of Gram-negative bacteria, the most frequently occurring of which are *E. coli* and *Klebsiella* spp. 'spp.' stands for 'species'(plural).

rise in its use from 2014 to 2015 (The Bureau of Investigative Journalism 2017)—
colistin-resistant bacteria are inevitably appearing (Mohanty et al. 2013; Balaji et al.
2011; Marchaim et al. 2011; Lesho et al. 2013).

## MCR-1

Concerns about the growing number of different bacteria resistant to colistin were
heightened by the publication of a study in *The Lancet Infectious Diseases* in
February 2016 (and online in November 2015), 'Emergence of plasmid-mediated
colistin resistance mechanism MCR-1 in animals and human beings in China: a
microbiological and molecular biological study' (Liu et al. 2015). A group of
Chinese and British researchers discovered a new colistin resistance mechanism,
'(plasmid-) mediated colistin resistance' (mcr-1) in both animals and humans, which
was transferred between *Enterobacteriaceae* spp.—including some that were
(highly) pathogenic—via a plasmid. The researchers found mcr-1 in 21% of all
animal samples, and 15% of raw meat samples. Although only relatively low
numbers of invasive isolates in humans carry the mcr-1 gene—1.4% of *E. coli*,
0.4% of *K. pneumoniae*, 0.1% of *E. cloacae* and 0.6% of *E. aerogenes*—in their
article the authors issue a clear warning. 'The rapid dissemination of previous
resistance mechanisms (e.g. NDM-1) indicates that, with the advent of transmissible
colistin resistance, progression of *Enterobacteriaceae* from extensive drug resistance to pan-drug resistance is inevitable and will ultimately become global. In this
context the emergence of transmissible, plasmid-mediated colistin resistance in the
form of mcr-1 is a finding of global significance'. Shortly after the publication of the
first study on the mcr-1 gene, mcr-1 genes were found in human, animal and
environmental samples in more than 30 countries on all continents during retrospective analyses of microbial isolates (Skov and Monnet 2016). Since the discovery of
mcr-1, comparable mcr-2 and mcr-3 genes have been found, which also make
bacteria resistant to colistin (CIDRAP 2017).

In January 2017, *The Lancet Infectious Diseases* published a further study, partly
authored by the same researchers. Among other topics, it looked into the molecular
epidemiology of mcr-1 positive *Enterobacteriaceae* (MCRPE) (Wang et al. 2017).
The authors identified an 'extreme divergence of *E. coli* strains carrying mcr-1 not
only between Zhejiang and Guangdong [the provinces where the study was carried
out], but also within each hospital'. The different *E. coli* strains carrying mcr-1 genes
came from patients with bloodstream infections. In a second study published in
January 2017, a Chinese group collected invasive isolates of *Escherichia coli* and
*Klebsiella pneumoniae* from patients with bloodstream infections at 28 hospitals in
seven Chinese provinces. Of 1495 *E. coli* isolates, 20 (1%) carried mcr-1 and were
resistant to colistin. According to the researchers, the study demonstrates the mcr-1
is still rare in Chinese healthcare settings and the community in general, but also that
a certain amount of transfer to different regions had already taken place (Quan et al.
2017). This finding was confirmed by the first, slightly more extensive study: '[...]
MCRPEC [mcr-1 positive *Enterobacteriaceae*] are diversely spread throughout

China and pervasive in Chinese communities' (Wang et al. 2017). These researchers also investigated the main risk factors for infection and colonisation by mcr-1 positive *E. coli*. Being a male was one risk factor for infection, as was being immunosuppressed, while the use of antibiotics during a hospital stay—particularly carbapenems—was a major risk factor. For colonisation, the risk factor was exposure to antibiotics. To the authors' surprise, living near a farm was not. 'Antibiotic use before hospital admission was associated with MCRPEC carriage in 35 patients compared with 378 patients with *mcr-1*-negative *E. coli* colonisation, whereas living next to a farm was associated with *mcr-1*-negative *E. coli* colonisation'. In their first study, on the discovery of mcr-1, the authors had written: 'Colistin has not yet been approved for use in human beings in China, but it has been used in animals as a therapeutic drug and feed additive since the early 1980s. Thus, we speculated that the emergence and spread of *mcr-1* probably occurred first in animals and spread to human beings (Liu et al. 2015)'.

Since the publication of the study on the discovery of mcr-1, China has banned the use of colistin in livestock farming and permitted its use for the treatment of human infections by highly resistant microbes. The scientists predict a reduction of colistin resistance rates in the community and an increase in hospitals due to more intensive use of the drug. 'Our study suggests that there are already significant risk factors for MCRPEC infections and these are likely to be exacerbated when colistin is used clinically. Furthermore, the carriage of MCRPEC as normal flora does not seem to be associated with rural living or diet, suggesting other factors, including environmental dissemination of MCR-1, might be associated with MCRPEC carriage' (Wang et al. 2017). Some data presented by the authors in the first study on mcr-1 possibly support this thesis that environmental dissemination can play a role in the spread of mcr-1 (Liu et al. 2015).

## World Number One

China is the world's number one producer of both poultry (17.5 million tonnes) and pigs (56.7 million tonnes), of which about 10% are for export. In addition, China is one of the biggest users of colistin for agricultural purposes. By the end of 2015, global agricultural use of colistin was estimated to be almost 12,000 tonnes, which was expected to rise to 16,500 tonnes by 2021. This increase in the use of colistin is mainly driven by China. Moreover, as the researchers note, 'of the top ten largest producers of colistin for veterinary use, one is Indian, one is Danish and eight are Chinese'. The European Union and the United States both imported hundreds of tonnes of Chinese colistin in 2015. Asia is responsible for almost three-quarters of global colistin production. China's decision to ban colistin as an animal feed additive in October 2016, and allow it for human use, could potentially have a huge impact. According to Timothy R. Walsh and Yongning Yu, two scientists closely involved in mcr-1 research, 'this seminal event will lead to the withdrawal of more than 8000 tonnes of colistin as a growth promoter from the Chinese veterinary sector' (Walsh and Wu 2016). In the summer of 2019, the Indian government followed the Chinese example (Poultry World 2019b) and banned colistin for veterinary use as, for example Argentina did before (Poultry World 2019a).

The high proportion of mcr-1 in samples taken from animals (21%), suggests that manure and wastewater may be ways in which the plasmid-mediated colistin resistance gene is disseminated in the environment. Colistin entering the environment through farming, industry wastewater and manure can be picked up by microbes that subsequently find their way to humans and animals. Another potentially vast source of colistin in the environment—and hence in plants, animals and humans—is the huge Chinese pharmaceutical industry, which is famous for its poor treatment of industrial wastewater. (Just like the important Indian pharmaceutical industry, it should be noted in passing.) In June 2015, SumOfUs, who describe themselves as 'a global consumer watchdog', published a report called *Bad Medicine*: *How the pharmaceutical industry is contributing to the global rise of antibiotic-resistant superbugs*. Based on research by the Changing Markets Foundation and Profundo Research and Advice, the report says that 'most of the world's antibiotic drugs are manufactured in China and India. China is now the top producer of penicillin industrial salts, a vital building block in the production of many antibiotics, and produces 80–90% of antibiotic active pharmaceutical ingredients (APIs)'. The Indian pharmaceutical industry is the third largest in the world, and focuses on the production of finished antibiotics using active ingredients imported mainly from China (SumOfUs 2015). The value of China's exports of organic chemicals—the kind most commonly used in pharmaceuticals—grew from $5.3 billion in 2004 to $36.5 billion in 2013 (Report to the Congress of the U.S. - China Economic and Security Review Commission 2014). 'The pharmaceutical industry', say the authors of *Bad Medicine*, 'has long maintained that antibiotic manufacturing does not play a significant role in fuelling drug resistance, arguing that the final product is so valuable that it would not be economically rational to discharge vast quantities of it as waste'. However, revelations by Chinese TV in 2014, and some scientific studies, have demonstrated that pollution by antibiotic factories is a very real phenomenon. Basically, a study carried out in 2013 showed that very few pharmaceutical industries in China and other Asian countries treat the wastewater of their production processes before it is discharged into rivers or canals (Zhang et al. 2013). 'The application of untreated wastewater (industrial and domestic) and biosolids (sewage sludge and manure) in agriculture causes the contamination of surface water, soil, groundwater and the entire food web with pharmaceutical compounds (PCs), their metabolites and transformed products (TPs) and multidrug-resistant microbes'. The researchers believe that 'this pharmaceutical contamination in Asian countries poses global risks via product export and international' (SumOfUs 2015).

The findings of these scientists were confirmed by another Changing Market study published in 2016 (Changing Markets and Ecostorm 2016) and by an earlier study on pharmaceutical contamination in highly populated developing countries (Rehman et al. 2013).

## Chinese River Basins

A group of researchers led by Professor Guang-Guo Ying, of the Institute of Geochemistry in Guangzhou and the Chinese Academy of Sciences, investigated the antibiotic pollution of Chinese river basins. They studied the usage of 36 antibiotics that are frequently detected in the environment, and commonly given to animals and humans, over the course of 2013. Their study (Zhang et al. 2015), published in *Environmental Science and Technology* in May 2015, did not take into account the possible role of the pharmaceutical industry, but concentrated on the use of antibiotics for animals and humans. In an interview for the Dutch public broadcaster NOS at the end of March 2016, Professor Ying stated: 'Personally, I think pharmaceutical factories are an isolated problem. Not like animal waste or human waste. The population is so large, and there are so many animals in China. In Guangzhou, for example, we have only three large factories producing ATB [...] We have done a lot of surveys, and the pharmaceutical factories are not a main contributor to antibiotics contamination. The chief factor is animal waste'. In their study, the scientists emphasise the poor management of wastewater containing antibiotics. 'In the majority of rural areas in China in particular, the rate of sewage treatment is quite low owing to the limited infrastructure. Additionally, in China there are as yet no specific requirements for treatment of livestock waste before discharge. Direct discharge into rivers and utilisation of livestock waste on agricultural lands are common practice' (NOS 2016).

And not just in China, one might add—in India, too, the situation is scarcely any different. In a study published in November 2017, researchers at the Centre for Disease Dynamics, Economics and Policy (CCDEP) wrote: 'Bacteria resistant to broad-spectrum (third generation) antibiotics have been found in poultry, cattle, pigs and fish. There are no set standards for antibiotic residues in pharmaceutical industrial pollution, and their effluents are therefore not monitored for these. Last-resort antibiotic resistance genes (NDM-1) have been identified in several major rivers in India' (Gandra et al. 2017). The consequences of this were presented in May 2019 by Jyoti Joshi during a conference of the CCDEP. *Klebsiella pneumoniae*, *Pseudomonas aeruginosa*, *Acinetobacter baumannii* and *Escherichia coli* show high levels of carbapenem resistance (Joshi 2019). The *Bad Medicine* report describes how 'in 2007, the first in a series of papers by Swedish researcher Joakim Larsson was published, showing very high emissions of pharmaceuticals from drug manufacturers in Patancheru, near the Indian city of Hyderabad. Tests on effluent from a treatment plant receiving wastewater from about 90 manufacturing plants showed that concentrations for some pharmaceuticals were greater than those found in the blood of patients undergoing treatment (Larsson 2014). The researchers told Bloomberg that concentrations of antibiotics in the river sediment further downstream were so high that if "ciprofloxacin [a type of antibiotic] were more valuable, we could mine it from the ground" (Bloomberg 2012).

The dumping of antibiotic waste by manufacturing plants creates ideal conditions for the massive proliferation of multidrug-resistant bacteria and the emergence of antibiotic resistance. Concentrations of antibiotics in effluent from manufacturing plants are much higher than those resulting from excretion (Leetz 2015). Antibiotic pollution therefore accelerates the spread of resistance genes and their transfer from environmental microbes to other species, and eventually to bacteria that are dangerous to humans (Kristiansson et al. 2011). Additionally, antibiotic pollution can harm environmental bacteria and algae present in water and soil, altering the distribution of species and causing harm to the ecosystem as a whole' (Lyons 2014).

## Production and Usage

Yings group estimated that, in 2013, the total production of all antibiotics in China was 248,000 tonnes. The total usage of all antibiotics in China during the same year was estimated to be 162,000 tonnes (48% for humans, 52% for animals), while exports were 88,000 tonnes and imports 600 tonnes. The level of antibiotics use in China is extremely high. In a personal email to the author Professor Ying writes that the global usage of antibiotics in 2013 was around 400,000 tonnes, so during that year China used more than 40% of all antibiotics used worldwide. According to the researchers led by Guang-Guo Ying, in terms of Defined Daily Doses per 1000 inhabitants per day (DID), China uses roughly five times more antibiotics for humans than the United Kingdom, United States, Canada and the EU (Zhang et al. 2015).

In the paper 'Review of antibiotic resistance in China and its environment' (Min et al. 2018), the total usage of 36 selected antibiotics was 92,700 tonnes, of which only 15.6% was used for humans, and the rest for veterinary purposes. Of these 92,700 tonnes, 54,000 tonnes were excreted via urine and faeces. Wastewater treatment plants removed an estimated 200 tonnes of antibiotics; the remaining 53,800 tonnes were discharged into the environment—almost half into water, the rest on soil. The emissions of antibiotics are at their highest in central and eastern China—roughly six times higher than in the west of the country. 'In general', says Yings team in their other quoted study (Zhang et al. 2015), 'the aquatic environment has relatively higher contamination levels when compared with other countries around the world'.

This can best be seen through the example of fluoroquinolones. On average, antibiotic pollution with fluoroquinolones in the 58 Chinese river basins is 303 nanograms per litre, but in seven rivers it was more than 1000 nanograms, and in one case even as much as 7560 nanograms per litre. In Italy, the average is 9 nanograms per litre, in Germany 20 and in the United States 120 nanograms per litre. Seventeen per cent of all antibiotics in China belong to the group of fluoroquinolones, compared with—for example—less than 10% in the United States. According to the researchers, 'the bacterial resistance rates in the hospitals and aquatic environments were found to be related to the predicted environmental concentrations and antibiotic usages, especially for those antibiotics used in the most recent period. This is the first comprehensive study which demonstrates the alarming usage and emission of various antibiotics in China'. Furthermore, they sound a note of warning: 'The results from the present study found an alarming nationwide overuse and emission of various antibiotics in China. This has resulted in relatively high environmental concentrations and increased antibiotic resistance in hospitals and receiving environments. In addition, animal use of various antibiotics has also been a serious concern as increased bacterial resistance and widespread presence of ARBs and ARGs[13] were reported in livestock farms and the surrounding environment. This could pose a great threat to human health when bacteria causing infections are no longer susceptible to antibiotic treatment; therefore, tight management measures are urgently needed to control the overuse of antibiotics in China. This could also be a reminder for other developing countries with similar situations. Rational use of antibiotics in humans and animals should be promoted around the world'.

Among 146 MCRPE isolates investigated for the study they carried out in Zhejiang and Guangdong provinces, the researchers who first discovered the mcr-1 gene found a total of five *E. coli* isolates from human infections and in chicken meat where mcr-1 coexisted with the carbapenem resistance genes NDM-5 (Yang et al. 2016), NDM-9 (Lai et al. 2017) and KPC-2 (Martins Aires et al. 2017). This coexistence, the Chinese scientists wrote, 'is of great concern, because the occurrence of the mcr-1 gene in CRE would seriously compromise treatment options not only in China but also globally' (Wang et al. 2017).

## India's Sore Point

We have already mentioned 'NDM'—which stands for 'New Delhi metallo-beta-lactamase'—on a couple of occasions. The enzyme was first identified in a *Klebsiella pneumoniae* bacterium infecting a Swedish patient of Indian origin (Yong et al. 2009. The man travelled to India in 2008 and contracted an infection of the urinary tract there. The *Klebsiella* that had caused the infection possessed a hitherto unknown resistance gene. The new enzyme was discovered by Professor Timothy Walsh, Head of the Department of Medical Microbiology at the Cardiff University School of Medicine. As was customary at the time, he named it after the place it first appeared: New Delhi. By so doing, he touched a sore point for the Indian authorities. After publishing a second study in *The Lancet* (Kumarasamy et al. 2010), where he described how he and his team had found bacteria with the NDM-1 enzyme in several places in India, Pakistan and the United Kingdom, Walsh began receiving hate mail from India. He was more or less declared persona non grata there. But Walsh—who was also one of the discoverers of the mcr-1 gene—does not regard himself as the culpable party.

'I would gladly have helped the Indian government to tackle this problem, but they were not prepared to talk to me', he told me at a meeting on the topic of antibiotic resistance organised during the Danish EU presidency in March 2012. 'By refusing to collaborate, India is violating the rules of the World Health Organisation

---

[13]ARBs = antibiotic resistant bacteria, ARGs = antibiotic resistance genes.

(WHO), which it actually committed to complying with. I would be truly happy to set up a research centre together with Indian colleagues. Instead of getting worked up about the name "New Delhi metallo-beta-lactamase", they should rather concentrate on developing antibiotics guidelines, and setting up a network of public lavatories to improve hygiene. The sanitary facilities in India are a nightmare. I am very glad that the WHO highlights so emphatically the connection between hygiene and clean drinking water on the one hand, and infectious diseases and antibiotic resistances on the other. But of course, something should have been done about this matter much earlier'. The British professor emphasised the importance of an international action plan for this problem. 'In Europe, we are still too much concerned with national solutions for this problem. But actually we should proceed on a European level or even a global one. Globalisation is making antibiotic resistance a worldwide problem. Therefore, we can only fight it on that same level. We must think globally'.

In his lecture at the conference in Copenhagen, Walsh referred to a bus accident in Switzerland, which killed 22 Belgian and Dutch children and six adults. 'That is a horrifying tragedy—but during the 15 minutes this presentation will last, 120 children in India will die from a preventable infectious disease'. In October 2011, Walsh's Flemish colleague Herman Goossens presented nine lectures in 1 week in six different Indian cities. He spoke to dozens of Indian doctors. 'In India, people are in fact primarily concerned about the effects of the NDM-1 story on medical tourism to the country', he says. 'Many private hospitals have made massive investments to attract patients from outside India. Financially speaking, many hospitals in India are only just keeping their heads above water and trying to make some profit from medical tourism. From an economic point of view, therefore, medical tourism is very important. Many people come from Pakistan and other neighbouring countries, but they also come from the Middle East, the US and, of course, from the UK with its large Indian community. For them, it is purely a matter of economic considerations. They are not so concerned about questions of public health. 'Oh,' they say, 'if a couple of hundred or thousand people out of a population of 1.2 billion die of treatable infections, what's that?' This is also because it is primarily a matter of poor people, who are treated in state hospitals. So they certainly worry about their money, but not about the health of the general population that is threatened by NDM. Many doctors there have asked me why the West gets so worked up about the NDM-1 bacterium. Ultimately, children die much more frequently of malaria and tuberculosis, which could be prevented by vaccination. NDM-1 causes far fewer fatalities. But they all confirm that patients die from non-treatable infections; they just do not want to publish any figures about it. And then, if you hear these figures from the people who are involved with them, you scarcely want to believe them', Goossens said.

'Between 60 and 80 per cent of *E. coli* and *Klebsiella* bacteria produce ESBL. And a substantial number of bacteria—around 20 to 30 per cent—are already resistant to carbapenems. In such cases, only tigecycline and colistin are of any use. They do not use tigecycline, as it is reputed to be a poor product, and therefore only colistin is left. Therefore in India, too, it is available on the market in a whole range of generic versions. Colistin is in fact administered a great deal, and it has been shown that, as a result, resistances against it also arise. Soon it will be "burnt-out" as a product, and then we won't have anything anymore'. Many outbreaks of carbapenem- and colistin-resistant *Klebsiella pneumoniae* in Italy (Mammina et al. 2012), Greece (Kontopoulou et al. 2010) and the United States (Marchaim et al. 2011), and of *Acinetobacter baumannii* in India (Taneja et al. 2011), had already been identified early in the second decade of this century and many more have been since (Bardhan et al. 2020; Palmieri et al. 2020; Lalaoui et al. 2019; Balkhair et al. 2019; Kalem et al. 2016).

## Combinations with Colistin

Stuart Cohen is of the same opinion as Goossens and several of his other colleagues. 'We're standing with our backs to the wall, there are only a few treatment options left. But we still know too little about the possibilities that might arise if we combine the available drugs. Research into this question is still in its infancy. However, it is only recently that it has become necessary to conduct research in this field, since before then effective medicines were still available'. At ECCMID 2012, the annual European conference for microbiologists, one workshop was devoted to the application of colistin.

A study from Israel presented at the workshop had established that colistin is increasingly being used as a last resort to treat patients suffering from infections caused by carbapenem-resistant bacteria. The study found that there was a greater beneficial effect when colistin was administered in combination with other agents. According to Israeli scientists, treatments with colistin monotherapy still have lower mortality rates than those using ineffective antibiotics or prescribing the wrong ones. In the case of critically ill patients infected with carbapenem-resistant bacteria, colistin monotherapy resulted in a higher mortality rate. The Israeli study came to the conclusion that colistin did not cause substantially more cases of renal toxicity than other antibiotics. If an equivalent side-effect occurs all the same, it is usually reversible. If high doses are used, then resistances to colistin appear in certain cases (Akova et al. 2012).

At the same workshop, Professor Yehuda Carmeli of the Tel Aviv Medical Centre and the Israeli National Centre for Antibiotic Resistance presented other data supporting the conclusion that colistin is a useful medicine. Above all, a combination of colistin and carbapenem antibiotics can help against bacteria that are resistant to carbapenems. Such combination treatments seem to be much more effective than monotherapy with colistin only. To illustrate this, James Stuart Cohen gives the example of vancomycin. This is an antibiotic that is ineffective against Gram-negative bacteria, such as *Klebsiella* or *Acinetobacter,* because it cannot penetrate their external cellular membrane. 'However, if you combine it with colistin, it clearly produces a synergistic effect. The colistin produces holes in the outer cell wall, which enables the vancomycin to penetrate it and thus take effect. If no new drugs become available, then at the moment it seems as though this is the way we're going to have to go. I'm convinced of that'. Stuart Cohen is researching new options to enable the continuing use of existing antibiotics.

In an e-mail sent to the author at the end of October 2017, James Stuart Cohen wrote that a small clinical trial involving twelve patients had yielded 'encouraging results'. Mr. Stuart Cohen had been preparing an article on the trial to submit for publication but unfortunately, he said, a pharmaceutical company had suddenly stopped production of one of the compounds used in it.

## References

Akova, M., Daikos, G. L., Tzouvelekis, L., et al. (2012). Interventional strategies and current clinical experience with carbapenemase-producing Gram-negative bacteria. *Clinical Microbiology and Infection, 8*(5), 439–448. https://doi.org/10.1111/j.1469-0691.2012.03823.x.

Balaji, V., Jeremiah, S. S., & Baliga, P. R. (2011). Polymyxins: antimicrobial susceptibility concerns and therapeutic options. *Indian Journal of Medical Microbiology, 29*(3), 230–242. https://doi.org/10.4103/0255-0857.83905.

Balkhair, A., Al-Muharrmi, Z., Al'Adawi, B., et al. (2019). Prevalence and 30-day all-cause mortality of carbapenem-and-colistin-resistant bacteraemia caused by *Acinetobacter baumannii*, *Pseudomonas aeruginosa*, and *Klebsiella pneumoniae*: Description of a decade-long trend. *International Journal of Infectious Diseases, 85*, 10–15. https://www.ijidonline.com/article/S1201-9712(19)30210-3/pdf.

Bardhan, T., Chakraborty, M., & Bhattacharjee, B. (2020). Prevalence of colistin-resistant, carbapenem-hydrolyzing proteobacteria in hospital water bodies and out-falls of West Bengal, India. *International Journal of Environmental Research and Public Health, 17*(3), 1007. https://doi.org/10.3390/ijerph17031007.

BBC News. (2019). *India's toilets: Report questions claims that rural areas are free from open defecation*. Accessed October 18, 2020, from https://www.bbc.com/news/world-asia-india-46400678

Bhullar, K., Waglechner, N., Pawlowski, A., et al. (2012). Antibiotic resistance is prevalent in an isolated cave microbiome. *PLoS One, 7*(4), e34953. https://doi.org/10.1371/journal.pone.0034953.

Blaak, H., Van Rooijen, S. R., & Schuijt, M. S. (2011). *Prevalence of antibiotic resistant bacteria in the rivers Meuse, Rhine, and New Meuse*. RIVM Report 703719071/2011. Accessed October 18, 2020, from http://www.rivm.nl/bibliotheek/rapporten/703719071.pdf

Bloomberg. (2012). *Drug-defying germs from India Speed post-antibiotic era*. Accessed October 22, 2020, from https://www.bloomberg.com/news/articles/2012-05-07/drug-defying-germs-from-india-speed-post-antibiotic-era

BMJ. (2007). *Shortlist medical milestones*. Accessed from https://www.bmj.com/content/medical-milestones

Cars, O., Hedin, A., & Heddini, A. (2011). The global need for effective antibiotics—Moving towards concerted action. *Drug Resistance Updates, 14*(2), 68–69. https://doi.org/10.1016/j.drup.2011.02.006.

Changing Markets and Ecostorm. (2016). *Superbugs in the supply chain: How pollution from antibiotics factories in India and China is fueling the global rise of drug-resistant infections*. Accessed from http://health21initiative.org/wp-content/uploads/2017/08/2016-Changing-Markets-Superbugs-in-the-Supply-Chain.pdf

CIDRAP (Center for Infectious Disease Research and Policy). (2017). *More colistin-resistance genes identified in Europe*. Accessed from https://www.cidrap.umn.edu/news-perspective/2017/08/more-colistin-resistance-genes-identified-europe

Clean India Mission. (2020). *Swachh Bharat Mission. Government of India, Department of Drinking Water and Sanitation*. Accessed October 19, 2020, from https://sbm.gov.in/sbmdashboard/IHHL.aspx

D'Costa, V., King, C., Kalan, L., et al. (2011). Antibiotic resistance is ancient. *Nature, 477*, 457–461. https://doi.org/10.1038/nature10388.

De Jonge, E., De Boer, M. G. J., Van Essen, H. E. R., et al. (2019). Effects of a disinfection device on colonization of sink drains and patients during a prolonged outbreak of multidrug-resistant *Pseudomonas aeruginosa* in an intensive care unit. *The Journal of Hospital Infection, 102*(1), 70–74. https://doi.org/10.1016/j.jhin.2019.01.003.

Devos, I. (2006). *Allemaal beestjes: mortaliteit en morbiditeit in Vlaanderen*, 18de-20ste eeuw, Academia Press Gent, p. 29 (in Dutch). Accessed from http://bit.do/fHkQE

ECDC (European Centre for Disease Prevention and Control). (2011). *Antimicrobial resistance surveillance in Europe 2010. Annual Report of the European Antimicrobial Resistance Surveillance Network (EARS-Net)*. https://doi.org/10.2900/14911. Accessed October 19, 2020, from https://bit.ly/3pNuKEP

ECDC (European Centre for Disease Prevention and Control). (2012a). *Antimicrobial resistance surveillance in Europe. Annual Report of the European Antimicrobial Resistance Surveillance Network (EARS-Net)*. https://doi.org/10.2900/6551. Accessed October 19, 2020, from https://bit.ly/35bNKVr

ECDC (European Centre for Disease Prevention and Control). (2012b). *Response plan to control and manage the threat of multidrug-resistant gonorrhoea in Europe*. https://doi.org/10.2900/60053. Accessed October 18, 2020, from https://bit.ly/3pJhVeG

ECDC (European Centre for Disease Prevention and Control). (2013). *Antimicrobial resistance surveillance in Europe 2012. Annual Report of the European Antimicrobial Resistance Surveillance Network (EARS-Net)*. https://doi.org/10.2900/93403. Accessed October 19, 2020, from https://bit.ly/3b5ginw

ECDC (European Centre for Disease Prevention and Control). (2015). *Antimicrobial resistance surveillance in Europe 2014. Annual Report of the European Antimicrobial Resistance Surveillance Network (EARS-Net)*. https://doi.org/10.2900/23549. Accessed October 19, 2020, from https://bit.ly/3ohlqbH

ECDC. (2018). European Centre for Disease Prevention and Control. In *ECDC study protocol for genomic-based surveillance of carbapenem-resistant and/or colistin-resistant Enterobacteriaceae at the EU level*. Version 2.0. Accessed March 28, 2021, from https://bit.ly/31sUZWN

ECDC (European Centre for Disease Prevention and Control) (2019). *Campylobacteriosis. Annual epidemiological report for 2017*. Accessed January 5, 2021, from https://bit.ly/2XcHubM

ECDC (European Centre for Disease Prevention and Control). (2020a). *Surveillance Atlas of Infectious Diseases*. Accessed January 5, 2021, from https://bit.ly/2Mq3zRV

ECDC (European Centre for Disease Prevention and Control). (2020b). *Antimicrobial resistance in the EU/EEA (EARS-Net) – Annual Epidemiological Report for 2019*. Accessed January 5, 2021, from https://bit.ly/2JMOTeT

Ferriman, A. (2007). BMJ readers choose the "sanitary revolution" as greatest medical advance since 1840. *BMJ, 334*, 111. https://doi.org/10.1136/bmj.39097.611806.DB.

Gakidou, E., Afshin, A., Abajobir, A. A., et al. (2017). Global, regional, and national comparative risk assessment of 84 behavioural, environmental and occupational and metabolic risks or clusters of risks, 1990-2016: A systematic analysis for the Global Burden of Disease Study 2016. *The Lancet, 390*(10100), 1345–1422. https://doi.org/10.1016/S0140-6736(12)61728-0.

Gandra, S., Joshi, J., Trett, A. et al. (2017). *Scoping report on antimicrobial resistance in India*. Center for Disease Dynamics, Economics & Policy. Accessed October 22, 2020, from https://bit.ly/38hFhlz

IHME. (2018). *Institute for health metrics and evaluation. Findings from the Global Burden of Disease Study 2017*. Seattle, WA: IHME. Accessed from https://bit.ly/3pS0mJw

Joshi, J. (2019). Scoping report on antimicrobial resistance in India - Key findings. In *Paper presented at the UK-India tackling AMR in the environment from antimicrobial manufacturing waste - Partnership workshop*. New Delhi India 15–17 May 2019. Accessed October 22, 2020, from https://bit.ly/3hMNcdU

Kalem, F., Ergun, A. G., Ertugrul, Ö., et al. (2016). Colistin resistance in carbapenem-resistant Klebsiella pneumoniae strains. *Biomedical Research, 27*(2). Accessed from https://bit.ly/359Lk9N

Kalpoe, J. S., Al Naiemi, A., Poirel, L., et al. (2011). Detection of an Ambler class D OXA-48-type β-lactamase in a Klebsiella pneumoniae strain in The Netherlands. *Journal of Medical Microbiology, 60*(5), 677–678. https://doi.org/10.1099/jmm.0.028308-0.

Kirby, W. M. M. (1945). Properties of a penicillin inactivator extracted from penicillin-resistant staphylococci. *The Journal of Clinical Investigation, 24*(2), 170–174. https://doi.org/10.1172/JCI101594.

Knapp, C. W., Dolfing, J., Ehlert, P. A. I., et al. (2010). Evidence of increasing antibiotic resistance gene abundances in archived soils since 1940. *Environmental Science & Technology, 44*(2), 580–587. https://doi.org/10.1021/es901221x.

Knox, R. (1961). Letter to the editor of the BMJ. *Association Medical Journal, 1961*(1): 126. Accessed October 19, 2020, from https://doi.org/10.1136/bmj.1.5219.126

Kontopoulou, K., Protonotariou, E., Vasilakos, K., et al. (2010). Hospital outbreak caused by Klebsiella pneumoniae producing KPC-2 beta-lactamase resistant to colistin. *The Journal of Hospital Infection, 76*(1), 70–73. https://doi.org/10.1016/j.jhin.2010.03.021.

Kristiansson, E., Fick, J., Janzon, A., et al. (2011). Pyrosequencing of antibiotic-contaminated river sediments reveals high levels of resistance and gene transfer elements. *PLoS One*. https://doi.org/10.1371/journal.pone.0017038.

Kumarasamy, K. K., Toleman, M. A., Walsh, T. R., et al. (2010). Emergence of a new antibiotic resistance mechanism in India, Pakistan, and the UK: A molecular, biological, and epidemiological study. *The Lancet Infectious Diseases, 10*(9), 597–602. https://doi.org/10.1016/S1473-3099(10)70143-2.

Lai, C. C., Chuang, Y. C., Chen, C. C., et al. (2017). Coexistence of MCR-1 and NDM-9 in a clinical carbapenem-resistant *Escherichia coli* isolate. *International Journal of Antimicrobial Agents, 49*(4), 517–518. https://doi.org/10.1016/j.ijantimicag.2017.02.001.

Lalaoui, R., Bakour, S., Livnat, K., et al. (2019). Spread of carbapenem and colistin-resistant *Klebsiella pneumoniae* ST512 clinical isolates in Israel: A cause for vigilance. *Microbial Drug Resistance, 25*(1). https://doi.org/10.1089/mdr.2018.0014.

Larsson, D. G. J. (2014). Pollution from drug manufacturing: Review and perspectives. *Philosophical Transactions of the Royal Society B.* https://doi.org/10.1098/rstb.2013.0571.

Leetz, A. (2015). *Uppsala Health Summit 2015: A world without antibiotics.* 2–3 June 2015 Uppsala. Paper presented at the Uppsala Health Summit (2015). Accessed October 18, 2020, from https://bit.ly/38jhL82

Lesho, E., Yoon, E. J., McGann, P., et al. (2013). Emergence of colistin-resistance in extremely drug-resistant *Acinetobacter baumannii* containing a novel *pmrCAB* operon during colistin therapy of wound infections. *The Journal of Infectious Diseases, 208*(7), 1142–1151. https://doi.org/10.1093/infdis/jit293.

Liu, Y. Y., Wang, Y., Walsh, T. R., et al. (2015). Emergence of plasmid-mediated colistin resistance mechanism MCR-1 in animals and human beings in China: A microbiological and molecular biological study. *The Lancet Infectious Diseases, 16*(2), 161–168. https://doi.org/10.1016/S1473-3099(15)00424-7.

Lopez, A. D., Mathers, C. D., Ezzati, M., et al. (2006). *Global burden of disease and risk factors, Washington (DC): The International Bank for Reconstruction and Development/The World Bank.* New York: Oxford University Press.

Lozano, R., Naghavi, M., Foreman, K., et al. (2012). Global and regional mortality from 235 causes of death for 20 age groups in 1990 and 2010: A systematic analysis for the global burden of disease study 2010. *Lancet, 380*(9859), 2095–2128. https://doi.org/10.1016/S0140-6736(12)61728-0.

Lyons, G. (2014). *Pharmaceuticals in the environment: A growing threat to our tap water and wildlife. A CHEM Trust report.* Accessed October 22, 2020, from https://bit.ly/392ZcE5

Mackenbach, J. P. (2007). Sanitation: pragmatism works. *BMJ, 2007*, 334. https://doi.org/10.1136/bmj.39044.508646.94.

Mammina, C., Bonura, C., Di Bernardo, F., et al. (2012). Ongoing spread of colistin-resistant Klebsiella pneumoniae in different wards of an acute general hospital, Italy, June to December 2011. *Eurosurveillance, 17*(33), 20248. Accessed from https://pubmed.ncbi.nlm.nih.gov/22913977/.

Marchaim, D., Chopra, T., Pogue, J. M., et al. (2011). Outbreak of colistin-resistant, carbapenem-resistant klebsiella pneumoniae in Metropolitan Detroit, Michigan. *Antimicrobial Agents and Chemotherapy, 55*(2), 593–599. https://doi.org/10.1128/AAC.01020-10. Accessed from https://aac.asm.org/content/55/2/593.

Martins Aires, C. A., da Conceição-Neto, O. C., Tavares de Oliveira, T. R., et al. (2017). Emergence of plasmid-mediated mcr-1 gene in clinical KPC-2-producing *Klebsiella pneumoniae* ST392 in Brazil. *Antimicrobial Agents and Chemotherapy*. https://doi.org/10.1128/AAC.00317-17. Accessed from https://bit.ly/3noAtPW

Min, Q., Ying, G. G., Singer, A., et al. (2018). Review of antibiotic resistance in China and its environment. *Environment International, 110*, 160–172. https://doi.org/10.1016/j.envint.2017.10.016.

Mohanty, S., Maurya, V., Gaind, R., et al. (2013). Phenotypic characterization and colistin susceptibilities of carbapenem-resistant of Pseudomonas aeruginosa and Acinetobacter spp. *The Journal of Infections in Developing Countries, 7*(11), 880–887. https://doi.org/10.3855/jidc.2924.

NARSS. (2019). *National Annual Rural Sanitation Survey (NARSS 2018-19)*. Accessed October 19, 2020, from https://bit.ly/2XfTvgs

Nobel Prize Committee. (1945). *The nobel prize in physiology or medicine 1945*. Accessed October 19, 2020, from https://www.nobelprize.org/prizes/medicine/1945/summary/

NOS. (2016). Accessed 22 October 2020. See the videoclip at https://bit.ly/3rZzhFQ

NSO. (2019). *Government of India, Ministry of Statistics and Programme Implementation, National Statistical Office. Drinking water, Sanitation, Hygiene and Housing Condition in India NSS 76th Round, July 2018–December 2018*. Accessed October 19, 2020, from https://bit.ly/35dLgpJ

Palmieri, M., D'Andrea, M. M., Pelegrin, A. C., et al. (2020). Genomic epidemiology of carbapenem- and colistin-resistant *Klebsiella pneumoniae* isolates from Serbia: Predominance of ST101 strains carrying a Novel OXA-48 plasmid. *Frontiers in Microbiology, 11*, 294. https://doi.org/10.3389/fmicb.2020.00294.

Pharmafilter. (2012). *Results of the demonstration project at Reinier de Graaf hospital, Delft, the Netherlands, in April 2012*. Accessed October 18, 2020, from https://reinierdegraaf.nl/linkservid/44B7C459-F836-4817-8B4D731173A37E73/showMeta/0/

Poultry World. (2019a). *Argentina: no more colistin in veterinary products*. Accessed October 22, 2020, from https://www.poultryworld.net/Health/Articles/2019/2/Argentina-No-more-colistin-in-veterinary-products-395426E/

Poultry World. (2019b). *Indian government bans Colistin*. Accessed October 22, 2020, from https://www.poultryworld.net/Health/Articles/2019/8/Indian-government-bans-Colistin-457309E/

Prasad, P., Sun, J., Danner, R. L., et al. (2012). Excess deaths associated with tigecycline after approval based on noninferiority trials. *Clinical infectious Diseases, 54*(12), 1699–1709. https://doi.org/10.1093/cid/cis270.

Quan, J., Li, X., Chen, Y., et al. (2017). Prevalence of *mcr-1* in *Escherichia coli* and *Klebsiella pneumoniae* recovered from bloodstream infections in China: a multicenter longitudinal study. *The Lancet Infectious Diseases, 17*(4), 400–410. https://doi.org/10.1016/S1473-3099(16)30528-X.

Rehman, M. S. U., Rashid, N., Ashfaq, M., et al. (2013). Global risk of pharmaceutical contamination from highly populated developing countries. *Chemosphere, 138*, 1045–1055. https://doi.org/10.1016/j.chemosphere.2013.02.036.

Report to the Congress of the U.S. - China Economic and Security Review Commission. (2014). *113th Congress Session 11-2014*. https://www.uscc.gov/sites/default/files/annual_reports/ Complete%20Report.PDF. See Chapter 1, Section 3: 127-182. Direct link. Accessed from http://bit.do/fHsUo

Riley, J. C. (2005). Estimates of regional and global life expectancy, 1800-2001. *Population and Development Review, 31*(3), 537–543. Accessed from https://www.jstor.org/stable/3401478.

Sissoko, B., Sütterlin, R., Blaschke, M., et al. (2004). *Conference paper on the 12th GHU Conference and the 8th ISEM Conference, 3–5 October 2004 in Halle(Saale) published in Hygiene & Medizin 29–12*. Accessed from https://www.cleanside.fi/wp-content/uploads/2019/ 09/sissoko-b.-et-al.-2004-hygiene-medizin-29-12.pdf

Skov, R. L., & Monnet, D. (2016). Plasmid-mediated colistin resistance (mcr-1 gene): Three months later, the story unfolds. *Euro Surveillance, 21*(9): https://doi.org/10.2807/1560-7917. ES.2016.21.9.30155. Accessed from https://www.eurosurveillance.org/docserver/fulltext/ eurosurveillance/21/9/eurosurv-21-30155-1.pdf?expires=1603218416&id=id& accname=guest&checksum=0780E43680858ADC1BC3451588137928

Smith, J. T., Hamilton-Miller, J. M. T., & Knox, R. (1969). Bacterial resistance to penicillins and cephalosporins. *Journal of Pharmacy and Pharmacology, 21*: 337–358. Accessed from https:// onlinelibrary.wiley.com/doi/pdf/10.1111/j.2042-7158.1969.tb08267.x

SumOfUs. (2015). Bad Medicine. *How the pharmaceutical industry is contributing to the global rise of antibiotic-resistant superbugs*. Accessed October 22, 2020, from https://bit.ly/2Xc7hAG

Taneja, N., Singh, G., Singh, M., et al. (2011). Emergence of tigecycline & colistin resistant *Acinetobacter baumanii* in patients with complicated urinary tract infections in north India. *Indian Journal of Medical Research, 133*(6), 681–684. Accessed from https://www.ncbi.nlm. nih.gov/pmc/articles/PMC3136000/.

The Bureau of Investigative Journalism. (2017). *Use of 'last hope' antibiotics soaring in Enmglish hospitals*. Accessed October 20, 2020, from https://bit.ly/2LiPTYt

The Lancet. (2012). *Global Burden of Disease 2010. 380*(9859), 2053–2260. Accessed from https://bit.ly/3bd6ckj

The Lancet. (2017). *Global burden of disease 2016. 390*(10100), 1083–1464. Accessed from https://bit.ly/395D5g9

The Lancet. (2020). Global health: Time for radical change? *The Lancet, 396*(10258), 1129–1306. Accessed from https://doi.org/10.1016/S0140-6736(20)32131-0

UNICEF and WHO. (2019). *United Nations Children's Fund (UNICEF) and World Health Organization. Progress on household drinking water, sanitation and hygiene 2000-2017*. Special focus on inequalities. Accessed October 20, 2020, from https://uni.cf/3rYFMJ1

Vandenbroucke-Grauls, C. (2018). Oud en Nieuw, Afscheidsrede. *Nederlands Tijdschrift voor Medische Microbiologie, 26*(4), 259–267. In Dutch. Accessed from https://bit.ly/3pPTwUM.

Walsh, T., & Wu, Y. (2016). China bans colistin as a feed additive for animals. *The Lancet Infectious Diseases, 16*(10), 1102–1103. https://doi.org/10.1016/S1473-3099(16)30329-2.

Wang, Y., Tian, G. B., Zhang, R., et al. (2017). Prevalence, risk factors, outcomes, and molecular epidemiology of *mcr-1* positive Enterobacteriaceae in patients and healthy adults from China: An epidemiological and clinical study. *The Lancet Infectious Diseases, 17*(4), 390–399. https:// doi.org/10.1016/S1473-3099(16)30527-8.

WHO. (2012). *World Health Organization. WHO: Urgent action needed to prevent the spread of untreatable gonorrhea*. Accessed October 18, 2020, from https://bit.ly/3pRXAUn

Willmann, M., Bezdan, D., Zapata, L., et al. (2015). Analysis of a long-term outbreak of XDR *Pseudomonas aeruginosa*: A molecular epidemiological study. *Journal of Antimicrobial Chemotherapy, 70*(5), 1322–1330. https://doi.org/10.1093/jac/dku546.

World Bank. (2020). Accessed October 18, 2020, from https://datahelpdesk.worldbank.org/ knowledgebase/articles/906519-world-bank-country-and-lending-groups

Yang, R. S., Feng, Y., Lu, X. Y., et al. (2016). Emergence of NDM-5- and MCR-1-producing *Escherichia coli* clones ST648 and ST156 from a Single Muscovy Duck (*Cairina moschata*).

*Antimicrobial Agents and Chemotherapy, 60*(11), 6899–6902. https://doi.org/10.1128/AAC. 01365-16. Accessed from https://aac.asm.org/content/60/11/6899.full.

Yong, D., Toleman, M. A., Giske, C. G., et al. (2009). Characterization of a new metallo-β-lactamase gene, $bla_{NDM-1}$, and a novel erythromycin esterase gene carried on a unique genetic structure in *Klebsiella pneumoniae* sequence type 14 from India. *Antimicrobial Agents and Chemotherapy, 53*(12), 5046–5054. https://doi.org/10.1128/AAC.00774-09.

York University. (2019). *Antibiotics found in some of the world's rivers exceed 'safe' levels, global study finds.* Accessed October 18, 2020, from https://bit.ly/3bbSBtR

Zhang, R., Tang, J., Li, J., et al. (2013). Antibiotics in the offshore waters of the Bohai Sea and the Yellow Sea in China: Occurrence, distribution and ecological risks. *Environmental Pollution, 174*, 71–77. https://doi.org/10.1016/j.envpol.2012.11.008.

Zhang, Q. Q., Ying, G. G., Pan, C. G., et al. (2015). Comprehensive evaluation of antibiotics emission and fate in the River Basins of China: Source analysis, multimedia modeling, and linkage to bacterial resistance. *Environmental Science & Technology, 49*(11), 6772–6782. https://doi.org/10.1021/acs.est.5b00729.

# Human and Economic Costs

**3**

At the beginning of 2011, Walther Kattner and his wife were expecting a child. Mid January, in the 28th week of her pregnancy, his wife had to go to the hospital for a check-up. She went to the nearest hospital. The gynaecologist there wanted to admit her for observation. But the clinic was not in a position to look after a premature infant in the 28th week of pregnancy. For safety's sake, Frau Kattner was transferred to the Bremen-Mitte clinic. A couple of days later, Walther Kattner's telephone rang. The call was from his wife. She asked if he could come to the hospital at once. She had a fever, and the baby was going to be delivered as soon as possible by caesarean section. The Kattners' son came into the world shortly after midnight, and was transferred to neonatal ward 4027.

A few months later, an outbreak of ESBL-producing *Klebsiella pneumoniae* was to occur in this department. Three newly born babies were to die of infection from this bacteria.[1] Mrs. Kattner's son was doing fine. But she herself was lying in the women's ward, and was not quite so well. This, however, is not uncommon after a caesarean. On 19 January, Walter Kattner was informed that his son was infected with MRSA. His wife would also need to be tested. One day later, it was found that she too was infected with MRSA. A course of treatment had no effect. It did not help rid her of the MRSA germs—in contrast to her son, whose bacteria soon disappeared again.

Mr. Kattner and his wife had to follow strict hygienic precautions if they wanted to visit their son. They had to wear hospital overalls, gloves and protective masks. Mrs. Kattner repeatedly contracted fever, and after a few days no longer wished to visit her son anymore. Her state of health was getting worse and worse. Since she was allergic to penicillin, it was not easy to treat her. When the MRSA finally disappeared, her kidneys and liver were already damaged irreparably. She died from the consequences of the MRSA infection with which she had become infected in

---

[1]More information on this outbreak of an ESBL-producing *Klebsiella pneumoniae* at the Bremen-Mitte Clinic can be found in Chap. 7, 'The end in sight?'

© The Author(s), under exclusive license to Springer Nature Switzerland AG 2021
R. van den Brink, *The End of an Antibiotic Era*,
https://doi.org/10.1007/978-3-030-70723-1_3

hospital. The Kattners' little boy became infected with MRSA once again on 8 March 2011, along with two other babies in the same ward. The boy was able to overcome this MRSA infection too, and was allowed home at the end of March 2011. But without his mother (Mayr 2012).

## Kim's Newborn Son

Among Gram-negative bacteria, attention is often focused on *Klebsiella pneumoniae,* because it has a virulent nature and can propagate itself relatively quickly. But even the less virulent *E. coli* can wreak considerable havoc. The parents of a baby born in a hospital in western Holland at the end of 2006 can confirm this. He came into the world as a spontaneous premature birth. It was too late for tocolytics: the birth could no longer be stopped, and therefore had to take place at the nearest hospital. The hospital had only a simple intensive care unit. The little boy, therefore, had to be transferred to a university clinic, since only university clinics are allowed to have a neonatal intensive care unit. When examined at the teaching hospital, the baby seemed healthy. Nevertheless, as a matter of standard procedure he was given an antibiotic, since this was a premature birth of unclear origin, which could indicate infection. His lungs had to be inflated after birth,[2] and later he had to be intubated and given artificial respiration. The inflation helps the lungs to expand, but can also result in air sacs rupturing. This can cause a so-called pneumothorax, in which air accumulates in the space between the chest wall and the lung. The baby was examined several times for suspected pneumothorax, but nothing was established. The child was transferred to a third hospital in the parents' hometown. One day later, they had to return to the university clinic after a pulmonary haemorrhage. 'Our son therefore had to be transferred yet again, with all the additional risks this involved,' says Kim, his mother. 'And yet all the necessary equipment and expertise had been available in the hospital he would be in to start with. I ask myself whether perinatal mortality was possibly increased by the stipulation that only university clinics could have neonatal intensive care units, rather than reduced as had been intended'. On the third day after the child's readmission to the university clinic, multiresistant *E. coli* was identified in a blood culture. Three days later, it was clear that the *E. coli* was also ESBL positive. The next day, the baby died of blood poisoning and/or meningitis caused by multiresistant ESBL-producing *E. coli.* The baby had become infected with this multiresistant *E. coli* in one of the three hospitals, or at some point during transport between them. He died 9 days after its birth, before his life had even really begun.

---

[2]Oxygen can be administered via a face mask by pressing a balloon. This is referred to as 'inflation'.

## Without Proper Surveillance Resistant Bugs Rapidly Spread

The death of Kim's newborn son is an example of the personal price people sometimes have to pay because of antibiotic resistance. In the big picture, the situation looks like this: According to the study 'State of Newborn Health in India', published in *The Journal of Perinatology* in December 2016 (Sankar et al. 2016; CDDEP 2012), India's neonatal mortality rate (NMR) is the highest in the world. This is mainly due to the fact that the early neonatal mortality rate (ENMR), the rate of mortality within the first 4 weeks, has been reduced far less this century than the late NMR (mortality after the first 4 weeks and before the first 5 years). 'Globally, India contributes one-fifth of live births and more than a quarter of neonatal deaths. In 2013, nearly 0.75 million neonates died in India—the highest figure for any country in the world. [...] There has been a significant reduction in the quantum of neonatal and child deaths in the past two decades. The annual burden of neonatal deaths has reduced from 1.35 million in 1990 to 0.75 million in 2013. [...] The NMR has declined from 44 per 1000 live births in 2000 to 28 per 1000 live births in 2013. [. . .] The projected rates for ENMR for 2017 and 2020 are 20 and 18 per 1000 live births, whereas those for late NMR are 4 and 4 per 1000 live births, respectively'. UNICEF data (UNICEF 2020) published in September 2020 shows that India's neonatal mortality rate decreased further to 22.7 per 1000 live births in 2018. At that time India was no longer the country where the NMR was the highest in the world. Pakistan, Afghanistan, Turkmenistan, Myanmar and many African countries did (far) worse. A large study published in The Lancet in the spring of 2020 confirms the strong decrease in this century of neonatal mortality and under 5 mortality in India (Kumar and Singhal 2020). The authors of the 2016 study in *The Journal of Perinatology* single out preterm birth complications as by far the most important cause of neonatal death (44%), followed by sepsis and other infections (21%). The first 24 h account for more than a third of all neonatal deaths, and the first week for approximately three quarters. Neonatal sepsis is a huge problem in India. According to the authors, 'hospital-based studies suggest an incidence of 30 per 1000 live births, whereas community-based studies indicate an incidence of 2.7–17% of all live births'(Sankar et al. 2016).

When Pakistani professor Zulfiqar A. Bhutta, of the Aga Khan University in Karachi, presented similar research findings at the 'Global Threat of Antibiotic Resistance' conference in Uppsala on 6 September 2010, I was present in the audience. 'Infections that develop around the time of birth, pneumonias and diarrhoea are responsible for almost 40 per cent of total child mortality globally', he said. According to him, an estimated 368,000 newborns die of sepsis every year in Afghanistan, Bangladesh, India, Nepal and Pakistan. And in around a quarter of these cases, sepsis is caused by multiresistant bacteria (Bhutta 2010).

But multiresistant bacterial infections do not only claim victims in poor or emerging countries. In 2009, the ECDC published a study which shows that at least 25,000 people in the European Union, Iceland and Norway die annually from the most significant infections caused by multiresistant bacteria (ECDC/EMEA 2009). These were: MRSA, VRSA (vancomycin-resistant *staphylococcus aureus*),

VRE (vancomycin-resistant enterococci), penicillin-resistant *Streptococcus pneumoniae* (PRSP), bacteria with ESBL, and two types of carbapenem-resistant bacteria. What these bacteria have in common is that all of them frequently cause sepsis, and that they are protected by a resistance mechanism that makes them multiresistant. Infections caused by the multiresistant bacteria named above are responsible for 2.5 million additional days of hospitalisation—and also for considerable extra costs in terms of healthcare and lost productivity. The ECDC estimates that these amount to at least 1.5 billion euros per year.

## Attributable Deaths

It took 9 years after the ECDC study before *The Lancet* published a similar one on the burden of disease caused by antimicrobial resistance—the number of attributable deaths, attributable DALYs (Disability Adjusted Life Years) and years of health lost as a result (Cassini et al. 2019). The authors of *The Lancet* article used data on 16 different resistance-bacterium combinations from the European Antimicrobial Resistance Surveillance Network (EARS-Net), as well as data from an ECDC point prevalence survey of healthcare-associated infections. With the aid of these data, they estimated the number of bloodstream and non-bloodstream infections in the EU and European Economic Area during 2015. The authors then 'developed disease outcome models for five types of infection on the basis of systematic reviews of the literature'. Five types of infection were included: bloodstream (BSIs), urinary tract, respiratory tract and surgical site infections, and others.

On the basis of the EARS-Net data collected throughout 2015, the authors of the *Lancet* study estimated that the number of infections with antibiotic-resistant bacteria was 671,689, of which 426,277 (63.5%) were associated with healthcare. These infections accounted for an estimated 33,110 attributable deaths and 874,541 DALYs. According to the researchers, 'the burden for the EU and EEA was highest in infants (aged <1 year) and people aged 65 years or older, had increased since 2007, and was highest in Italy and Greece. Our results present the health burden of five types of infection with antibiotic-resistant bacteria expressed, for the first time, in DALYs. The estimated burden of infections with antibiotic-resistant bacteria in the EU and EEA is substantial compared with that of other infectious diseases, and has increased since 2007. Our burden estimates provide useful information for public health decision makers prioritising interventions for infectious diseases'.

According to the study, the incidence of infections caused by (multi)resistant microbes was 131 per 100,000 members of the population, and the estimated attributable mortality was 6.44 per 100,000. The attributable DALYs per 100,000 members of the population were estimated to be 170. The study comes up with some remarkable points. 'Despite its relatively low incidence, carbapenem-resistant *K. pneumoniae* had a high burden of disease because of its high attributable mortality, whereas vancomycin-resistant *E. faecalis* and *E. faecium* (which had a similar incidence to carbapenem-resistant *K. pneumoniae*) was associated with a low burden of disease'. Moreover, 'Italy and Greece had a substantially higher estimated burden of antibiotic-resistant bacteria than other EU and EEA countries, with carbapenem-resistant or colistin-resistant bacteria causing a larger proportion of the total burden in Greece than in Italy.

In 2015, in addition to a substantial burden due to infections with carbapenem-resistant or colistin-resistant bacteria, Portugal and Malta had a substantial burden due to MRSA infections'. Despite the clear decrease in the population-weighted proportion of MRSA among *S. aureus* isolates—from 26.6% in 2007 to 16.8% in 2015—the authors of the *Lancet* study estimated that MRSA infections had increased by a factor of 1.28. This means that there are fewer carriers of MRSA, but it is clear that more people are contracting an MRSA infection (Cassini et al. 2019).

This study is based on disease models, into which the available data were fed. In terms of quality, availability and representativeness, these data differ widely. Moreover, it is widely recognised that attributing deaths or DALYs to infections is hard to substantiate. And estimates imply uncertainties in either direction: they might overestimate a problem or, on the contrary, underestimate it—as Mirjam Kretzschmar stresses. Professor of the Dynamics of Infectious Diseases at the University Hospital in Utrecht, she is one of the authors of the *Lancet* study. Kretzschmar is very conscious of its limitations. 'Surveillance is undoubtedly better than it was a decade ago', she says 'When you look harder, you see more. This may have influenced the fact that we now estimate the number of attributable deaths due to infections with antibiotic-resistant bacteria to be higher than we did before'. But surveillance data do not tell the whole story either', she argues. 'They only reveal part of the problem. So we continue to need estimates of the actual size of these problems. And estimating remains very difficult. The risks of under- or over-estimating are real, especially when the surveillance data are not collected in a standardised way in all countries'.

And attributing deaths and DALYs remains a huge problem too. 'Patients, especially older ones, are often hospitalised with a number of diseases. They have an incurable cancer, maybe a heart disease too, and then they get a severe infection. When they pass away, which is the cause of death? Moreover, which is registered as the cause of death?' The researchers based their estimates of attributable deaths and DALYs on the number of infections by antibiotic-resistant bacteria reported to EARS-Net. 'Our model used these reported cases of infections to estimate the number of attributable deaths and DALYs', explains Kretzschmar. This process was then repeated for all five types of infection, plus the 16 different combinations of resistance genes and bacteria. Such a procedure can lead to findings that are simply wrong.

## 'Figures That Raise Questions'

According to the estimates of the *Lancet* study, in 2015 there were almost 5000 infections caused by (multi)resistant bacteria in the Netherlands, causing an estimated 206 deaths. 'These figures raise questions', says Marc Bonten, Head of the Department of Medical Microbiology at the university hospital in Utrecht—both in personal conversation with the author, and in his online blog (Bonten 2018). 'In these estimates for the Netherlands, we find deaths from infections caused by resistant bacteria we have never seen in infected patients until now'. Among the estimated 206 annual deaths caused by such infections in the Netherlands, 24 patients die each year from infections by colistin- and/or carbapenem-resistant *E. coli*. 'To the best of my knowledge', says Bonten, 'we haven't identified such bacteria in infected patients up to now'. His colleague, Professor Alex Friedrich of the Groningen university hospital, in the north of the Netherlands, confirms this. According to the *Lancet* study, out of 3500 infected Dutch patients, an estimated 107 die each year from infection by an *E. coli* bacterium resistant to third-generation cephalosporins. Bonten agrees that these infections are not rare but, according to him, 'our estimates of attributable mortality due to these infections are close to zero'.

The PhD thesis *Quantifying the burden of antibiotic resistance in the Netherlands* that clinical microbiologist Wouter Rottier defended in February 2019 at the University Hospital in Utrecht supports the observations of both professors Bonten and Friedrich. Rottiers main finding is that in the Netherlands the attributable mortality of infections caused by (multi-)resistant microbes is not higher than the attributable mortality due to infections by susceptible microbes. 'The studies in this thesis provide evidence' writes Wouter Rottier, 'that the burden of antimicrobial resistance is currently manageable within the Netherlands. These conclusions may generalize to some other high-income, mainly Northern European countries. At the same time, they may serve as an incentive to study the burden of the global antibiotic resistance crisis in those settings where it is more likely to manifest itself, especially in low and middle income countries. Whereas it is essential to remain vigilant in the Netherlands with regard to the potential threat, resources spent globally on antibiotic resistance should take into account the extremely skewed distribution of its burden, and the scarcity of information on it in many settings' (Rottier 2019).

## Annual Number of HAIs

In a report published in July 2013, the ECDC estimated that the total number of patients who succumb to healthcare-associated infections—by both resistant bacteria and those susceptible to antibiotics—was about 3.2 million annually (ECDC 2013). This means that every day there are 80,000 patients lying in European hospitals who are suffering from an infection they acquired there. That is almost 6 per cent of all cases. The figures are based on a reference measurement carried out on 230,000 patients at 947 hospitals in the EU plus Norway and Iceland.[3] 'We can produce

---

[3]The margin of error for these figures remains large, since it is a reference measurement. The number of patients with healthcare-associated infections is between 4.5 and 7.4 per cent. On the basis of studies in the literature, in 2008 the ECDC estimated that 37,000 people died of HAIs every year in the EU, Norway and Iceland, of which 25,000 died of infections through multiresistant germs (ECDC 2008). In its first report, published in 2014, the O'Neill Commission estimates that

figures as evidence', said Marc Sprenger, at the time Director of the ECDC. 'We hope that the figures that we publish at the ECDC – the rankings of countries, antibiotic use and frequency with which antibiotic resistances occur – will make it clear to the governments of the European Union that something finally needs to be done about antibiotic resistance'.

More than 5 years later, in mid-November 2018, the ECDC published in *Eurosurveillance,* the scientific magazine published by the ECDC, a second point prevalence survey on antimicrobial use and healthcare-associated infections (HAIs) at acute care hospitals in 28 out of the 31 EU/EEA countries (Plachouras et al. 2018). The data were collected in 2016 and 2017. The researchers included 310,755 patients in the survey, from 1209 hospitals. On any given day, 1 in every 15 patients in European hospitals acquires an HAI.

The ECDC carried out a similar study at long-term care facilities (Ricchizzi et al. 2018). It included data from 102,301 eligible residents at 1788 long-term care facilities in 24 countries. On any given day, 1 out of every 26 residents has at least one healthcare-associated infection. According to these two studies by ECDC, every year, 8.9 million HAIs are being contracted in European hospitals and long-term care facilities. Among other things, in both studies the researchers stress that the surveys are limited because they were carried out on a single day, which 'can be prone to variation', as they put it.

Twenty nine per cent of all antibiotics administered in long-term care facilities were prescribed for prophylaxis. Three out of every four of these courses were prescribed to prevent urinary tract infections. Overall, on any given day 4.9% of residents were prescribed at least one antimicrobial agent. According to the authors of the study, 'overall the urinary tract was the most common body site for which antimicrobials were prescribed (46.1%), followed by the respiratory tract (29.4%) and skin or wounds (12.6%). In combination, these sites accounted for 88.0% of all antimicrobial prescriptions. When stratified by indication, the most common sites for antimicrobial treatment were the respiratory tract (37.2%), the urinary tract (34.4%), skin or wounds (15.8%) and the gastrointestinal tract (2.8%). The most common body site for prophylaxis was the urinary tract (74.0%), followed by the respiratory tract (11.3%), skin or wounds (4.8%), another non-specified body site (3.4%) and the gastrointestinal tract (2.4%)'.

The prevalence of antimicrobial use—reported as the percentage of patients receiving at least one antimicrobial agent on the day of the survey—was 30.5%. In their article for *Eurosurveillance* the researchers (Plachouras et al. 2018) state that 'the most common indication for prescribing antimicrobials was treatment of community-acquired infection, followed by treatment of HAI and surgical prophylaxis (preventive use of antibiotics to avoid infections of surgical sites). Over half (54.2%) of antimicrobials for surgical prophylaxis were prescribed for more than 1 day. The most common infections treated by antimicrobials were respiratory tract

---

the total global death toll due to antimicrobial resistance is 700,000 deaths a year (O'Neill 2014). For further information on the O'Neill Commission, see Chap. 11.

infections, and the most commonly prescribed antimicrobial agents were penicillins with beta-lactamase inhibitors'. The researchers found wide variation between countries in the selection of the antimicrobials they used, the resources for antimicrobial stewardship and the prevalence of antibiotic usage. The observed prevalence of antimicrobial use in the acute care hospitals varied between 15.9% in Hungary and 19.7% in France at the lower end, 30.5% in the EU/EEA, 33.1% in the Netherlands and 37.4% in the United Kingdom in the middle ground, and 44.5% in Italy, 46.3% in Spain and—last but not least—55.6% in Greece at the upper end of the scale. The study also revealed improper and unnecessary use of antibiotics in acute care hospitals.

The use of broad-spectrum antibiotics varied from 16% in Lithuania to 62% in Bulgaria. The use of these antibiotics—which are drivers for antimicrobial resistance—is not always necessary. Well targeted small-spectrum antibiotics are often preferable for the treatment of a specific infection, since they only attack the pathogen causing it. In the WHO List of Essential Medicines, certain broad-spectrum antibiotics appear on either the 'watch' list ('be careful when using') or the 'reserve' list ('don't use unless you have no other option') (WHO 2019). And yet they are intensively used in many countries. According to the researchers, 'this could in part be explained by the high prevalence of resistance among a number of reported microorganisms, e.g. MRSA, vancomycin-resistant enterococci or third-generation cephalosporin-resistant *Enterobacteriaceae*. However, many of these antibacterials are also associated with both the emergence and the spread of healthcare-associated Clostridium difficile and multidrug-resistant microorganisms'. In particular, 'third-generation cephalosporins, fluoroquinolones and carbapenems' are associated with 'the emergence of multidrug-resistant Gram-negative bacteria, which are currently among the most important public health threats related to AMR. The wide variation and sometimes extensive use of broad-spectrum antibacterials indicate the need to review their indications in many countries and hospitals. Antimicrobial stewardship programmes must be designed to take into account both the risk of emergence of AMR and patient safety. Ensuring that broad-spectrum antibacterials are used appropriately is a key element of any strategy against AMR' (Plachouras et al. 2018).

In the view of the study's authors, 'surgical prophylaxis is recommended for the prevention of surgical site infections. For the majority of surgical procedures, one preoperative dose is sufficient. In this PPS (Point Prevalence Study, RvdB), however, more than half of the antimicrobial courses for surgical prophylaxis lasted more than 1 day. Although this proportion slightly decreased since the first survey in 2011–12 (54% versus 59%), it remains very high and outside the recommended duration, in common with other studies where it ranged from 40.6% to 86.3%. This is an important source of unnecessary use of antimicrobials and should be a priority target for future efforts on antimicrobial stewardship in many European acute care hospitals.

## The Financial Burden

Calculating the costs caused by antibiotic resistance is very complicated. Regardless of whether they are caused by resistant or susceptible bacteria, infections generally befall weak patients: newborns, older people and patients who are already severely ill. 'Identifying the additional costs caused by antibiotic resistance – both in terms of human lives, and financially – is one of the greatest challenges that we have to overcome', says Andreas Heddini. Director and driving force behind 'ReAct – Action on Antibiotic Resistance' at the University of Uppsala until the spring of 2012, he then moved to GlaxoSmithKline, one of the world's major pharmaceutical companies, where he works since the summer of 2018 as Cluster Medical Director, Nordic Region.

'If you want to convince people that they need to solve this problem', he continues, 'costs are an important argument. But how can you determine the additional costs of antibiotic resistance if, in many cases, we don't even know whether antibiotic resistance is present? Or if we don't notice that the meningitis that has ended the life of a young patient is caused by a resistant bacterium? We are constantly getting better at recognising and monitoring resistance problems, at least in our part of the world. Or surveillance systems are getting ever better, but we still have far too few data – and those we have actually, we don't know how reliable they are. The ECDC data which everyone uses are based on only five pathogens. These are really just estimates, nothing more than very rough estimates. We still need to do a lot more surveillance work.[4] That's exactly what it's all about: surveillance, surveillance and surveillance'. Because it is so hard to obtain reliable estimates regarding the costs of antibiotic resistance and nosocomial infections, Heddini welcomes every initiative in this sphere. That is why he is excited by the BURDEN study.

## High Costs

In October 2011, the BURDEN study group, headed by Hajo Grundmann, then Professor of Medical Microbiology at the University Medical Centre Groningen published a Europe-wide study on the costs of infections caused by MRSA and *E. coli* that were resistant to third-generation cephalosporins.[5] The latter are usually resistant because they produce the ESBL enzyme. However, there are also some cases where another resistance mechanism is at work.

---

[4] By 'surveillance' we mean collecting data on the prevalence of resistant bacteria.

[5] Particularly for the epidemiology of infectious diseases. Since 2016, Professor Grundmann has been responsible for infection prevention and hospital epidemiology at the University Hospital of Freiburg, Germany. He is Honorary Professor of Infectious Disease Epidemiology at the University of Groningen in the Netherlands.

Grundmann and his team estimated that MRSA and *E. coli* resistant to third-generation cephalosporins cause 43,000 infections annually in Europe, resulting in the death of 8200 patients and in 376,000 extra days of hospitalisation. For the treatment of sepsis cases caused by these two resistant bacteria alone, the additional treatment costs amounted to 62 million euros. 1380 hospitals and 774 laboratories in 33 countries took part in the study. The data used came from 2007. The researchers foresaw a decline in the number of MRSA infections, from 28,000 in 2007 to 10,000 in 2015. But in the case of resistant *E. coli*, the trend was going in precisely the opposite direction, and much faster at that. The number of infections here would rise from 15,000 in 2007 to 86,000 in 2015. The total number of sepsis cases caused by these two bacteria would rise from 43,000 to 96,000, and the number of deaths from 8200 to 17,000, which would result in the associated costs rising to 120 million euros (De Kraker et al. 2011).

'However, we have to remember that we used the price levels of 2007 for our calculations, although the prices have probably increased', says Marlieke de Kraker, who worked on the BURDEN study as part of her doctoral programme at the University Medical Centre Groningen in the summer of 2012. 'And we assumed that the spread of infections in the 33 countries would remain the same until 2015. If we assume that there are fewer infections in the United Kingdom and more in Romania, then this naturally affects the calculation of costs, since the daily costs of a hospital stay are a lot higher in the United Kingdom.'

In an American study published in 2009, the costs of infection by multiresistant bacteria in 2000 were calculated with the aid of a large case study at a Chicago hospital (Roberts et al. 2009; Illinois Department of Public Health 2020). Scaled up for the entire United States, the figures showed that, in 2000, infections caused by multiresistant bacteria resulted in additional medical costs of over 20 billion in the United States, and lost production added a further 15 billion in social costs. Since 2000, the number of infections by multiresistant bacteria in the United States has more or less doubled, and the costs have also increased considerably. Eli Perencevich, a specialist in infectious diseases and epidemiology based in Iowa City, has been writing a blog about healthcare-associated infections for several years. Here, on Wednesday, 13 June 2012, he published a neat graphic representation of the additional costs caused by the two most important healthcare-associated infections: sepsis and pneumonia (Eber et al. 2010).

For his calculations, Perencevich used the data from 58.7 million hospital stays in 40 US states between 1998 and 2006. In more than 8.5 million of these hospital admissions, invasive procedures were used—i.e. surgical interventions. Afterwards, nearly half a million patients developed blood poisoning, and almost 80,000 pneumonia. This considerably increased mortality: nearly 18 per cent of the patients who developed sepsis died of the consequences. The same applied to more than 8 per cent of the patients who developed pneumonia in the hospital after their operation. In all, 20 billion in extra costs were spent in these 9 years as a result of these two nosocomial (hospital acquired) infections. Projecting these data onto the entire United States, Perencevich arrives at figures of 2.3 million extra days at American hospitals, 8.1 billion dollars of extra expenses, and 43,000 avoidable deaths through sepsis and pneumonia alone in 2006.

In an information sheet produced in 2012, ReAct—Action on Antibiotic Resistance—summarises a number of studies on the costs of antibiotic resistance (ReAct 2012). Here is a small selection. A US study put all healthcare-associated infections caused by Gram-negative bacteria between 2000 and 2008 under the microscope (Mauldin et al. 2010). An infection caused by a (multi)resistant bacterium resulted in 30 per cent higher costs than an infection caused by non-resistant bacteria. The main reason for this was that patients infected by resistant bacteria stay in hospital a quarter longer than patients with an infection caused by a non-resistant bacterium. Studies carried out in Israel show that blood infections caused by ESBL-producing bacteria not only strongly increase the mortality risk by a factor 3.6, but also increase the duration of hospital stays and costs per patient by more than a half (Schwaber et al. 2006). A more recent Brazilian study on the economic burden of hospitalized patients infected with a carbapenemase-producing *Klebsiella pneumoniae* gives a similar picture (Mombaque dos Santos and Secoli 2019).

In September 2013, the US Center for Disease Control (CDC) published a report, *Antibiotic resistance threats in the United States, 2013*. It estimated that the annual number of clinical cases caused by multiresistant Gram-negative bacteria was more than 2 million. At least 23,000 of these patients die every year. Moreover, every year there are between 250,000 to 1 million infections by the Gram-positive intestinal bacterium *Clostridium difficile* in the United States.[6] Fourteen thousand people die of it annually. The CDC estimates that extra healthcare costs due to these infections run to 20 billion dollars per year. According to the CDC, days off sick, loss of production and extra fatalities cost society up to 35 billion dollars a year (CDC 2013). In the 2019 version of the same report, the CDC estimates the total number of infections caused by (multi)resistant bacteria to be 2.8 million resulting in the death of more than 35,000 people annually. In addition to that in 2017 almost 224,000 *Clostridium difficile* infections occurred causing 12,800 deaths (CDC 2019). The very alarming CDC reports seem to have had a positive impact. In the period between the 2013 and the 2019 report, the number of deaths due to infections caused by antibiotic-resistant bugs decreased by 18% and the in-hospital mortality even by 28%. This seems to be in contradiction with the death toll from the 2013 report but that figure was estimated too low, in fact the number of infections by multiresistant Gram-negative bacteria was 2.6 million in 2013 and the death toll 44.000 according to the new report that does not give new estimations of the extra healthcare and societal costs of antimicrobial resistance.

---

[6] *Clostridium difficile* (*C. diff.*) is a Gram-positive, bacillary intestinal bacterium. Disturbances to the intestinal flora caused by the use of antibiotics can lead to excessive growth of *C. diff.*, which can cause severe diarrhoea. At the VUmc in Amsterdam, a dog (beagle) was trained to smell the bacteria. A smaller study (Bomers et al. 2012) has yielded very promising results. The dog proved a good bloodhound.

## PREZIES Network

The Netherlands National Institute for Public Health and the Environment (RIVM) in Bilthoven collects data on the incidence of healthcare-associated infections in the Netherlands. For this purpose, it set up the PREZIES[7] Network, which has been carrying out a 'national prevention study of healthcare-associated infections' every 6 months since March 2007. This means that, every March and October, it determines the number of patients who have contracted one or more healthcare-associated infections (HAI). In July 2019, the RIVM published the relevant data for the period 2014–2018 (PREZIES 2019). The data shows a decreasing trend in the prevalence of healthcare-associated infections from 5.1% in 2014 to 4.6% in 2018. There are huge differences between participating hospitals. The prevalence of HAIs varies from 0.0% to 10%. Over the years, the number of participating hospitals has sharply decreased from 51 institutions with 75 locations to 33 with 41 locations. The most common infections are postoperative wound infections, respiratory infections, sepsis and urinary tract infections. In September 2020 the RIVM published data on the prevalence of HAIs in the Dutch hospitals. They showed an increase in the number of HAIs to 5.4% in 2019 (PREZIES 2020). The report gives no information on the supplementary costs of these HAIs.

In Germany, too, studies on the costs of hospital infections are thin on the ground. In an article published in January 2016, Professor Klaus-Dieter Zastrow from the Institute for Hygiene and Environmental Medicine of the Vivantes Hospitals in Berlin mentions an annual figure of 900,000 healthcare-associated infections in Germany, which included at least 30,000 deaths (Zastrow 2016). On average, a patient with an HAI in Germany spends 10 days longer in hospital. Zastrow estimates the annual costs of HAIs in Germany to be 'billions of euros'. In August 2010 Matthias Schrappe, Director of the Institute for Patient Safety at the Friedrich-Wilhelm University in Bonn, quoted a figure of 2.5 billion euros in the *Kölner Stadt-Anzeiger* newspaper. He based this on an estimated 500,000 HAIs per year[8] and additional costs of 5000 euros per case (Kölner Stadt Anzeiger 2010).

In November 2016, at the University of Groningen, Jan-Willem Dik gave a defence of his thesis 'Impact of Medical Microbiology: a clinical and financial analysis'. Part of his work consisted of a comparative analysis of several nosocomial outbreaks in terms of per diem costs per patient. All seven of the outbreaks studied

---

[7]PREventie van InfectieZIEkten door Surveillance (Prevention of infectious diseases by surveillance).

[8]The Robert Koch Institute estimated in 2011 that the number of healthcare-associated infections is between 400,000 and 600,000 per year. In May 2011, the German Society of Hospital Hygiene, the Society of Hygiene, Environmental Medicine and Preventative Medicine, and the Federal Association of Public Health Service Doctors declared in a report for the Bundestag Health Committee that the figures quoted by the RKI were far too low. These professional associations assume that the figure is at least 700,000 HAIs annually (Bundestag 2011). November 2019 the RKI again estimated the annual number of HAIs between 400,000 and 600,000 and the number of attributable deaths between 10,000 and 15,000 (Zacher et al. 2019).

occurred between 2012 and 2014 at the Groningen University Hospital (UMCG), and were analysed using the same method. The costs varied enormously, depending e.g. on the type of ward in which the outbreak occurred, and whether the ward had to be temporarily closed or not. The costs of the seven outbreaks Dik studied ranged from €10,778 for a Norovirus outbreak to €356,754 for an outbreak of *Serratia marcescens* in a neonatal ICU. The per diem costs per positive patient ranged from €10 for a patient with Norovirus to €1369 for a patient with an ESBL+ *Klebsiella pneumoniae,* with an average cost of €546.

As Jan-Willem Dik argues in his thesis, since the costs of nosocomial outbreaks are high, and since the number of high-risk microorganisms is increasing, there may be a good business case for infection prevention measures that 'are vital to prevent nosocomial outbreaks'. According to Dr. Dik, financial evaluations of this kind are scarce, which is why he carried out one for the Infection Prevention Unit of the Groningen University Hospital. Dr. Dik calculated the predicted number of patients who would succumb to outbreaks on the basis of the (increasing) numbers of the following high-risk microorganisms: MRSA, ESBL and/or carbapenemase-producing *Klebsiella pneumoniae,* multi-resistant *Pseudomonas aeruginosa, Serratia marcescens, Acinetobacter baumannii* and Norovirus. He compared the figure, he had calculated to the number of patients that he actually found. Then, using the same dataset he had used to determine the costs of nosocomial outbreaks, he calculated that the return of investment was 1.94. This means that every euro invested in infection prevention saves costs of 1.94 euros through prevention of outbreaks alone (Dik 2016).

## References

Bhutta, Z. A. (2010). *Millennium development goals and child survival: Does antimicrobial resistance matter?* In Presented at the conference global need for effective antibiotics – Moving towards concerted action, Uppsala, 6–8 September 2010. Accessed from https://bit.ly/394Vz0l

Bomers, M. K., Van Agtmael, M. A., Luik, H., et al. (2012). Using a dog's superior olfactory sensitivity to identify *Clostridium difficile* in stools and patients: Proof of principle study. *BMJ, 345,* e7396. https://doi.org/10.1136/bmj.e7396.

Bonten, M. (2018). *AMR deaths in Europe. Reflections on infection prevention and control.* Accessed from https://bit.ly/35g5T4N

Bundestag. (2011). *Grundsätzliches Ja zum Infektionsschutzgesetz.* Accessed October 25, 2020, from https://bit.ly/35hpt0h

Cassini, A., Högberg, L. D., Plachouras, D., et al. (2019). Attributable deaths and disability-adjusted life-years caused by infections with antibiotic-resistant bacteria in the EU and the European Economic Area in 2015: A population-level modelling analysis. *Lancet Infectious Disease, 19,* 56–66. https://doi.org/10.1016/S1473-3099(18)30605-4.

CDC (Centers for Disease Control and Prevention). (2013). *Antibiotic resistance threats in the United States, 2013.* Accessed October 18, 2020, from https://www.cdc.gov/drugresistance/pdf/ar-threats-2013-508.pdf

CDC (Centers for Disease Control and Prevention). (2019). *Antibiotic resistance threats in the United States.* Accessed October 18, 2020, from www.cdc.gov/DrugResistance/Biggest-Threats.html

CDDEP (The Center for Disease Dynamics, Economics & Policy). (2012). *The burden of antibiotic resistance in Indian neonates*. Accessed October 24, 2020, from https://cddep.org/tool/burden_ antibiotic_resistance_indian_neonates/

De Kraker, M. E. A., Davey, P. G., & Grundmann, H. (2011). Mortality and hospital stay associated with resistant *Staphylococcus aureus* and *Escherichia coli* bacteremia: Estimating the burden of antibiotic resistance in Europe. *PLoS Medicine*. https://doi.org/10.1371/journal.pmed.1001104.

Dik, J.-W. (2016). *Impact of medical microbiology: A clinical and financial analysis*. University of Groningen. Accessed from https://bit.ly/2HABfK8

Eber, R., Laxminarayan, R., Perencevich, E. N., et al. (2010). Clinical and economic outcomes attributable to health care-associated sepsis and pneumonia. *Archives of Internal Medicine, 170* (4), 347–353. Accessed October 25, 2020, from https://bit.ly/3s1Z1BN

ECDC (European Centre for Disease Prevention and Control). (2008). *Annual epidemiological report on communicable diseases in Europe 2008*. Accessed October 25, 2020, from https://bit. ly/3nebiPS

ECDC (European Centre for Disease Prevention and Control). (2013). *Point prevalence survey of healthcare associated infections and antimicrobial use in European acute care hospitals*. https://doi.org/10.2900/86011 Accessed October 25, 2020, from https://bit.ly/2LliJHH

ECDC/EMEA (European Centre for Disease Prevention and Control/European Medicines Agency). (2009). *Joint technical report. The bacterial challenge: Time to react A call to narrow the gap between multidrug-resistant bacteria in the EU and the development of new antibacterial agents*. https://doi.org/10.2900/2518. Accessed October 25, 2020, from https://bit.ly/3q7JjmX

Illinois Department of Public Health. (2020, permanently updated). *llinois Hospital Report Card and Consumer Guide to Health Care Health Care-associated infections*. Accessed October 25, 2020, from https://bit.ly/2XiIXND

Kölner Stadt Anzeiger. (2010). *Hygienemängel 5000 vermeidbare Todesfälle*. Accessed October 25, 2020, from https://bit.ly/3opEdBS

Kumar, P., & Singhal, N. (2020). Mapping neonatal and under-5 mortality in India. *The Lancet, 395* (10237), 1591–1593. https://doi.org/10.1016/S0140-6736(20)31050-3.

Mauldin, P. D., Salgado, C. D., Hansen, I. S., et al. (2010). Attributable hospital cost and length of stay associated with health care-associated infections caused by antibiotic-resistant gram-negative bacteria. *Antimicrobial Agents and Chemotherapy, 54*(1), 109–115. https://doi.org/10. 1128/AAC.01041-09.

Mayr, G. (2012). *Die Spur der Keime*. Accessed October 24, 2020, from https://archive.org/details/ diespurderkeime-gabymayr2012

Mombaque dos Santos, W., & Secoli, S. R. (2019). Economic burden of inpatients infected with *Klebsiella pneumoniae carbapenemase*. *Einstein São Paulo, 17*(4). https://doi.org/10.31744/ einstein_journal/2019GS4444.

O'Neill, J. (2014). Antimicrobial resistance: Tackling a crisis for the health and wealth of nation. *Review on Antimicrobial Resistance*. Accessed 25 October 2020, from https://bit.ly/2IXcCIk

Plachouras, D., Kärki, T., Hansen, S., et al. (2018). Antimicrobial use in European acute care hospitals: Results from the second point prevalence survey (PPS) of healthcare-associated infections and antimicrobial use, 2016 to 2017. *Eurosurveillance, 23*(46). https://doi.org/10. 2807/1560-7917.ES.23.46.1800393.

PREZIES. (2019). *Referentiecijfers 2014 t/m 2018: Prevalentieonderzoek ziekenhuizen*. In Dutch. Accessed October 25, 2020, from https://bit.ly/3hPJDn3

PREZIES. (2020). *Referentiecijfers 2015 t/m 2019: Prevalentieonderzoek zorginfecties ziekenhuizen*. In Dutch. Accessed October 25, 2020, from https://bit.ly/398kAHX

ReAct. (2012). *Health care-associated infections*. Accessed October 25, 2020, from https://bit.ly/ 3s1oU4E

Ricchizzi, E., Latour, K., & Kärki, T. (2018). Antimicrobial use in European long-term care facilities: Results from the third point prevalence survey of healthcare-associated infections and antimicrobial use, 2016 to 2017. *Eurosurveillance, 23*(46). https://doi.org/10.2807/1560-7917.ES.2018.23.46.1800394.

Roberts, R. R., Hota, B., Ahmad, I., et al. (2009). Hospital and societal costs of antimicrobial-resistant infections in a Chicago Teaching Hospital: Implications for antibiotic stewardship. *Clinical Infectious Diseases, 49*(8), 1175–1184. https://doi.org/10.1086/605630.

Rottier, W. C. (2019). *Quantifying the burden of antibiotic resistance in the Netherlands.* Dissertation UMC Utrecht. Accessed October 25, 2020, from https://dspace.library.uu.nl/handle/1874/375834

Sankar, M. J., Neogi, S. B., Sharma, J., et al. (2016). State of newborn health in India. *Journal of Perinatology, 36*(3), 3–8. https://doi.org/10.1038/jp.2016.183.

Schwaber, M. J., Navon-Venezia, S., Kaye, K. S., et al. (2006). Clinical and economic impact of bacteremia with extended-spectrum-β-lactamase-producing *Enterobacteriaceae. Antimicrobial Agents and Chemotherapy, 50*(4), 1257–1262. https://doi.org/10.1128/AAC.50.4.1257-1262.2006.

UNICEF. (2020). *Neonatal mortality.* Accessed October 24, 2020, from https://bit.ly/39moPA7

WHO (World Health Organization). (2019). *WHO model lists of essential medicines.* Accessed October 25, 2020, from https://bit.ly/2XhNT5q

Zacher, B., Haller, S., Willrich, N., et al. (2019). Application of a new methodology and R package reveals a high burden of healthcare-associated infections (HAI) in Germany compared to the average in the European Union/European Economic Area, 2011 to 2012. *Eurosurveillance, 24* (46). https://doi.org/10.2807/1560-7917.ES.2019.24.46.1900135.

Zastrow, K.-D. (2016). Krankenhausinfektionen – ein medizinisches, soziales und ökonomisches Problem. *Passion Chirurgie, 6*(1), 13–16. Accessed from https://bit.ly/3pZTRV3

# Major Outbreak at Maasstad Hospital

**4**

On Friday, 27 May 2011, the public relations department of Dutch broadcaster NOS[1] received an e-mail. Since it was already after office hours, I did not get to see the mail until shortly after 11 o'clock the following Monday. The mail came from an anonymous whistle-blower and had been sent via a secure e-mail address to guarantee the writer's anonymity. In a few sentences, it explained that 'an extremely lethal and incurable superbug' had already been spreading for a considerable time at the Maasstad Hospital in Rotterdam. The anonymous source also knew which bacterium was involved. 'This OXA-48-producing *Klebsiella pneumoniae* can be compared with the NDM-1 bacteria', the e-mail said. 'You will know, therefore, how serious this is'. I did indeed know. NDM-1 is a killer.[2]

The anonymous whistle-blower also reported that the hospital had kept the outbreak secret. Neither patients nor GPs were informed, and other hospitals and nursing homes in Rotterdam and the rest of the country did not know anything about this either. But infected patients were certainly being transferred to them. 'Only now', wrote my informant, 'is an investigation of the outbreak beginning—after the alarm was raised by several hospitals that had admitted patients from the Maasstad Hospital infected with the bacterium. Meanwhile several patients have died of infections by this bacteria, and there are still many more who have become infected by it'.

This brief e-mail marked the beginning of the story of the Klebsiella outbreak at the Maasstad Hospital, which was to have major repercussions: not just at the

---

[1]NOS (Nederlandse Omroep Stichting): the largest public radio and television broadcaster (news broadcaster) in the Netherlands.

[2]NDM-1 and OXA-48 are carbapenemases—enzymes that possess the ability to neutralise the effects of antibiotics belonging to the class of carbapenems. Carbapenems are potent antibiotics with few side effects. They are used as last resort drugs. Resistance to carbapenems is often combined with resistance to other beta-lactam antibiotics such as penicillin and cephalosporins. In case of carbapenem resistance, there are only a few medicines left, which are either much more toxic, less effective, or both.

© The Author(s), under exclusive license to Springer Nature Switzerland AG 2021
R. van den Brink, *The End of an Antibiotic Era*,
https://doi.org/10.1007/978-3-030-70723-1_4

hospital itself—where the consequences were vast—but also far beyond. The lessons of the tragedy that played out at the Rotterdam hospital have, in part, already been translated into new guidelines. In 2013, Achmea, the largest health insurer in the Netherlands, began to lay down specific conditions regarding matters of infection prevention when concluding new contracts with hospitals. For the most part, these demands stem from the report by an inquiry committee named after his President, the Lemstra Commission, which investigated the Klebsiella outbreak at Maasstad. There is now a registration service for outbreaks of particularly resistant microorganisms (BRMO), which was one of Lemstra's demands. In the light of the major consequences of the Klebsiella outbreak, it seems logical to take a detailed look at what actually occurred in the Rotterdam hospital.

## Tightrope Walk with the Truth

The outbreak became known to a small number of people outside the hospital after the Maasstad Hospital transferred a patient to the Slotervaart Hospital in Amsterdam at the beginning of April 2011. On the very same day that I received the tip-off mail, I sent the hospital an e-mail with eight questions. The Maasstad Hospital answered my questions by e-mail on the same evening. To at least three of my questions I received an answer that did not correspond with the truth. These were questions about the start date of the outbreak and at what point it became clear that, among other things, this was an outbreak involving an OXA-48-producing *Klebsiella pneumoniae*.

On 31 May, I sent another e-mail with a series of questions, in which I confronted the Maasstad Hospital with its lies—stating that the hospital knew it was dealing with an OXA-48-producing *Klebsiella pneumoniae* much earlier than it had claimed. The outbreak of ESBL-producing *Klebsiella pneumoniae* had begun much earlier than the hospital stated, and had infected many more patients than the Maasstad Hospital admitted. The answers that I received a couple of hours later were, in part, completely rewritten versions of the previous untruths. 'Here', wrote the press spokesperson for the Maasstad Hospital, 'are the figures showing how many patients tested positive for ESBL-Klebsiella between 2008 and 2011:

2008—not known.
2009—four out of approx. 1000 patients staying in the intensive care unit in this year.
2010—32 out of approx. 1000 patients staying in the intensive care unit in this year.
2011—39 out of approx. 1000 patients staying in the intensive care unit in this year.

OXA-48 was identified in retrospective tissue analyses in October 2010, and therefore not as early as 2009, let alone 2008. The intensive care unit has been closed once since 2008 due to *acinetobacter baumannii*. That was in 2010. On that occasion the unit was cleaned using a gas exposure technology'.

## Inadequate Response

On the evening of the 31st of May, NOS broadcast the first report on the Klebsiella outbreak at the Maasstad Hospital (Van den Brink 2011a). The key message was that the hospital had already been battling against a 'very dangerous and almost untreatable bacterium' for 7 months, and had only started investigating the appearance of these bacteria a few days earlier. And this was despite the fact that the hospital had already been twice informed which bacteria was causing so many problems. The hospital's managing director, Paul Smits, admitted that the Maasstad Hospital's response to these problems had been inadequate. 'We should have reported the matter to the health authority sooner', he said during this first broadcast, 'and requested the help of the RIVM'.[3] By this time the hospital had identified OXA-48-producing Klebsiella in 34 patients.

Nothing was yet known about the extent of the outbreak or whether it might have spread to other healthcare facilities.[4] At the time of the outbreak, the Maasstad Hospital was split between two different sites: the Zuiderziekenhuis and the Clara Hospital, which were both outdated. On 17 May 2011, both hospitals moved into a handsome new building in the Lombardijen district of Rotterdam. The Maasstad Hospital is one of three centres for severe burns patients in the Netherlands, and patients are very often transferred from it to other hospitals. The patient transferred from the Maasstad Hospital to the Slotervaart in Amsterdam had become infected in the intensive care unit of the Zuiderziekenhuis. When the patient was transferred to Amsterdam the Maasstad Hospital sent a report along with him, containing the most important information about the man's medical history, and also mentioning that he was infected with an unknown multiresistant Klebsiella.

At that time, Jayant Kalpoe was Clinical Microbiologist at the Slotervaart Hospital. He placed the patient in strict isolation and launched an investigation to find out which second, additional multiresistant ESBL-producing Klebsiella was involved. 'Mid-April I phoned my colleague at the Maasstad Hospital', Kalpoe told me, 'and informed him that the unknown multiresistant Klebsiella was resistant against carbapenems, the most effective class of antibiotics'. A few days later, Kalpoe knew that he was dealing with an OXA-48-producing *Klebsiella pneumoniae*. To confirm this, he sent the strain to the RIVM, where the national reference laboratory for investigating this type of multiresistant bacteria is also housed. The RIVM confirmed Kalpoe's findings. 'On 29 April I rang my colleague at the Maasstad Hospital again. I informed him that the unknown multiresistant Klebsiella produced

---

[3]RIVM (Rijksinstituut voor Volksgezondheid en Milieu, National Institute for Public Health and the Environment), comparable to the Public Health England (PHE) Centre of Disease Surveillance and Control (EPIET) in the United Kingdom and the CDC in the United States.

[4]In an e-mail to the author, Winfred Schop, at the time teammanager infectious diseases at the local health authority (GGD) in Rotterdam writes: 'The GGD in Rotterdam-Rijnmond received seven reports about patients who were transferred from the Maasstad Hospital to other healthcare institutions, and who also proved to be infected with OXA-48 Klebsiella afterwards. In two cases a hospital was involved, the other five affected retirement homes and nursing homes'.

the OXA-48 enzyme and was therefore resistant to carbapenem antibiotics'. The RIVM also contacted the Maasstad Hospital to offer help and to obtain the bacteria strains, which would enable them to validate a test[5] that was being developed and a procedure for identifying OXA-48.

'But we did not receive the strains', says one of the RIVM staff who was intensively involved with the case at the time. 'We received hardly any information, and we weren't welcome'. A written request for delivery of the bacteria strains was again sent in mid-May. The Maasstad Hospital did not exactly seem overjoyed by the RIVM's offer of help. It was ignored for 5 weeks. When the hospital learned that NOS News was going to report the outbreak, however, they quickly established contact with the RIVM and accepted the offer of help. On 1 June, a team from the RIVM in Rotterdam arrived on their doorstep. But even then the Maasstad staff were none too eager to collaborate with the RIVM.

## Harsh Judgement by Inspectorate

In their interim report of 2 November 2011, *The avoidable Klebsiella outbreak at the Maasstad Hospital,* the IGZ (Dutch Health Care Inspectorate) wrote: 'Even after the full extent of the outbreak had become clear no measures were taken, owing to a lack of understanding for the emergency and failures at management level'. The IGZ passed judgement on the events at the Maasstad Hospital in no uncertain terms. The overall conclusion was: 'Because the Maasstad Hospital did not act adequately, many patients were exposed to considerable risks over a long period. The fact that patients (among others) died as a result of infection by the Klebsiella OXA-48 bacterium shows how great these risks were. Since the outbreak was inadequately resisted for months, over 4000 patients came into unnecessary contact with infected patients. If the hospital had followed the guidelines of the national working group for infection prevention (WIP—Werkgroep voor Infectie Preventie),[6] the outbreak would have been brought under control sooner, would not have occurred on such a large scale, and the consequences would also have been less serious' (Schippers 2011).

On 21 June 2011, the NOS broadcast a second news report (Van den Brink 2011b). The Maasstad Hospital was very keen to be involved, 'in order to show that we have nothing to hide, as the NOS claims'—as the Managing Director at the time,

---

[5]This involved a PCR test. PCR stands for 'polymerase chain reaction'. With the aid of the test, enough material can be extracted from a few DNA molecules to analyse it.

[6]The WIP was a joint venture between the Netherlands Society for Clinical Microbiology, the Society for Infectious Diseases and the Society for Hygiene and Infection Prevention in Healthcare. It ceased its activities on 1 June 2017, after struggling financially for over 2 years. Neither hospitals nor the Ministry were willing to give the WIP sufficient funding. The Minister of Health—at that time Ms. Edith Schippers—asked the national health institute, the RIVM, to create a new structure for the work that the WIP had done up till then, and to coordinate the efforts of all parties involved. End March 2021 the WIP still not has been replaced by a new structure.

Paul Smits, put it. Besides Smit, we also spoke to the acting Head of Clinical Microbiology, Tjaco Ossewaarde, and the Head of the Communications Department, Dick Berkelder. 'After we had identified the first 34 patients', explains Ossewaarde, 'we analysed the data and established that the outbreak in the intensive care unit had actually come to a standstill. After that, we began to look retrospectively at old patients. In a short time we investigated 3500 samples'.

In the meantime, more and more patients colonised by an OXA-48 Klebsiella were being identified: both old patients that had been identified in the retrospective tests, and new ones that were staying in the Maasstad Hospital during June and July 2011. According to Ossewaarde, three patients were identified who had been transferred, while infected with OXA-48, to other healthcare facilities: one to the Slotervaart Hospital in Amsterdam, one to a retirement home in Rotterdam, and one who had spent months in the intensive care unit at the Maasstad Hospital and whose urine sample had been cultivated in March 2011 at a GP's laboratory in Etten-Leur. The culture gave grounds for suspecting that it was carbapenem-resistant. The laboratory at the Franciscus Hospital in Roosendaal confirmed the findings of the laboratory in Etten-Leur. It subsequently sent the strain to the RIVM. On 14 March 2011, the RIVM informed the laboratory in Etten-Leur that the bacteria strain found was a Klebsiella with OXA-48. In Etten-Leur, the microbiologist Ann Demeulemeester then called the doctor who had sent the urine sample to tell him that, if infections should occur, his patient could only be treated with intravenous antibiotics. When the doctor told her that he intended to have his patient readmitted to the Maasstad Hospital, Demeulemeester immediately called the Department of Clinical Microbiology there, in order to inform them of the upcoming arrival of a patient who had already been admitted before, and who was infected with an OXA-48-producing *Klebsiella pneumoniae*. This was in the middle of March, almost two and a half months before the hospital informed the GGD that it had bacteria with OXA-48 on its premises.

## Report the Deaths or Not?

On 21 June, Smits and Ossewaarde also said that, up to then, 47 patients with an OXA-48 Klebsiella had been identified. The first infection dated back to the end of October 2010. Twenty-one of these patients had died—as the Maasstad Hospital mentioned in the final sentences of a press release published the same day. What no one knew—apart from a few people directly involved and myself—was that, in the original version of the press release, the deaths had not been mentioned. The relevant passages were only included after the RIVM had threatened to publish their own press release instead. Some members of the external team that tried to bring the situation at the Maasstad Hospital back under control painted an unsettling picture of what they discovered there. By the beginning of July 2011, the number of patients with OXA-48 Klebsiellas had risen to approximately 65. The team members did not know how many of these patients had died. 'It's incredible', one of them said—'the hospital can't even tell us which patients the positive samples came from. They're unable to match the strains tested to the patients. Or perhaps they can—but don't want to'. The frustrations of the team from the RIVM and UMC Utrecht, which was trying to stop the outbreak and bring its effects under control, were now increasing. 'There were no guidelines for dealing with multiresistant bacteria in this hospital', said one of them. 'Absolutely nothing. They simply did nothing. They didn't even isolate the patients admitted from foreign hospitals'.

All suggestions to the Maasstad Hospital to communicate openly and honestly fell on deaf ears. It became clear from interviews with relatives of deceased patients and others involved, both inside and outside the hospital, that the Maasstad Hospital had trampled the basic rules of infection prevention and control underfoot (Van den Brink 2011c). Patients with multiresistant bacteria were not isolated at all, or not early enough. The hygiene regulations were not taken seriously: even when patients were placed in maximum isolation, staff went in and out without washing their hands or putting on protective clothing. Six months after my disclosure, the IGZ established that I had been right. Half a year later still, the Lemstra Commission came to exactly the same conclusion. The Maasstad Hospital had not adhered to the guidelines of the Working Group for Infection Prevention.

## 'New' Isn't Always New

The Maasstad Hospital plot continued to thicken. On 20 July 2011, the Head of the Communications Department announced that four more patients infected with OXA-48 Klebsiella had died (Van den Brink 2011d). What he didn't say—but what I found out a day later from one of the members of the RIVM/UMC Utrecht team—was that three of these cases were 'old' cases. 'We're still testing strains from the deep freeze. The positive strains are "newly discovered" infections—in other words, new additions to the list of infected patients'. But that is something quite different from new cases. This would refer to patients that become infected in the here and now. 'It is truly incredible that they could be so stupid as to announce this as well. But there you are, they're deciding what is communicated to the outside world'.

The Dutch Health Care Inspectorate (IGZ) reacted to the news of the 'new' fatalities as though thunderstruck (Van den Brink 2011e). Despite the strict agreements that had been made, the Maasstad Hospital had not informed the IGZ about the four additional deaths. The authority placed the Maasstad Hospital under strict supervision. A day later, at a press conference, the hospital announced that Professor Marc Bonten of UMC Utrecht had been appointed as supervisor (Van den Brink 2011f). This was one of the conditions laid down by the inspectorate.

The Head of the Intensive Care Unit and former Director of Medical Staff, Albert Grootendorst, explained that the hospital 'had always complied with the guidelines of the Working Group for Infection Prevention meticulously when Klebsiella with ESBL was diagnosed in an intensive care patient'. In their report, the Lemstra

Commission reproduced an e-mail from Grootendorst.[7] In this mail of 27 April 2011, Grootendorst informed the Managing Director, Smits, 'that the departments for clinical microbiology and hospital hygiene had failed', and concluded: 'It is no exaggeration to say that this threatens the continuing existence of the hospital' (Lemstra 2012). Managing Director Paul Smits did not react to this wake-up call from his Director of Medical Staff. And afterwards, Grootendorst did not do anything else either. He did not speak to Smits again, did not send any report to the Health Care Inspectorate, did not turn to the media, and did not inform his colleagues about his assessment.

## Considered Verdict

On 2 September 2011, Evert de Jonge, Professor for Intensive Medicine from the University Hospital in Leiden, presented the findings of his investigation into the actual role of OXA-48 *Klebsiella pneumoniae* in the deaths of the first 28 patients known to be infected with the bacterium. He arrived at a carefully considered and well-founded verdict. In three cases he considered it 'very probable' that the deaths of the patients had been caused by the bacteria. In the case of ten patients, it 'could not be ruled out' that the bacterium had played a role in their deaths, 'but not proven either'. However, these patients would have died anyway, owing to the severity of their original illness. In 14 cases, De Jonge came to the conclusion that it was 'highly unlikely' that the bacteria had contributed to the deaths of the patients. And in one case he was unable to make any statement, because he did not have enough data. This was the patient who had been transferred from the Maasstad Hospital to the Slotervaart in April 2011. At that time Jayant Kalpoe, the microbiologist who had diagnosed OXA-48 Klebsiella in this patient, told me that 'the patient died of heart failure. The infection with Klebsiella had nothing to do with it'.

Linda van Os is one of the relatives. Her mother was one of the ten patients whose deaths Professor De Jonge could not attribute with certainty to OXA-48 Klebsiella or to other causes. Linda's mother Riet van Os, 74 years old at the time, was admitted to the Zuiderziekenhuis on 20 December 2010 with enteritis. Her condition was pretty severe. The inflammation from which Riet van Os was suffering was accompanied by an abscess that pressed on her ureter. Her treatment with antibiotics ended successfully, and on 31 December she was sent home so that she could celebrate New Year with her family. Soon afterwards she became sick again, and after several visits to the hospital as an outpatient, she was readmitted on 20 January. On the same day, she started to go downhill.

Ms. Van Os became infected with several multiresistant bacteria. On 28 January, she was diagnosed as having multiresistant *Klebsiella pneumoniae*. Two months later it was established that she had also become infected by a multiresistant *E. coli*

---

[7]Grootendorst resigned from his posts as Director of Medical Staff and Head of the Intensive Care Unit in 2012. He has continued to work for several years in the hospital's intensive care unit.

and a multiresistant *Enterococcus faecium*. Both the Klebsiella germ and the *E. coli* germ produced ESBL. With disregard for the guidelines, she was not isolated until after 7 weeks. This can be seen in her medical records that her family shared with me. In the meantime she was going around the whole hospital as an ambulatory patient, seeing acquaintances from her days in hospital and before. But even when Riet van Os was finally isolated, other things still went wrong. According to her family, for the most part, the hygiene regulations were not observed.

'My mother's blood was sampled without gloves, even though she was in the isolation ward', says Linda van Os. 'People came in without protective clothing, while others only wore gloves and a face mask. I pointed out to several healthcare staff and even doctors that my mother had been placed in strict isolation, and that therefore they should wear protective clothing'. On 23 March 2011, Riet van Os had an operation. Afterwards her condition became even worse. For two days she was transferred to the intensive care unit as an emergency measure—with a double infection of the urinary tracts which developed into a sepsis, a so-called blood poisoning. 'Then they reacted just in time. She got better, and on 28 March was transferred back to the department. A couple of days later the wounds opened up again. On 6 April, they operated on her again. On 9 April she had to go back to the intensive care unit. It was there that she died, during the night between 9 and 10 April'. A second blood poisoning had proved fatal for Riet van Os.

'The doctor in the intensive care unit immediately told us that our mother had died of a very dangerous bacterium. In a later conversation, this statement was withdrawn. She had allegedly died of an intestinal problem. Later the Director of the hospital, Paul Smits, confirmed that my mother had died of a bacterium. He did not mention which. In any case that didn't really matter'.

## Respect or Otherwise

Jeanette Beuzenberg's mother is one of the three patients whose death, in Professor Evert de Jonge's opinion, had almost certainly been caused by the OXA-48 Klebsiella. Her mother was admitted to the Zuiderziekenhuis at the end of March 2011 with stomach problems. An exploratory operation found nothing. The clinical picture suggested an abscess, the doctors told her, but initially, they had not been able to find any. 'She became more and more unwell', says Jeanette Beuzenberg, 'and two weeks later was brought to the operating theatre as an emergency case'. During the preparations for the operation, she was told, her mother suffered a cardiac arrest and had to be resuscitated, probably as a result of a blood poisoning caused by the Klebsiella germ. That was on 13 April 2011. Despite this, the operation then went ahead, and an abscess and a piece of her intestine were removed. When she recovered, the doctors said, everything would be all right again. Unfortunately, this was not the case. A couple of days later, the doctors informed Jeanette that her mother was infected with the OXA-48 Klebsiella.

Sunday, 17 April was a day of hope. 'For the first time she came round again, fortunately without any brain damage. She recognised everybody and reacted quite normally'. But the family's joy was premature. Jeanette's mother remained severely ill. The infection became worse and worse, despite the doctors' assurances that 'her body was sound'. The doctors decided to discontinue the antibiotic treatment. They then decided to remove the abscess anally, and then puncture and drain any remaining abscesses. Just when a doctor wanted to perform the intervention, Jeannette's mother contracted pneumonia. 'The doctors presented us with a choice: either they could treat the pneumonia, as long as it hadn't been caused by the Klebsiella, since antibiotics wouldn't help in that case'. Or, they said, 'they could leave it to my mother's body to fight the infection by itself'. In view of their mother's overall weakness and the long ordeal of over 9 weeks, the family decided for the second option. Jeanette's mother died on the very same day, Monday 13 June 2011.

## Clear and Lucid Reports

The Lemstra Commission was set up on 13 September 2012. Previously, its director Professor Wolter Lemstra had already been Director of the Netherlands Association of Hospitals, State Secretary at the Ministry of Health, Welfare and Sport and Mayor of the town of Hengelo. The Lemstra Commission published its report roughly 6 months later, but the Dutch Health Care Inspectorate (IGZ) was on the case first. On 25 January 2012, the IGZ published their concluding report *Falen infectiepreventie in het Maasstad Ziekenhuis verwijtbaar* (Culpable negligence of hospital hygiene at the Maasstad Hospital). In it, the inspectorate announced that they would summon the hospital's microbiologists before the disciplinary committee (Van den Brink 2012). The IGZ regards them as the main culprits for the failure to manage the Klebsiella outbreak. According to the inspectorate, the hygiene professionals are 'directly responsible', but they are not subject to medical disciplinary law. The IGZ has therefore called for the Netherlands Health Minister, Edith Schippers, to change the laws accordingly. The managers, directors, doctors and care staff involved in the collapse of hospital hygiene were let off with the verdict that they were 'unprofessional'.

During the hearing of their case on 19 March 2013, the microbiologists disclaimed any responsibility for the breakdown of management during the Klebsiella outbreak (Van den Brink 2013a). They passed on the blame to a fourth microbiologist who did not have to appear before the disciplinary hearing because he was incurably sick, and to the specialist hygiene staff, who did not have to take responsibility because they were not subject to medical disciplinary law. However, this attitude did not get them any further. On 14 May 2013, the disciplinary court decided that the three microbiologists certainly did bear responsibility for the situation, even if they were not the only ones who had failed (Van den Brink 2013b). The disciplinary court reprimanded the three microbiologists. A reprimand of this kind is published in several newspapers, and a note of it remains inserted in the BIG register, which lists all doctors, for 5 years.

The Lemstra Commission published its report on 29 March 2012 (Lemstra 2012). Like the IGZ, they too praised the important role NOS News had played in this case.

And they passed a very severe judgement on the way the Maasstad Hospital had dealt with the Klebsiella outbreak. The commission came to the conclusion that there had been a 'collective failure' on the part of the management, supervisory board, microbiologists, hygiene specialists, doctors at the ICU and other medical specialists involved. 'Right from the beginning they failed to introduce appropriate measures to contain the outbreak in good time', the Lemstra Commission wrote. According to the commission's judgement, 'severely culpable behaviour' had occurred in many cases. In terms of quality and safety, the Maasstad Hospital had collectively failed in its handling of the crisis.

In the report, the commission recommended a number of measures. These were not just directed at the Maasstad Hospital but at all healthcare institutions and authorities, both in the Netherlands and abroad. In the commission's view, everyone could learn something from the breakdown at the Maasstad Hospital. The recommendations include reorganisation of hospital hygiene, introduction of quality and safety systems, and reinforcing the role of medical microbiologists and hygiene specialists. On top of this, the Lemstra Commission calls on professional scientific associations to make their guidelines for handling extremely resistant microorganisms more detailed and more binding. The commission also recommends that clinical microbiologists in hospitals should be salaried employees, even if the laboratory is no longer housed in the hospital as a result of mergers or amalgamations. Lemstra also calls on the authorities to carefully consider the risks posed by the increase in antibiotic resistance and the expected cuts in the healthcare budget.

A study published in March 2014 in *Eurosurveillance* gave a few more hard facts (Dautzenberg et al. 2014). During the outbreak, at least 128 patients became infected with an OXA-48-producing bacterium. Amongst this patient group, it was possible to establish the presence of the OXA-48 *Klebsiella pneumoniae* that caused the outbreak in 118 persons, and the presence of other OXA-48-producing bacteria in ten patients. By the end of April 2012, 36 of these 118 patients had died. According to Marc Bonten, who acted as supervisor, none of the eight newly discovered deceased patients had been infected by Klebsiella OXA-48. 'They did not have any of the associated symptoms, and the cases were identified in the course of the retrospective screening', he said. A total of 7527 patients were screened at the time, three times each. During the entire period of the outbreak, a total of 72,000 patients were admitted to the Maasstad Hospital. Four thousand, seven hundred and twenty-two of these were classified as 'at risk' patients. On average, the patients who had been infected with an OXA-48 were admitted to the Maasstad Hospital three times during the outbreak period, and almost half of them (44%) ended up in the intensive care unit. Many patients with OXA-48 Klebsiella also spent time in the surgical ward and the renal disease unit. Twenty patients actually developed an infection as a result of the bacterium. Only 10% of the 128 strains in which OXA-48 was identified were bacteria other than *Klebsiella pneumoniae*. 54 patients (also) carried *E. coli* with OXA-48. A further 12 types of bacteria were also found, which all produced the

OXA-48 enzyme.[8] The patients were colonised by various combinations of these bacteria. In 15 patients, Klebsiella, *E. coli* and a third bacteria with OXA-48 were all identified. The genetic information which encodes the production of the OXA-48 enzyme is stored in a location on the bacteria that makes it easy to transfer the information to other bacteria, and even to bacteria of other species.[9]

## Death Toll Higher in Retrospect

After 18 July 2011, no more new infections were identified. Therefore, in mid-September 2011, it was officially asserted that the outbreak was under control. The date given for the start of the outbreak was 1 July 2009. It is true that the patient with the earliest proven infection dated from September 2010, but there are clear indications that this was not the first infected patient. 'On the basis of the suscepti-bility data from the VITEK system,[10] we cannot exclude the possibility that patients had already been carriers prior to this', says Marc Bonten in a report on the outbreak (IGZ 2012). 'Therefore, for pragmatic reasons it was stated that the outbreak had begun on 1 July 2009'. In the VITEK data, there were a large number of resistance patterns that revealed considerable similarities with the resistance patterns identified in the bacteria of patients with OXA-48 Klebsiella. In all, there were 84 patients who were classified as 'dark grey suspicious cases'.[11] Marc Bonten spoke about this during a presentation on 17 April 2012 at the spring conference of the NVMM (Nederlandse Vereniging voor Medische Microbiologie = Netherlands Society for Medical Microbiology). 'We cannot prove that we are dealing with identical strains here', Bonten said, 'but because of the similarity, we have decided to play safe and backdate the start of the outbreak to 1 July 2009'. The reconstruction of events at the Maasstad Hospital carried out by Bonten and his team stretches back to week 31 of 2008. From this time onwards, the Maasstad Hospital began having problems with ESBL-producing Klebsiellas at its Zuiderziekenhuis site. This genetic type of ESBL occurs globally and can be passed on between different types of bacteria relatively easily.[12] In addition to OXA-48, the OXA-48 *Klebsiella pneumoniae* responsible for

---

[8]Six patients with *enterobacter cloacae* with OXA-48, six with *Klebsiella oxytoca* with OXA-48, five with *morganella morgannii* with OXA-48, three with *citrobacter freundii* with OXA-48. In addition to this, nine more types of bacteria with OXA-48 were identified, each of them in one or two patients. Forty-nine patients were carriers of more than one type of OXA-48 bacteria.

[9]The genetic information in which this form of antibiotic resistance is encoded is located on a plasmid, a separate, circular piece of DNA. This makes it possible to pass on the information to other bacteria, including those of other species.

[10]A VITEK is a system that makes it possible to test which antibiotics a bacterium is susceptible to.

[11]'Dark grey suspicious cases' are patients whose risk of infection with an OXA-48 Klebsiella was estimated to be the highest—in contrast to light grey suspicious cases, whose risk was lower. 'White patients' are not carriers. 'Black patients' are carriers, or infected with OXA-48 Klebsiella.

[12]The type in question is CTX-M-15. CTX-M-15 is also an enzyme.

the outbreak at the Maasstad Hospital also possessed an ESBL of the same genetic type as the ESBL Klebsiellas that had already been identified in the hospital in 2008.

## Competence Centres Needed

It was not easy to identify the OXA-48 strains, explains Marc Bonten, Supervisor of the Department for Clinical Microbiology and Hospital Hygiene at the Maasstad Hospital since 23 July 2012. 'OXA-48 is quite hard to identify, but at the Maasstad Hospital it went on for far too long. Half of the strains we were able to identify would certainly not have been found by any other laboratory. We screened for OXA-48, because otherwise it wouldn't have been possible. But half the strains possessed MIC values[13] that we would not normally have classified as resistant. As a result of the outbreak, therefore, the procedure took on proportions that were double those of other screening processes. For example, if the OXA-48 gene is present in an *E. coli,* then the *E. coli* is susceptible as usual. But when an ESBL is added as well, then it can suddenly become resistant to the beta-lactam antibiotics in standard use, and even to carbapenems. If new resistance mechanisms develop at the tempo we've seen in recent years, we are going to have more problems in the years ahead. I therefore believe that we need to establish a number of reference centres in the Netherlands, which must keep up with the rest of the world in the field of resistance problems at the highest level. These centres must constantly keep up to date, in order to be able to advise other hospitals and healthcare institutions. Believe me, the smaller hospitals in particular cannot solve these problems under their own steam'.

## Silver Lining

Many of the people I spoke to, both at home and abroad, regard the events of the Maasstad affair as a convincing argument for the importance of a functioning system of clinical microbiology and hospital hygiene. 'This is therefore a blessing in disguise—as I always say', says James Cohen Stuart. 'But it is difficult to say that out loud, after all the pain and grief that the outbreak has caused'.

Professor Robert Skov is Head of the Infection Control Department at the Statens Serum Institut in Copenhagen, the Danish equivalent of the Centers for Disease Control and Prevention in the US. I spoke with him on 14 and 15 March 2012 at the European 'Combatting Antimicrobial Resistance' conference. 'As terrible as they are for those affected, events such as those at the Maasstad Hospital also have their useful side. They make it clear how important combatting and preventing infectious diseases is'. Until 1 March 2012, Andreas Heddini was Director of ReAct—'Action on Antibiotic Resistance'. In 2012 he moved to GlaxoSmithKline. 'In the last

---

[13]The minimum inhibitory concentration (MIC) is the lowest concentration of a medicine that can still inhibit the growth of a bacterium.

analysis, the outbreak at the Maasstad Hospital is turning out to be a kind of blessing. Such an event attracts a lot of attention, and this is sorely needed. We had a group of colleagues from Ghana visiting us at ReAct, and they told us that they'd recently had an outbreak of MRSA. During the outbreak, three small children lost their lives. Naturally this is terrible—but they also said that it had helped them to convince the people and government that antibiotic resistance posed a very grave threat to public health'.

Until the end of 2013, Edwin Boel was President of the Netherlands Society for Medical Microbiology (NVMM). At this time he heads the Taskforce molecular diagnostics founded in 2020 during the first wave of the SARS-CoV-2 pandemic. 'Maasstad shows us what happens when the system no longer functions', he said. 'The negative side of it is that, as a result, microbiologists had to be summoned before a tribunal. The positive side is that it made clear how important a well-functioning microbiological sector is. The problem with clinical microbiology is that people hardly notice it when everything is functioning smoothly. It only becomes visible when things go wrong. Then it becomes clear what it costs in terms of human suffering and money when it does not function properly. It's like the electricity supply. As long as you have electricity, you don't think about it. It's only when there's a power cut that you notice how important a functioning electricity supply system is'.

Discussed above in some detail are the human costs of the OXA-48 Klebsiella outbreak in the Maasstad Hospital. As for its financial consequences, they were also huge. According to the hospital itself, the outbreak cost them around 7 million euros. But these are only the direct costs related to massive extra testing of patients, the hiring of expertise and claims of patients or their relatives, to give a few examples. But the sum does not account for the considerable loss of income caused by patients avoiding the Maasstad Hospital after the outbreak became public. In 2010, the hospital realised a growth of 17% and a net benefit of 5 million euros (Maasstad Ziekenhuis 2011). In 2011—the year the outbreak was revealed by NOS News—the hospital showed a negative growth of 2.7% and a net loss of 14 million euros (Maasstad 2012). That same year the mean growth in the hospital sector was 6,8%. If the Maasstad had matched this mean growth factor, it would have had 29 million euros more in revenues. Consequently, the total financial burden of the Klebsiella outbreak in the Maasstad Hospital seems to be 6 or 7 times higher than the 7 million euros claimed by the hospital.

## References

Dautzenberg, M. J., Ossewaarde, J. M., de Kraker, M. E., et al. (2014). Successful control of a hospital-wide outbreak of OXA-48 producing Enterobacteriaceae in the Netherlands, 2009 to 2011. *Eurosurveillance, 19*(9). https://doi.org/10.2807/1560-7917.ES2014.19.9.20723.

IGZ Inspectie voor de Gezondheidszorg (Health Inspectorate). (2012). *Falen infectiepreventie in het Maasstad Ziekenhuis verwijtbaar* (Culpable negligence of hospital hygiene at the Maasstad Hospital). In Dutch. Accessed October 26, 2020, from https://bit.ly/3olseoW

Lemstra, W. (2012). *Oog voor het onzichtbare (An eye for the invisible)*. Available in Dutch https://
eursafety.eu/wp-content/uploads/maasstad.pdf or in German. Accessed November 16, 2020,
from https://eursafety.eu/wp-content/uploads/Maasstad-DE.pdf

Maasstad Ziekenhuis. (2011). *Annual Report 2010*. Accessed October 26, 2020, from https://bit.ly/
3pUPlXH

Maasstad Ziekenhuis. (2012). *Annual Report 2011 in Dutch*. Accessed October 26, 2020, from
https://bit.ly/3hM6Fvn

Schippers, E. I. (2011). Reactie op het IGZ-tussenrapport 'Klebsiella-uitbraak in Maasstad
Ziekenhuis vermijdbaar' Reaction of the Health Secretary to the preliminary IGZ-report *Klebsi-
ella-outbreak at the Maasstad Ziekenhuis avoidable*. Contains the report itself. In Dutch.
Accessed October 25, 2020, from https://bit.ly/2Xi1rhu

Van den Brink, R. (2011a). *Maasstad Ziekenhuis faalt bij aanpak resistentie*. NOS 31 May 2011. In
Dutch. Accessed October 25, 2020, from https://nos.nl/artikel/244894-maasstad-ziekenhuis-
faalt-bij-aanpak-resistentie.html

Van den Brink, R. (2011b). *21 doden met resistente bacterie Rotterdam*. NOS 21 June 2011. In
Dutch. Accessed October 25, 2020, from https://nos.nl/artikel/250081-21-doden-met-resistente-
bacterie-rotterdam.html

Van den Brink, R. (2011c). *Maasstad negeerde regels bacteriën. NOS 12 July 2011*. In Dutch.
Accessed October 25, 2020, from https://nos.nl/artikel/255447-maasstad-negeerde-regels-
bacterien.html

Van den Brink, R. (2011d). *Opnieuw besmette patiënten Rotterdam overleden. NOS 20 July 2011*.
In Dutch. Accessed October 25, 2020, from https://nos.nl/artikel/257549-opnieuw-besmette-
patienten-rotterdam-overleden.html

Van den Brink, R. (2011e). *Maasstad onder verscherpt toezicht*. NOS 20 July 2011. In Dutch.
Accessed October 26, 2020, from https://nos.nl/artikel/257654-maasstad-onder-verscherpt-
toezicht.html

Van den Brink, R. (2011f). *Maasstad Ziekenhuis stelt supervisor aan*. NOS 21 July 2011. In Dutch.
Accessed October 26, 2020, from https://nos.nl/artikel/258005-maasstad-ziekenhuis-stelt-
supervisor-aan.html

Van den Brink, R. (2012). *Microbiologen Maasstad voor tuchtrechter*. NOS 25 January 2012. In
Dutch. Accessed October 26, 2020, from https://nos.nl/artikel/333923-microbiologen-
maasstad-voor-tuchtrechter.html

Van den Brink, R. (2013a). *Microbiologen ontkennen schuld*. NOS 19 March 2013. In Dutch.
Accessed October 26, 2020, from https://nos.nl/artikel/486441-microbiologen-ontkennen-
schuld.html

Van den Brink R (2013b). *Berisping microbiologen Maasstad*. NOS 14 May 2013. In Dutch.
Accessed October 26, 2020, from https://nos.nl/artikel/506643-berisping-microbiologen-
maasstad.html

# A Thin Layer of Faeces on Everything You Touch

The screen shows a map of the United Kingdom. The hospitals are marked by black dots. One of these dots is white, because in this hospital an outbreak of MRSA (methicillin-resistant *staphylococcus aureus*) has occurred. It is a hospital in the eastern part of the Midlands, in the area around Leicester and Nottingham. Every now and then, a line shoots out from this white dot to one of the black dots in the region. Over time the number of lines increases, and so does the speed with which they appear. More and more black dots become white. This means that up to 10% of all patients there are now colonised. Within 2 years, MRSA can be identified in hospitals throughout the whole of Great Britain. Then the first yellow dots crop up. They mean that between 10 and 15% of the patients in these hospitals are colonised. And then the first red dot appears. It indicates a value of over 15% MRSA. The lines shoot out over the screen at a constantly increasing rate, and the dots change colour ever more rapidly. After two years, half of British hospitals are colonised with MRSA. After nearly 6 years, there are patients colonised with MRSA in every hospital. In dozens of hospitals, particularly teaching hospitals, more than 15% of patients are affected. There is no longer a single hospital in which fewer than 10% of the patients are colonised by MRSA (NOS 2012).

This model (Donker et al. 2012), created by scientists at the Groningen University Clinic and the RIVM, shows how MRSA would spread in Great Britain if no countermeasures were taken. It demonstrates that a proliferation of resistant bacteria can occur very quickly, and that it does not just depend on the quality of hospital hygiene. Movements of patients between hospitals seems to be a decisive factor for the spread of resistant bacteria. For their computer animation, the scientists used data on patient movements between hospitals over 1 year. Teaching hospitals play a decisive role in proliferation. As soon as they come into contact with MRSA, the process enters a new phase, since there is a lot of patient movement between teaching hospitals and other hospitals. Patients with complex diseases are transferred from other hospitals to teaching hospitals, and sent back to their hospital of origin as soon as possible.

© The Author(s), under exclusive license to Springer Nature Switzerland AG 2021
R. van den Brink, *The End of an Antibiotic Era*,
https://doi.org/10.1007/978-3-030-70723-1_5

What holds true for MRSA can be applied to other multiresistant bacteria. And what holds true for the UK also applies to other countries, such as the Netherlands. The same scientists had already carried out an earlier study there, which led to similar results. All Dutch hospitals are connected with one another either directly or indirectly, and the teaching hospitals are the points of intersection in this network (Donker et al. 2010). It is no different in Germany. There too, the hospitals are closely interlinked on a regional basis. In a study carried out in the border region of Gronau-Enschede, in the Dutch-German EUREGIO, scientists from Groningen, Münster and Berlin proved this very elegantly. The MRSA types occurring in different Dutch hospitals are closely related genetically, or even identical. In Germany, other types of MRSA are found, which are also identical to the MRSA types in other German hospitals, or closely related to them. 'There findings are in keeping with the fact that MRSA follows patients if they are transferred from hospitals in one country to a hospital in another', the EUREGIO research group reported. Whether a specific bacterium spreads within a population or not depends on various factors. The bacterium's pathogenic qualities, those of its host, and contacts between potential hosts all play a role. But the organisation of the healthcare system is also an important factor. The scientists give a neat example to illustrate this. In 2005, an MRSA of a new genetic type surfaced on both sides of the Dutch-German border—to be more precise, in a hospital in Enschede and one in Münster. On the Dutch side of the border, the MRSA type did not spread any further. On the German side of the border, the MRSA spread to 19 of the 39 hospitals in the regional hospital network. It even spread beyond the regional boundary of North Rhine-Westphalia to Lower Saxony. 'Patient movements are a significant player in the spread of MRSA', wrote the scientists. 'The latest efforts to facilitate cross-border access to medical care in the member states of the European Union, and in particular the EUREGIO, could lead to new challenges in the prevention of cross-border proliferation of multiresistant microorganisms. Therefore the hospitals which are practically situated in the same healthcare region—independently of administrative structures and across national borders—must come to an agreement on infection prevention, as though they were a single, common hospital' (Ciccolini et al. 2013). This idea of a modern infection prevention system, which underlies the study, was proposed by one of its authors, Tjibbe Donker, in his doctoral thesis *Disease transmission through hospital networks* (Donker 2014), which earned him a *summa cum laude*. 'Avoiding the spread of resistance takes priority', writes Donker, 'because the number of treatment options for bacterial infections is rapidly decreasing. By studying the contacts between patients inside the treatment networks, we can introduce a set of measures to avoid the proliferation of resistant bacteria and other pathogens in treatment institutions.

- Above all, investments must be made in infection prevention in those closely networked hospitals that form the intersection points of the healthcare provision.
- Infection prevention must be coordinated on a regional level.

- Of course existing healthcare regions should be maintained, so that patients are mainly treated in their home region, and no cross-border specialist treatment centres should be developed.
- Surveillance centres should be set up to monitor the appearance of new hospital germs or resistance mechanisms.
- Bacterial subtypes that might have a considerable impact on public health provision should be identified with the latest mathematical procedures and models on the basis of routinely gathered data'.

Mr. Donker's plea for a regionalisation of infection prevention in hospital referral networks, in his thesis *Disease transmission through hospital networks* (Donker 2014), found wide support amongst microbiologists in the Netherlands. Based on this idea, a task force led by Alex Friedrich developed a vision document to keep the Netherlands 'CRE-free' (NVMM 2015). The idea also won support from the Minister of Health, Ms. Edith Schippers. In a letter to Parliament in July 2016, the minister presented a plan to create regional referral networks between the best-connected hospitals and other healthcare institutions (Schippers 2016). She also proposed budgets for the years 2016–2019. Parliament approved the plans. Marc Bonten, Head of the Department of Medical Microbiology at the University Hospital in Utrecht, responded in a article in the NTvG—the magazine of the KNMG, the Royal Dutch Society of Doctors. 'Those networks do indeed make it possible to do extremely useful things such as improving cooperation between GPs, homes for the elderly and laboratories', he stated. 'But in the hands of the Health Ministry they have become a bureaucratic Moloch. My network coordinator spends most of his time bookkeeping'. His colleague Professor Jan Kluijtmans, Head of the Department of Medical Microbiology in Breda, near the Dutch-Belgian border, agrees. 'The ministry is looking for the right way to proceed. But I trust that they will find it' (De Vrieze 2018). The main objective of the regional referral networks is to keep carbapenemase-producing *Enterobacteriaceae* (CPE) out of the Netherlands. At the moment these are very rare—less than 1% of all isolates that cause an infection are CPEs. For the last 5 years, their number has been more or less stable at 0.7% of all invasive isolates (De Greeff et al. 2020).

Until now I have mainly been talking about MRSA—the resistant bacterium that is best known to the general public—as well as *E. coli* and Klebsiella with ESBL, or with the carbapenemases that have become increasingly common over recent years, such as OXA-48. But this is only a small segment of the resistant bacteria we have to deal with. Because of the selection process caused by the use of antibiotics, and as a result of horizontal and vertical gene transfer, new types are constantly being added.[1] Or somewhere a bacterium pops up that had hardly ever existed there before. VRE is one example. Vancomycin-resistant enterococci are a relatively harmless type of resistant bacteria. Enterococci are part of normal human intestinal flora and are easily passed on. VREs are harmless for healthy humans but can become dangerous for

---

[1]For information about horizontal and vertical gene transfer, please refer to Chap. 2.

people with weakened immune systems, for example patients in intensive care units. VREs are resistant to the first-choice antibiotics for the treatment of enterococci infections, making it hard to treat these types of infection. In a hospital environment, VREs can survive a pretty long time. This makes it extremely difficult to rid a hospital of them once they have found their way in. For hospitals, therefore, VRE outbreaks are often much harder to stop than outbreaks of bacteria that are more pathogenic. The financial and human costs of a VRE outbreak can assume considerable proportions.

## The First Outbreaks

The first VRE outbreaks in the Netherlands occurred in 1999 on the haematology ward[2] of the VU University Medical Centre (VUmc) in Amsterdam (Leavis et al. 2004). Prior to this, cases of VRE in humans had occurred only sporadically in the Netherlands (Endtz et al. 1997). The outbreak became known when three patients got ill as a result of a sepsis caused by a VRE. During checks, 23 carriers of the bacterium were identified. In two of them, it also caused a sepsis. In the case of one patient, the infection was not discovered until after his death. The remaining patients with sepsis were successfully treated. Strict measures were implemented at the VUmc to completely change working practices on the haematology ward. Infected patients were isolated in single rooms, or treated in multi-occupancy rooms by means of cohort care.[3] On top of this, they were are all given their own chemical toilet, and strict hygienic measures were put in place. Because the haematology ward itself was fairly well isolated, with a manageable group of patients, the staff succeeded in bringing the outbreak fully under control within a couple of months. 'But you must draw up very strict rules and implement them in order to keep VRE in check', says Christina Vandenbroucke-Grauls, Head of the Department for Medical Microbiology at VUmc until her retirement in October 2017. On top of this, negative cultures are not always reliable. 'In 1999 we discharged a patient whose control culture was negative, but when he returned to the clinic two weeks later, he was nevertheless carrying VRE. So a negative culture doesn't afford any guarantee'. A year after the outbreak at VUmc, the UMC Utrecht had to cope with VRE. The outbreak in Utrecht was the biggest VRE outbreak in the Netherlands up to 2012. In all, 84 patients carrying VRE were identified. This gave rise to infections in 14 haematology patients, but none of them suffered serious consequences.

---

[2]Haematology is concerned with diseases or disorders of the blood, the bone marrow, the spleen or the lymphatic system.

[3]In cohort care, one group of patients is treated in isolation as a group.

## Outbreak in Sweden

Some years later, an even bigger series of VRE outbreaks occurred just as suddenly in Sweden (Söderblom et al. 2010). They lasted from July 2007 to March 2009. In these 20 months, 760 cases of VRE colonisation were reported to the Swedish health authorities. During the previous 7 years, from 2000 to 2006, 194 VRE cases were reported in total. In Sweden, it is mandatory to report cases of VRE. The outbreaks began in a number of hospitals in the province of Stockholm. VRE then turned up in the provinces of Halland (in the extreme south-west) and Västmannland (north-west of Stockholm)—and not just in hospitals, but in care homes and retirement homes as well. Reports of isolated cases came from ten other provinces. In almost all these cases, the infection with VRE had occurred in Sweden, and in the vast majority of cases the patients had picked up the germ in institutions of the healthcare system. The three areas are geographically separate from one another, and yet in the majority of cases, the VRE strains were closely related genetically. Of the 760 patients colonised by VRE, 15 developed a sepsis.

In the Netherlands, after the outbreak at the UMC Utrecht, it took a further 10 years before another VRE outbreak occurred. From summer 2010 to May 2011, the University Medical Centre Groningen (UMCG) had to battle against an outbreak that came in several waves. In all, 139 patients became infected with VRE. Two of them developed severe sepsis. According to Professor Alex Friedrich, Head of the Department for Medical Microbiology at UMCG, in roughly 20% of the VRE cases the bacteria strain involved could not be identified by standard, conventional diagnostic methods. In the Ems Dollart Region (EDR),[4] the northeast of the Netherlands and the northwest of Germany, a collaborative study is now being carried out in general hospitals and three teaching hospitals in Groningen, Münster and Oldenburg. The hospitals are looking for people with highly resistant microorganisms (BRMO) in their intestines. So far the study has shown that there are only very limited cases of VRE in this northern region. 1.3 per cent of the 'at risk' patients examined are carriers of VRE. On the Dutch side of the border, only VRE from the genetical subtype VanB was identified, but on the German side, three-quarters of the VREs belonged to the VanA genotype.[5] Around 5% of all the genotype VanB VREs found remain below the detection threshold of conventional diagnostic procedures, as a result of their insufficiently pronounced resistance to vancomycin. Amongst the other highly resistant microorganisms, ESBL was the most common. It was detected more frequently on the Dutch side of the border. 8.8 per cent of all 'at risk' patients examined were carriers of an ESBL. In almost all

---

[4]The Ems Dollart Region (EDR) comprises the Dutch provinces of Groningen, Friesland, Drenthe and Overijssel, and the north-western part of the German states of Lower Saxony and North Rhine-Westphalia.

[5]The VRE genotype in question is VanB. The VanB genetic type makes a bacterium resistant to vancomycin, but not teicoplanin. The VanA genotype causes resistance to both antibiotics. VanB VRE sometimes possesses a low level of resistance to vancomycin that cannot be identified by traditional testing methods. This leads to underdiagnosis and spread of resistance.

cases it was *E. coli*. On the German side of the border, the percentage of ESBL carriers was lower, at 7.7 per cent. In Germany *E. coli* was identified most often, but also ESBL-positive *Klebsiella pneumoniae*.

Shortly after the outbreak at the UMC Groningen had been brought under control, VRE outbreaks occurred at the neighbouring Martini Hospital in Groningen and the Isala Clinics in Zwolle in the summer of 2011. This was followed by a series of VRE outbreaks at Dutch hospitals in spring and summer 2012. In these, hundreds of patients became colonised by VRE, and some of them developed an infection. Carriers of VRE can carry the bacterium around with them for months or even years. By the end of 2012 Rob Willems, VRE specialist at UMC Utrecht, had received 169 VRE strains from 18 hospitals, originating from 16 different clones. Ten clones were identified in various hospitals.[6]

## Important Consequences

The VRE outbreaks had far-reaching effects on the hospitals. Between February and July 2012, the Slingeland Hospital in Doetinchem—a city in the east of the Netherlands—recorded 63 confirmed VRE cases. Ten of these patients died, but none of them from a VRE infection. Five wards at the hospital were affected, as well as a division of a nursing home in the region. Swabs were taken from roughly 4000 patients. Four wards were closed for disinfection, and two others reserved for patients with VRE. For several weeks, the hospital had to carry out fewer operations and placed an admissions ban on a number of wards. Throughout the whole period, the Slingeland Hospital kept the public informed of the problems. This was also the case at the St. Antonius Hospital in Nieuwegein, one of the main centres for the treatment of heart diseases in the Netherlands. The VRE outbreak began at the end of April 2011 at a premises in Utrecht, but the Nieuwegein site was almost equally affected. By the middle of November 2012, the outbreak was under control. By that time, 140 patients had become colonised by VRE. Four wards were closed for a long period, operations were cancelled, and patients were isolated. More than 3000 patients were recalled to the hospital to be tested for VRE. Over 2000 actually went back and, after being tested five times, were declared clean. In all, 17,000 VRE tests were carried out. At the beginning of 2013, sporadic cases of VRE colonisation were still being detected. In the second half of this year, only one more colonised patient was found. The St. Antonius Hospital allowed the deaths of 12 patients with VRE to be investigated by a commission. In 11 of the 12 patients, there was no causal connection between their deaths and colonisation by VRE, but a possible causal connection was established in one patient. Every year since 2012 between 10 and 20 VRE-outbreaks are counted in Dutch hospitals. So, VRE-outbreaks seem here again to stay.

---

[6]Rob Willems presented the figures quoted here at the symposium 'VRE Wat moet je ermee' ('VREs: what is their significance?'), which took place in Nijmegen on 4 October 2012.

The University Hospital Tübingen (UKT) in Germany had also had to deal with VRE outbreaks several times already. Five patients were diagnosed with VRE in 2003, but in 2004 it really hit the university hospital. Between June 2004 and May 2005, 205 patients at the UKT became infected with VRE. The predominant strain involved in this outbreak surfaced simultaneously in several other south German hospitals and turned out to be much more virulent than enterococci usually are. Of the 105 patients, 75 developed an invasive infection. The costs of the outbreak were devastating. In an article in *Emerging Infectious Diseases,* they were estimated to be something between 1 and 1.6 million euros. This figure took 93 patients into account. But since, in the end, more patients were affected, the actual costs are higher still. Repeated use of the reserve drug linezolid to treat the VRE infections already led to the development of resistance to the drug during the campaign against the VRE outbreak itself (Sagel et al. 2008; Schulte et al. 2008).

The differences in VRE incidence across Europe are considerable. In Iceland, Luxembourg and Slovenia the incidence of vancomycin-resistant *Enterococcus faecium* is close to zero. In France, it is 0.7 and in the Netherlands 0.9%. In Croatia, Germany and Slovenia it is well above 20%. In Romania, Hungary, Ireland, Latvia and Lithuania it is close to 40%. Poland and Greece have a VRE-incidence of far beyond 40% and Cyprus holds the record with 50% (ECDC 2020a).

## The VRE Paradox

In 2000, shortly after taking up his post at UMC Utrecht, Professor Marc Bonten found himself dealing with a major VRE outbreak. Since then he has been regarded as one of the leading experts. 'It is strange that we're now seeing so many outbreaks of VRE suddenly appearing at the same time. In the United States there is a high prevalence[7] of VRE in hospitals. In Europe VRE was in fact hardly ever seen, although about 15 years ago there was a very large reservoir of it in livestock farming. In animals, it has disappeared. VRE was quickly linked to the use of avoparcin, an antibiotic used in livestock farming. This is so similar to vancomycin that vancomycin-resistant enterococci developed in animals as a result of it. These are passed on to human beings, who are admitted to hospitals and intensive care units, and then they lead to problems in them. But this argument was flawed in many respects. In the USA there were no VREs in animals or healthy humans, but nevertheless there were many cases in hospitals. In Europe it was precisely the other way around. The livestock stalls were full of VRE. It was even found in healthy people, but we never saw it in hospitals. We call this the VRE Paradox'. For a long time, antibiotics were used in intensive livestock farming as a growth promoter. In all the countries where avoparcin was used as a growth promoter, the animals were full of VRE. The VREs were living in the meat that came on the market, and they

---

[7]The prevalence of a condition describes the number of cases per 1000, 10,000 or 100,000 members of the population at a specific point in time.

were also found in the intestines of healthy people. In countries where avoparcin was not used in intensive livestock farming—like Sweden, where growth promoters have been banned since 1986—VRE was not identified in either animals, meat or healthy humans until the outbreak in 2007 (Van den Bogaard et al. 2000). As early as September 1998, the Netherlands Health Council (GR)[8] published a document addressing the issue of whether humans might acquire problems as a result of the antibiotic-resistant bacteria found in livestock farming (Gezondheidsraad 1998). Among other things, the GR referred to a report on avoparcin by the Scientific Committee for Animal Nutrition of the European Commission (SCAN 1996). 'Avoparcin is similar to vancomycin', the report of the Health Council said, 'at present the only available antibiotic that is still effective for patients with methicillin-resistant *staphylococcus aureus* (MRSA). We have already come across resistance to vancomycin in another germ that is responsible for healthcare-associated infections: *Enterococcus* spp.[9] Although the committee took the view that there were was no solid scientific evidence that pathogenic bacteria in humans could form resistances as a result of the use of avoparcin as a growth promoter in livestock farming, the factors pointing in this direction could not be sufficiently discounted either. One of the results of this conclusion was that the European Commission banned the use of avoparcin as a growth promoter in the EU until 1999'. In several countries, this immediately led to a sharp decline in the incidence of VRE. In Denmark, the prevalence of VRE in hens fell from more than 80% in 1995 to less than 5% in 1998. But in pigs, by far the most important sector of the Danish livestock industry, there was no change. Twenty per cent of the animals continued to be colonised by VRE. In Germany, the number of hens infected with VRE fell from 100 to 25% as a result of the ban. The number of VRE carriers amongst healthy people in Germany fell from 12% to 3%. In Italy, the number of hens infected with VRE fell from 15 to 8% as a result of the ban on growth promoters. In the Netherlands, the prevalence of VRE in healthy humans, pigs and hens was reduced by at least a half (Van den Bogaard et al. 2000).

On 1 January 2006, a Europe-wide ban was imposed on the use of antibiotics—or rather, antimicrobial drugs—as growth promoters. This led to a sharp decline in the use of antibiotics as growth promoters. However, it was accompanied by an equally pronounced increase in the therapeutic use of antibiotics. The animals were now given massive doses of antibiotics as a preventative measure.

---

[8]The government and parliament's independent advisory body on questions of public health.

[9]Enterococcus is the name given to a group of bacteria of several types (species), e.g. *Enterococcus faecalis* or *Enterococcus faecium*. *Enterococcus* spp. is the designation given to the whole group, without specifying which species is intended. The double 'p' indicates the plural. *Enterococcus* sp. with one 'p', means that a single *Enterococcus* is being referred to, but it is not clear which type.

## Human and Financial Costs

As already mentioned, enterococci are not particularly pathogenic bacteria, but VREs can survive on a hospital windowsill for a few years. 'They can't be killed off', says Bonten. 'Wherever you look in a patient's surroundings, they're there. On the toilet seat, the TV remote control, the tables—everywhere. My American mentor calls it a "faecal veneer": a graphene-thin[10] layer covering everything you touch. It's therefore very difficult to bring a VRE outbreak under control—much more difficult than an outbreak of MRSA or OXA-48'.

The practical consequences of a VRE outbreak reveal a second paradox. As already mentioned, the VRE outbreak that plagued the UMC Groningen in 2010 and 2011 resulted in the colonisation of 139 patients, of whom 2 developed severe sepsis. 'We spent 140,000 euros on additional diagnostic tests', recalls Alex Friedrich, Head of Microbiology and Hospital Hygiene. 'Our disinfection processes were adapted. We had to pay extra costs for the cleaning service, since it took two hours longer to disinfect a room. That costs us 30,000 euros a year. When we suspect infection with *Enterococcus faecium* we prefer to use teicoplanin as an antibiotic, rather than vancomycin. But to do this, the clinical microbiologist must always give the patient personal advice. Vancomycin costs six euros per patient per day. Teicoplanin costs 70 euros. We had several bans on admissions, we had to keep beds empty and postpone operations. All this resulted in a loss of income, which cost us an estimated 440,000 euros. We estimate the total costs of the outbreak to amount to around 700,000 euros'. The regulations for infection prevention prescribe isolating the patient and carrying out a contact investigation. In contact investigations, all the patients staying in the same room as a patient diagnosed as having multiresistant bacteria, and all patients who have stayed in that room since the first sample that tested positive was taken, must be investigated for the presence of the same bacterium. In some cases, the contact investigation may be extended to include even more patients. The guidelines of the working group for infection prevention (WIP), 'Measures against the transmission of highly resistant microorganisms (BRMO)' demand that a patient with VRE must always be isolated in a single room. Besides the isolation of the infected patients and the contact investigation, additional hygienic measures and, sometimes, the disinfection of entire wards are required (WIP 2011, 2018). 'And then the question always presents itself', says Bonten. 'Can we keep this up, can we afford the costs and—above all—are they worth it for the results?' Or as Christina Vandenbroucke-Grauls asked during the Symposium 'VRE Wat moet je ermee?' ('VRE: what must we do about it?) in Nijmegen at the beginning of October 2012: 'Is VRE sufficiently pathogenic to justify this expenditure? Do the costs and benefits of the measures still balance one another out?'

---

[10]Graphene consists of a single layer of carbon atoms.

## Immovable Protocols

'The Dutch guidelines for handling infectious diseases are famous all over the world, because they're so good', says Marc Bonten. 'But we pay too little attention to the costs. And by that I mean both the financial and the human costs. I know that Dutch hospitals have turned away patients whose admission was absolutely essential from a medical point of view because of the guidelines on prevention and control of infections. I've also seen this for myself. It even happened twice during our big VRE outbreak in 2000. We had a patient with VRE in the gastroenterology/nephrology department.[11] She wasn't getting any better, and in fact she ought to have been transferred to a nursing home. The first care home we contacted declined to admit her, and warned all the other nursing homes in the region. The nursing home said that their staff had too little experience in dealing with infections, and were afraid the pathogen might spread. This woman lay in a room on her own for months on end. She became psychotic, and died'.

Bonten then had to deal with the same problem all over again. This time it involved a patient needing neurosurgery, who was sent to the UMC Utrecht for the operation as an emergency patient. In Utrecht, the man became infected with VRE. He too could not be sent back to the general hospital in his home region again, near his family, even when his illness permitted it and it would have been desirable. Their arguments were similar to those of the nursing home I just mentioned: the fear of bringing a new problem into the hospital, a lack of hygiene specialists, as well as the fear that his stay could turn out to be a long one. The result was that this patient had to be treated in Utrecht, more than 100 km from his home town, for several months. On top of this, the patient was occupying a bed in a university clinic unnecessarily. This impeded the flow of patients and represented an additional risk of infection by a resistant bacterium for the highly susceptible patients. In addition, several tedious preventative hygienic measures became necessary in the university clinic as a result. On several occasions, Bonten also had to deal with the precise opposite of this, when patients were not admitted into his own hospital because of multiresistant bacteria. This came about as a result of the almost immovable protocols of the MRSA guidelines. A woman was admitted to a hospital in Bruges after a brain haemorrhage. The haemorrhage had been caused by an aneurysm—a bulge in one of the brain's arteries. This can be treated by interrupting the blood supply of the aneurysm with a clip. 'The woman, who came from Utrecht, had to be transferred to Utrecht for the operation', says March Bonten. 'At that time we were one of the few clinics who could carry out this intervention'. The case occurred in 2005, just after Bonten had become Head of the Department for Hygiene and Infection Prevention at UMC Utrecht. Although her situation was life-threatening, at first UMC Utrecht declined to accept the patient. 'According to protocol, she had to be admitted to a single room in the intensive care unit. She could be infected with

---

[11]Gastroenterology is concerned with diseases of the gastrointestinal tract; nephrology is concerned with kidney diseases.

MRSA. But there were no single rooms available. So they absolutely refused to accept her'. The neurosurgeon who was supposed to operate on the woman wouldn't accept this, and called Bonten. He gave permission for the woman to be admitted, and placed her on her own in a multi-bed room. 'Otherwise, everyone would have obediently followed the protocol, but the patient would be dead'. This is a good example of the conflict between the patient's individual interests and the importance of public safety, of which Jan Kluijtmans spoke.

## Infection Prevention Under Discussion

In an article dramatically entitled 'The lepers of the new century' Mascini and colleagues wrote already in 2001 about the conflict between the impact on the individual patient and the collective interests of public health (Mascini et al. 2001). 'The upshot of all this is that the debate about the priority of infection prevention quickly flares up in hospitals, and that doctors and care staff become heated when patient care is at risk'. The authors emphasise that the Dutch Health Care Inspectorate supports their point of view. 'The inspectorate holds the view that the contagiousness of a bacterium should never be a reason for an institution to refuse a patient. Unfortunately the inspectorate's authority does not extend beyond exercising an advisory function, and they cannot demand any admissions.'

From November 2013 until December 2018 Professor Jan Kluijtmans has been Director of the Dutch Society for Medical Microbiology (NVMM). 'Our guidelines do not stipulate how far we have to go when screening patient contacts. The guidelines define our thought patterns. A hospital must decide for itself how many patients to recall for the appropriate examinations. It is important to assess the risks correctly. Oncology patients are usually at greater risk than ENT patients.[12] You could also see it this way. The Klebsiella outbreak at the Maasstad Hospital and, above all, the public discussion of their inadequate response to it has triggered a reflex response, so that the reaction to any outbreak is now the maximum possible. And normally it's also true that a problem can be solved more quickly if you immediately react to it with maximum force. A weaker or slower reaction has often caused many problems. But I sometimes wonder whether a little too much energy isn't being expended on certain VRE outbreaks, since for the vast majority of patients the bacteria aren't all that dangerous. On the other hand, the Isala Clinics in Zwolle reacted to their maximum extent in summer 2011, and as a result they are now free from VRE'.[13]

Up to now, the same way of proceeding has also prevailed in Germany. The consensus recommendation published in Baden-Württemberg in 2006 (Von Baum et al. 2006), recommending the maximum level of reaction to VRE, is still in force.

---

[12]ENT, ear, nose and throat.

[13]At the end of September 2012, VRE was once again diagnosed in some patients in the Isala Clinics. The conversation with Kluijtmans had already taken place by this time.

But Bonten's views are supported by a more recent study published in the *Deutsches Ärzteblatt* (Mutters et al. 2013). 'The transfer of vancomycin-resistant enterococci (VRE, in particular *E. faecium*)', say the authors, 'mainly causes a large number of colonisations in hospitals, but only sporadic infections'. To optimise protection from infection for patients at risk, a detailed, valid risk assessment is needed. The foremost concern must be to effectively reduce VRE-related morbidity and lethality rates in patients at risk, but also to inhibit unnecessary infection prevention measures for patients not at risk. [...] In specific clinical situations it is therefore necessary to comply rigidly with tighter hygienic measures (contact isolation) in order to optimally protect "at risk" patients from infection'. Alex Friedrich takes a similar view. 'What I say is, "search and relax". We must keep our monitoring of VRE in place, because without it we won't find any other virulent pathogens. But then we must decide what to do on a case-by-case basis. It's a good idea to practise in a situation involving fewer risks so that then, in a crisis, we're well equipped to combat it successfully. In the end, it's much more often about how the bacteria spread than about the pathogens themselves'.

Dr. Guido Werner is Head of the Unit for Nosocomial Pathogens and Antibiotic Resistances at the Robert Koch Institute in Wernigerode, and an expert on VRE. 'In everyday hospital life today, it's becoming increasingly difficult to implement the strict guidelines established 10 years ago to the highest standard. At least, this is what the hygienists responsible tell us. Nevertheless there is general agreement that the standard hygienic measures, if consistently implemented, would actually result in major successes. In many cases however, particularly with pathogens like VRE, basic hygienic measures are decisive factors for preventing them from spreading in clinics. Everyone's thoroughly familiar with these measures, but in practice they're often hard to implement. We can definitely identify differences between individual European countries here, for example regarding the staffing ratio, the time available for each patient, or the spatial layout of the hospitals.' Werner's colleague Professor Markus Dettenkofer—Head of the Hospital Hygiene Section at the University Medical Centre Freiburg until the end of 2014—is intensively involved with VRE and since 2015 has been the Head of the Institute for Hospital Hygiene and Infection Prevention of the Constance Region Healthcare Network. 'For me, this as an extremely exciting topic that gives me a few headaches. At the Basel University Hospital, for example—only 50 kilometres south of Freiburg—there have so far been almost no cases of VRE. At Freiburg, a major healthcare centre with a large haematological department, such cases have been increasingly identified for the past 3 or 4 years.[14] At present, however, we're seeing a slight decline in the figures. And then there are certainly smaller clinics in Germany, but also larger ones such as Aachen, where there have been hardly any VRE cases to date. However, they also don't look for them and aren't carrying out any VRE screening. VREs are problematic, because they are remarkably stable, proliferate very easily, and can easily be passed on. I'm sceptical whether we can succeed in ridding Central Europe of these

---

[14]This conversation with professor Dettenkofer took place late 2014.

pathogens again. There are however examples, such as Switzerland, where they are attempting to do this strictly and consistently by means of very intensive checks, screenings in risk areas and, naturally, isolation. When you first encounter a major VRE problem, it's naturally very hard to invest enough and be strict enough to lower the number of cases again. For Germany this would certainly be very, very expensive, and it's not realistic to isolate so many patients. In German clinics, there aren't enough specialised staff or single rooms to do this. I've already spoken to the Robert Koch Institute several times, because in Germany there still aren't any national guidelines on this at present (Klare et al. 2012). In France there's been a national guideline for years, and it works relatively well. The French have succeeded in creating a significantly lower nationwide VRE rate than Germany. So obviously, with investment and consistency you can achieve something'.

---

## VRSA

Enterococci are able to pass on the genetic information that makes them resistant to vancomycin to other bacteria species. If this should happen with MRSA bacteria, we have a major problem. Vancomycin is the preferred medicine for treating MRSA. If the VRE bacteria pass on the genetic information that makes them resistant to vancomycin to MRSA, it produces the 'superbug' VRSA. This can cause infections that are very difficult to treat with the two remaining antibiotics.[15] Reports of reduced susceptibility of MRSA to vancomycin are still rare. A report of a vancomycin-resistant *Staphylococcus aureus* (VRSA) surfaced for the first time in 1997, in Japan (Hiramatsu et al. 1997). Reports from India (Bhateja et al. 2005), South Korea (Song et al. 2004) and Thailand (Trakulsomboom et al. 2001) followed. Since 2002, a dozen patients with VRSA have been identified in the USA (Sievert et al. 2002; Kest and Kaushik 2019). VRSA cases have also been identified in several other countries such as France, Italy and Brazil. (Hiramatsu 2001).

In the EARSS[16] annual report for 2008, two cases of VRSA were reported in the European Union (both in Austria), and 11 cases of MRSA that were less susceptible to vancomycin. Of those 11, eight came from Austria, two from Hungary and one from the United Kingdom (EARSS 2009). On 20 July 2013, *The Lancet* published a description of one of the first VRSA infections in Europe, involving a Portuguese patient (Melo-Christino et al. 2013). The authors of this article were clearly very concerned about this VRSA case, since Portugal is one of the top-ranking countries in terms of MRSA and VRE percentages.[17]

---

[15]Linezolid and the new drug telavancin.

[16]European Antimicrobial Resistance Surveillance System.

[17]According to the annual ECDC figures, in 2013, 46.8% of all invasive *S. aureus* isolates in Portugal were MRSA. By 2019 it had decreased to 34.8%. In 2013, 23.3% of invasive isolates of *Enterococcus faecium* in Portugal were resistant to vancomycin. After a remarkable reduction in 2019 the number of invasive *E. faecium* isolates resistant to vancomycin in Portugal had decreased to 9% (ECDC Surveillance Atlas – Antimicrobial resistance 2020b).

Jan Kluijtmans thinks that the danger of VRSA is not yet so great. 'If VRE were able to transfer its genetic information to MRSA bacteria so easily, then in my opinion this would certainly have happened already. In particular, there would have to be many thousands of patients infected with VRE and MRSA in the US; but up to now there have only been a few reports of VRSA.' Alex Friedrich shares this view. 'There are some obvious hurdles standing in the way of stable exchange of genetic information between VRE and MRSA. With enterococci, even now we can often no longer prescribe vancomycin; and if soon this won't be effective against *Staphylococci* either, then there are only a few medicines left. And then comprehensive chemotherapy or organ transplants will be very risky'.[18] Despite the comforting words of Kluijtmans and Friedrich, in June 2013 the WHO published an epidemiological warning against VRSA (PAHO/WHO 2013). But in a review of global cases published in 2020, the authors establish a total of 52 isolated VRSA strains worldwide up till then (Cong et al. 2020).

## Registration Service for Nosocomial Infections and Antibiotic Resistance

After the outbreaks at VUmc in Amsterdam and UMC, nothing more was heard about VRE in the Netherlands for several years. All this changed in spring 2010. It was then that the first case of VRE in a patient at the University Medical Centre Groningen surfaced, leaving the clinic to battle against the bacterium well into spring 2011. After this, the Martini Hospital in Groningen and Isala Clinics in Zwolle were next in line. At the time, the UMC Groningen had informed the Martini Hospital— 'but more on an informal basis, by telephone and apparently not thoroughly enough', says Alex Friedrich, who came to the UMCG while the outbreak was in progress. Since 2012, regular and intensive meetings have been taking place between clinical microbiologists and hygiene specialists in the region. 'Prior to that, we set up the "Regional microbiological and infectiological symposium (REMIS)" in autumn 2011, which allows us to discuss these problems as quickly as possible (REMIS 2018). These enable communication regarding outbreaks to occur on a regular basis.' Clinical microbiologists, infectious disease specialists, German public health service doctors and hygiene specialists from the provinces of Groningen, Friesland, Drenthe and Overijssel take part in REMIS. In a way, REMIS became the model used to build the regional referral networks of interconnected hospitals and healthcare institutions.

In order to better understand what is happening in the area of multiresistance and how outbreaks are connected with one another or not, in 2012 a registration service for nosocomial infections and antibiotic resistance was set up in the Netherlands by the RIVM and the Dutch Society for Medical Microbiology (NVMM). Hospitals are

---

[18]The University Medical Centre Groningen is the largest transplant centre in the Netherlands, and the only centre where transplants of all organs are carried out.

supposed to report outbreaks of multiresistant bacteria to this service. The registration service must also enable hospitals to react adequately when they admitted a patient from a hospital that was dealing with a multiresistance problem. Setting up the registration service, which until July 2019 operated on a voluntary basis, is one of the recommendations that the Lemstra Commission made in its report *Oog voor het onzichtbare* ('An eye for the invisible') on the management of the Klebsiella outbreak at the Maasstad Hospital (Lemstra 2012). Such a registration service is all the more important because the probability of outbreaks involving multiresistant bacteria is more likely to increase than decrease in future. But there is a further important reason, and it is to be found in the changes in the organisational structure of the healthcare system. In their efforts to improve the quality of provision, hospitals are becoming more and more specialised. This results in ever more frequent contacts between hospitals via patients. And this, in turn, increases the risk of spreading multiresistant bacteria and infectious diseases. The same applies, of course, to the spread of viruses and fungal infections. As per July 1, 2019 the recommendation of the Lemstra Commission has resulted in the obligation to report outbreaks of Carbapenemase Producing Enterobacteriaceae (CPE).

## Warning System

Concentration of healthcare provision ought to go hand in hand with a tightening up of infection prevention and control. In the Netherlands, there is already a network to which laboratories can send positive cultures of multiresistant bacteria. Additionally, there is now the partly mandatory registration service for outbreaks of multiresistant bacteria and the obligation to report CPE-outbreaks. 'We're all lying in the same hospital bed', is how Gijs Ruijs describes the close connections between all the hospitals in the Netherlands. 'There are many transfers of patients from one site to another. And they're always taking their intestinal flora with them, including their multiresistant bacteria, which we're coming up against over and over again'. Ruijs is the former President of the NVMM and was until 2020 clinical microbiologist at the Isala Clinics in Zwolle. 'It is important for hospitals to recognise that any problem they have with multiresistant bacteria is also the problem of other hospitals, nursing homes and even people at home', says Roel Coutinho, who until August 2013 was the Director of the Centre for Infectious Disease Control at the RIVM. 'This means that they must be much more transparent in their handling of them'. And often there are still problems with this, says Edwin Boel, who was replaced by Jan Kluijtmans as President of the NVMM at the end of November 2013. 'Sometimes hospitals want to conceal an outbreak because they think it's bad publicity for them'.

It is precisely because of this that, in addition to the registration service for outbreaks of multiresistant bacteria, a second initiative was launched. As Coutinho says: 'The most important lesson that we have learned from the Klebsiella outbreak at the Maasstad Hospital is that, for far too long, one person alone was able to determine how to react to an outbreak. That is completely wrong. That's why we've introduced a warning system. There was also resistance to this, on the lines of "that means we're being controlled, then". Of course people don't like that. What we want is openness: we want them to develop a willingness to say what's going on and talk to one another. In my opinion, something's really going wrong in this area. And not only where clinical microbiologists are concerned. It's all connected with the idea that a medical specialist is some kind of god. This has to stop, but that would entail a very fundamental change. With our warning system, we're trying to achieve a kind of breakthrough in this area. And we have a strong argument for it—because what happens in one hospital has consequences for others. More and more contacts between hospitals are taking place, because the hospitals are becoming increasingly specialised in order to improve the quality of their treatment. Previously', says Coutinho, 'healthcare-associated infections were a problem of the hospital where they occurred. Now they've become a problem for all hospitals—and the more dealings they have with one another, the bigger the problem becomes. This means that hospitals must also inform one another reciprocally. And that's just what until 2020 they didn't do—or at least, not enough. This kind of openness is not taken for granted in hospitals, and the way the market functions it isn't going to get any better either. At present, many hospitals see themselves as competitors. But on the other hand, they recognise that their reputation is seriously damaged if they don't behave properly. That's the other side of the coin. So the Maasstad disaster has actually led to hospitals realising they need to be more open. But that's not easy'.

## Reporting: Mandatory or Not?

Coutinho is no supporter of mandatory reporting of outbreaks. Vandenbroucke-Grauls shares this opinion. 'Since 1987, reporting MRSA infections has always been voluntary.[19] In this way we've become the best in the world', she says. The Lemstra Commission, which investigated the Klebsiella outbreak at the Maasstad Hospital, has spoken out in favour of mandatory reporting (Lemstra 2012). The commission's view is supported by the European Centre for Disease Prevention and Control. In a report on carbapenem resistance from November 2011, the ECDC endorsed this kind of obligation to report (ECDC 2011). And from July 2019 CPE-outbreaks in the Netherlands must be mandatory reported. 'Only a small portion of our information comes from diseases subject to mandatory reporting', says Coutinho. 'A considerably larger proportion comes from various information systems in which people participate voluntarily'. Inge Gyssens concurs with Coutinho. 'Acting voluntarily is part of Dutch medical culture. Powerful professional groups act on their own initiative with the support of the government, but without compulsion'.

---

[19]Nonetheless, since the introduction of the Dutch Public Health Act on 1 December 2008, which replaced the infection legislation (among other things), an obligation to report MRSA infections has indeed existed.

And yet it sounds strange. An obligation to report meets with resistance, whereas a voluntary reporting system is supposed to work. 'You report the things you have to, but there's a high probability that extraordinary things which occur will no longer be reported, because there is no obligation to report them', says Christina Vandenbroucke-Grauls. 'Does every case of resistance have to be reported, then, or not? And if not, which resistance mechanisms must be reported? Why resistance to carbapenems, but not others? All that can become very complicated. For me it's a question of getting an overview of the problem. At the moment, we're only inadequately achieving this. Thanks to ISIS-AR and NethMap,[20] we have very good information about the use of antibiotics in the Netherlands and their resistance, though we don't know how many outbreaks there are' (SWAB 2020).

According to the most recent data, from summer 2017, more than 40 laboratories participated in the ISIS-AR network—more than half of all 60 laboratories for clinical microbiology and, according to the RIVM, almost three-quarters of all hospital laboratories for clinical microbiology.

'The hospitals who still aren't participating are more or less operating under the radar', says James Cohen Stuart. 'We have no idea what is going on in these hospitals. ISIS-AR is a wonderful system in which somebody from outside is watching to see if patterns of resistance in a hospital are changing in a strange way. If the Maasstad Hospital in 2010 and 2011 had taken part in ISIS-AR, then we would have found out about the Klebsiella outbreak there very much sooner. Months sooner. And we would also have noticed that they had an ESBL problem much earlier as well'.

But whether healthcare institutions are going to report their outbreaks—voluntarily or mandatory depending on the kind of outbreak—remains to be seen. So, for the time being, it is uncertain what the usefulness of a register of outbreaks will be in the daily practice of infection prevention.

## References

Bhateja, P., Mathur, T., Pandya, M., et al. (2005). Detection of vancomycin resistant *Staphylococcus aureus*: A comparative study of three different phenotypic screening methods. *Indian Journal of Medical Microbiology, 23*(1), 52–55. Accessed from http://www.bioline.org.br/pdf?mb05012.

Bonten, M. J. M., Friedrich, A., Kluytmans, J. A. J. W., et al. (2014). Infectiepreventie in Nederlandse ziekenhuizen. *Nederlands Tijdschrift voor Geneeskunde (NTVG), 158,* A7395. Accessed from https://bit.ly/38oFt2K English abstract https://bit.ly/35ibrf2

Ciccolini, M., Donker, T., & Köck, R. (2013). Infection prevention in a connected world: The case for a regional approach. *International Journal of Microbiology, 303*(6-7), 380–387. https://doi.org/10.1016/j.ijmm.2013.02.003.

---

[20]A report appears annually (NethMap) presenting data on the current use of antibiotics and the development of resistance in the Netherlands. In 2012, for the first time, this appeared simultaneously with the MARAN Report covering the veterinary sector. The Stichting Werkgroep Antibioticabeleid (SWAB) publishes the report annually in English.

Cong, Y., Yang, S., & Rao, X. (2020). Vancomycin resistant *Staphylococcus aureus* infections: A review of case updating and clinical features. *Journal of Advanced Research, 21*, 169–176. https://doi.org/10.1016/j.jare.2019.10.005.

De Greef, S. C., Schoffelen, A. F., & Verduin, C. M. (2020). *NethMap 2020: Consumption of antimicrobial agents and antimicrobial resistance among medically important bacteria in the Netherlands in 2019/MARAN 2020: Monitoring of antimicrobial resistance and antibiotic usage in animals in the Netherlands in 2019.* https://doi.org/10.21945/RIVM-2020-0065

De Vrieze, J. (2018). Antibioticaresistentie in Nederland. Alles uit de kast? *Nederlands Tijdschrift voor Geneeskunde (NTvG), 162*, C3994. Accessed from https://www.ntvg.nl/artikelen/antibioticaresistentie-nederland

Donker, T. (2014). *Disease transmission through hospital networks.* Thesis. Accessed November 12, 2020, from https://bit.ly/2Uniygq

Donker, T., Wallinga, J., & Grundmann, H. (2010). Patient referral patterns and the spread of hospital-acquired infections through National Health Care networks. *PLoS Computational Biology.* https://doi.org/10.1371/journal.pcbi.1000715.

Donker, T., Wallinga, J., Slack, R., et al. (2012). Hospital networks and the dispersal of hospital-acquired pathogens by patient transfer. *PLoS One.* https://doi.org/10.1371/journal.pone.0035002.

EARSS. (2009). EARSS Annual Report 2008. *On-going surveillance of S. Pneumoniae, S. aureus, E. coli, E. faecium, E. faecalis, K. pneumoniae, P. aeruginosa.* Accessed November 16, 2020, from https://bit.ly/2UtY6u3

ECDC (European Centre for Disease Prevention and Control). (2011). *Updated ECDC risk assessment on the spread of New Delhi metallo-β-lactamase and its variants within Europe.* https://doi.org/10.2900/14890. Accessed from https://bit.ly/39enL17

ECDC (European Centre for Disease Prevention and Control). (2020a). *Additional tables EU/EEA population weighted mean 2019.* Accessed January 7, 2021, from https://bit.ly/35jUHEa

ECDC (European Centre for Disease Prevention and Control). (2020b). *Surveillance Atlas – Antimicrobial resistance; permanently updated.* Accessed November 16, 2020, from https://bit.ly/38ozxq8

Endtz, H. P., Van den Braak, N., & Van Belkum, A. (1997). Fecal carriage of vancomycin-resistant enterococci in hospitalized patients and those living in the community in The Netherlands. *Journal of Clinical Microbiology, 35*(12), 3026–3031. Accessed from https://bit.ly/398xt54.

Gezondheidsraad. (1998). *Health Council of the Netherlands: Committee on Antimicrobial growth promotors. Antimicrobial growth promotors.* In Dutch with English summary. Accessed November 14, 2020, from https://bit.ly/3ktZjwc

Hiramatsu, K. (2001). Vancomycin-resistant *Staphylococcus aureus*: A new model of antibiotic resistance. *The Lancet Infectious Diseases, 1*(3), 147–155. https://doi.org/10.1016/S1473-3099(01)00091-3.

Hiramatsu, K., Aritaka, N., Hanaki, H., et al. (1997). Dissemination in Japanese hospitals of strains of *Staphylococcus aureus* heterogeneously resistant to vancomycin. *The Lancet, 350*(9092), 1670–1673. https://doi.org/10.1016/S0140-6736(97)07324-8.

Kest, H., & Kaushik, A. (2019). Vancomycin-resistant *Staphylococcus aureus*: Formidable threat or silence before the storm? *Journal of Infectious Diseases and Epidemiology, 5*(5). https://doi.org/10.23937/2474-3658/1510093.

Klare, I., Witte, W., Wendt, C., et al. (2012). Vancomycin-resistente Enterokokken (VRE). *Bundesgesundheitsblatt, 55*(11/12), 1387–1400. https://doi.org/10.1007/s00103-012-1564-6.

Leavis, H. L., Willems, R. J., & Mascini, E. M. (2004). Vancomycin resistant enterococci in the Netherlands (Abstract). *Nederlands Tijdschrift voor Geneeskunde (NTvG), 148*(18), 878–882. Accessed from https://bit.ly/35lcKtH.

Lemstra, W. (2012). *Oog voor het onzichtbare (An eye for the invisible).* Accessed November 16, 2020, in Dutch https://bit.ly/3hQF9g8 or in German https://bit.ly/3pYYIG4

Mascini, E. M., Bonten, M. J. M., Troelstra, A. et al. (2001). *De melaatsen van de nieuwe eeuw*. Medisch Contact. Accessed March 31, 2021, from https://www.medischcontact.nl/nieuws/ laatste-nieuws/artikel/de-melaatsen-van-de-nieuwe-eeuw.htm

Melo-Christino, J., Resina, C., Manuel, V., et al. (2013). First case of infection with vancomycin-resistant *Staphylococcus aureus* in Europe. *The Lancet, 382*(9888), 205. https://doi.org/10. 1016/S0140-6736(13)61219-2.

Mutters, N. T., Mersch-Sundermann, V., Mutters, R., et al. (2013). *Kontrolle von Vancomycin-resistenten Enterokokken im Krankenhaus. Epidemiologischer Hintergrund und klinische Relevanz*. In German. https://bit.ly/35BUxsp English abstract: *Control of the spread of vancomycin-resistant enterococci in hospitals—Epidemiology and clinical relevance*. Accessed from https://bit.ly/2LrnoYP

NOS. (2012). *Video*. Accessed November 12, 2020, from https://bit.ly/3i2YvyV

NVMM. (2015). *Nederlandse Vereniging voor Medische Microbiologie - Dutch Society for Medical Microbiology*. In Dutch. Accessed November 12, 2020, from https://bit.ly/3bfjPj1

PAHO/WHO. (2013). *Pan American Health Organization/World Health Organization Epidemiological Alert: Vancomycin-resistant Staphylococcus aureus*. Accessed November 16, 2020, from https://bit.ly/38odVdE

REMIS. (2018). *Regionaal Microbiologisch-Infectiologisch Symposium (Regional microbiological and infectiological symposium)*. In Dutch. Accessed November 16, 2020, from https://www. remis-plus.net/over-remis/

Sagel, U., Schulte, B., & Heeg, P. (2008). Vancomycin-resistant enterococci outbreak, Germany, and calculation of outbreak start. *Emerging Infectious Diseases, 14*(2), 317–319. https://doi.org/ 10.3201/eid1402.070752.

SCAN. (1996). *Report of the Scientific Committee for Animal Nutrition (SCAN) on the possible risk for humans of the use of avoparcin as feed additive*. Opinion expressed 21 May 1996. Accessed November 14, 2020, from https://bit.ly/2LdVXBI

Schippers, E. I. (2016). *Kamerbrief over voortgang aanpak antibioticaresistentie*. In Dutch. Accessed November 12, 2020, from https://bit.ly/35mtPDY

Schulte, B., Heininger, A., & Authenrieth, I. B. (2008). Emergence of increasing linezolid-resistance in enterococci in a post-outbreak situation with vancomycin-resistant *Enterococcus faecium*. *Epidemiology and Infection, 136*(8), 1131–1133. https://doi.org/10.1017/ S0950268807009508.

Sievert, D. M., Boulton, M. L., & Stoltman, G. (2002). *Staphylococcus aureus resistant to Vancomycin – United States, 2002*. Morbidity and Mortality Weekly Report (MMWR) of the Centers for Disease Control and Prevention (CDC), 51(26), 565–567. Accessed from https://bit. ly/2L2sg6V

Söderblom, T., Aspevall, O., & Erntell, M. (2010). Alarming spread of vancomycin resistant enterococci in Sweden since 2007. *Eurosurveillance, 15*(29). https://doi.org/10.2807/ese.15. 29.19620-en.

Song, J. H., Hiramatsu, K., Suh, J. Y., et al. (2004). Emergence in Asian countries of *Staphylococcus aureus* with reduced susceptibility to vancomycin. *Antimicrobial Agents and Chemotherapy, 48*(12), 4926–4928. https://doi.org/10.1128/AAC.48.12.4926-4928.2004. Accessed from https://aac.asm.org/content/48/12/4926.

SWAB – Stichting Werkgroep Antibioticabeleid. (2020). *Nethmap/Maran annual reports*. Accessed November 16, 2020, from https://swab.nl/nl/nethmap

Trakulsomboom, S., Danchaivaijitr, S., Rongrungruang, Y., et al. (2001). First report of methicillin-resistant *Staphylococcus aureus* with reduced susceptibility to vancomycin in Thailand. *Journal of Clinical Microbiology, 39*(2), 591–595. https://doi.org/10.1128/JCM.39.2.591-595.2001.

Van den Bogaard, A. E., Bruinsma, N., & Stobberingh, E. E. (2000). The effect of banning avoparcin on VRE carriage in The Netherlands. *Journal of Antimicrobial Chemotherapy, 46* (1), 146–148. https://doi.org/10.1093/jac/46.1.146.

Von Baum, H., Dettenkofer, M., Fahr, A.-M., et al. (2006). Konsensusempfehlung Baden-Württemberg. Umgang mit Patienten mit Glykopeptid-resistenten Enterokokken (GRE)/Vancomycin-resistenten Enterokokken (VRE). *Hygiene & Medizin, 31*(1/2), 30–32. Accessed from https://bit.ly/38M8jui.

WIP – Werkgroep Infectie Preventie Working Party on Infection Prevention. (2011, 2018). *WIP-Richtlijn BRMO (Ziekenhuizen)*. In Dutch. Accessed November 14, 2020, from https://bit.ly/3s52qzN

WIP – Werkgroep Infectie Preventie Working Party on Infection Prevention. (2011, 2018). *WIP-Richtlijn BRMO (VWK)*. In Dutch. Accessed November 14, 2020, from https://bit.ly/2LrqPyH

# The Beginning of the End

## 6

I can still remember the situation very clearly. Along with a colleague, I was in the middle of preparing a news feature on the sale of medicines, particularly antibiotics, by veterinarians. It was Friday afternoon, 5 March 2010. Following a study (Beemer et al. 2010) by the management consultancy Berenschot, the Dutch Agriculture Minister at the time, Verburg, considered that it was unnecessary to distinguish between prescribing veterinary drugs and selling them. Berenschot expressed concerns about uncoupling the two things in this way. It would not lead to the desired results and would entail too much bureaucracy and major problems of implementation. Nevertheless, the minister demanded that veterinary surgeons should prescribe fewer antibiotics. An agreement was therefore made with veterinarians and representatives of the livestock sector. Farmers and veterinarians promised to use 20% fewer antibiotics in 2011 compared to 2009. On this same Friday, we were also busy finishing another feature on this same topic that was supposed to be broadcast the same day. Verburg was weighing up the idea of banning the use of cephalosporins of the third and fourth generation in livestock farming,[1] since they are very important antibiotics for humans. 'The excessive use of these drugs in breeding broiler chickens', the article we published on the NOS-website stated, 'was, among other things, being linked to the increase of ESBL[2] in the poultry sector. A large proportion of poultry are infected with ESBL'. This was the first time the NOS used the term 'ESBL'.

---

[1]Like penicillins, cephalosporins belong to the class of beta-lactam antibiotics. Cephalosporins are bactericidal medicines, i.e. they kill bacteria. They are used to treat pyelonephritis, infections of the respiratory tract and skin infections. Over the course of the years, four generations of cephalosporins have been launched on the market. Cephalosporins are reserve medicines, which are only used in hospitals when the bacteria are resistant to other drugs. They are usually administered via an infusion.

[2]The term 'extended spectrum beta-lactamases' (ESBLs) is used to describe a group of enzymes that make penicillins and cephalosporins ineffective (the antibiotics most frequently used to treat enterobacterial infections).

The next morning the telephone rang. The caller introduced himself as Mr. Koos. 'You have no idea what's going on', he said, in a pretty indignant tone of voice. Then he showered me with a flood of information. It concerned ESBLs, an enormous increase of them in animals and humans, and plasmids,[3] which have made the spread of ESBLs very easy, and about the percentage of Dutch hens—almost 100%—and an increasing number of humans who are carrying multiresistant ESBL bacteria. He spoke about infections for which, in around 15 years, there would no longer be any effective treatment, because the bacteria would be resistant against all antibiotics. There were ministers who were hurriedly getting briefed about this matter. He spoke about sick people and deaths. It was more than enough to make me listen very attentively. It was clear that I had someone on the line who knew what he was talking about. This became all the more clear to me when my caller began to read out some passages from a document unknown to me. 'Enterobacteriaceae are a group of (Gram-negative) bacteria, of which E. coli[4] and Klebsiella spp. are the best-known representatives. These bacteria are the main pathogenic agents of urinary tract infections, and they are also responsible for a considerable percentage of the bacterial infections in hospitals and nursing homes. In recent years, an alarming increase of resistance to several of the available antibiotics has been observed in these bacteria worldwide. It would appear that the rapid increase of resistance to penicillins and cephalosporins can, to a considerable extent, be traced back to the production of extended spectrum beta-lactamases (ESBLs)'. And: 'Particularly alarming is the increasing rate of ESBL-positive isolates in the general practices[5] that are resistant to all available oral antibiotics. Infections caused by ESBL-producing bacteria are also associated with higher morbidity,[6] mortality,[7] length of hospital stay and costs than those caused by bacteria without ESBL. Moreover there is a close connection between ESBL-producing strains and the occurrence of epidemics in healthcare institutions'. The caller also quoted the most incendiary part of the document: 'Although the worldwide intestinal colonisation of poultry by ESBL-positive bacteria and the high percentage of contaminated meat allow one to infer a causal connection between poultry and humans, these findings afford no proof of this'.

---

[3] A plasmid is a circular strand of DNA that is mobile, which therefore enables it to transfer genetic material between bacteria of the same or different species. Besides ESBLs, other resistance genes are often found on these plasmids as well.

[4] Escherichia coli or E. coli, named after the German microbiologist Theodor Escherich, is a Gram-negative bacterium of the enterobacteriaceae family. E. coli exists in several different forms. For example, EHEC is an E. coli. EHEC is described in detail in Chap. 9.

[5] An isolate is a bacteria culture that derives from a single bacterium.

[6] The term 'morbidity' describes the number of clinical cases, in this case caused by a bacterium.

[7] The term 'mortality' describes the death rate, in this case caused by an infection triggered by a bacterium.

## Heavily Protected

Naturally, I wanted to meet Mr. Koos at once, so that I could read for myself the document from which he was quoting. But Mr. Koos was not interested. No meeting, no phone number, and certainly no document. In an attempt to locate this unknown document, I started phoning up microbiologists. These included Paul Gruteke, from the Onze Lieve Vrouwe Gasthuis hospital in Amsterdam. He confirmed the information about the increasing ESBL problem. 'We see it in the urinary tract infections which can't be treated by GPs or nursing homes anymore because the bacteria are resistant to the conventional orally administered antibiotics. These patients then come to us at the clinic'. Like Paul Gruteke, Ellen Stobberingh, medical microbiologist at the University Hospital Maastricht, referred me to Maurine Leverstein-van Hall, who was working for the RIVM at the time. 'I think it was she who wrote this document', she said. Stobberingh made some further remarks. 'An enzyme such as ESBL can't be destroyed by roasting the meat. The genetic material is consumed along with the chicken leg. It can then encounter a bacterium that can host these genes, and there they can reproduce themselves. This is certainly a potential risk'.

## A Breakthrough

And so I went on, talking to one person after another. But nobody I spoke to knew about this document. Suddenly, after 2 days' searching, someone knew what I was talking about. More than this—this person even wanted to let me read the document. What I had come across was a document by Maurine Leverstein-van Hall entitled *Significance of ESBL for public health*. It was a report to the Ministers for Health and Agriculture dated 5 March 2010. Later I learned that Leverstein had been commissioned to write this note for the ministers within a few hours on that same Friday afternoon. Unfortunately, that report is no longer publicly accessible. But a study the same Leverstein published a year later gives a good idea of the content of the note to the Ministers (Leverstein-Van Hall et al. 2011). The subject itself had already given rise to considerable disquiet; our broadcast did the rest. Members of Parliament urged the responsible Ministers to answer a series of questions (Klink 2010). The story actually begins in summer 2009, at the Amphia Hospital in Breda. It was then that Jan Kluijtmans received a visit from 17-year-old Jasper Bastiaansen, a school student who wanted to do an internship in the Department of Medical Microbiology, in order to see whether studies in the medical field might interest him.

'At the back of my head', recalled Kluijtmans, 'for a long time I'd already had the idea of investigating what was causing the big increase in ESBL in our patients someday. In the literature, meat was repeatedly mentioned as a possible source. We decided there and then to carry out a cost-effective and practical study, since we had more or less no financial means at our disposal. All the analysts in the five hospitals[8]

---

[8]The Amphia Hospital in Breda, the Lievensberg Hospital in Bergen op Zoom, the Franciscus Hospital in Roosendaal and the St. Elisabeth and TweeSteden hospitals, both in Tilburg.

of our network were asked to cut off a small piece of raw, unprocessed meat for our study after purchase. My internee Jasper then carried out the tests in the laboratory. To our surprise, almost 90 per cent of the chicken meat was contaminated with ESBL-producing bacteria. And they were very similar to the types that we had also found in human beings. After this we took samples from all the inpatients in our hospitals, in order to investigate whether they were also contaminated with ESBL. And once again we found an unexpectedly high number of ESBLs'. Kluijtmans discussed his findings with some colleagues who were working in the interface between human and animal medicine. These confirmed that the high rate of infection with ESBL in hens was nothing new. 'However, the high percentage of contaminated meat was something new to them. But they assured me that I need not worry about it, because the ESBL genes in chickens and in people were completely different'.

This occurred in January 2010. Not really satisfied, Kluijtmans decided to compare the ESBL genes and properties of the bacteria strains from the meat samples with those from his patients. He did this in collaboration with a group of British scientists. 'I was forced to conclude that there were more similarities than differences between the ESBLs from the meat samples and those from my patients. I then called Roel Coutinho,[9] who immediately shared my concerns. He decided to convene a panel of experts to assess the situation and, if necessary, establish what measures were needed. The report that Maurine Leverstein-van Hall wrote was based on the original message in which I reported my findings'.

## Negligent and Excessive

Leverstein's message hit the nail on the head. In particular, the section marked 'confidential', 'Is poultry a source of ESBL for humans?', which Mr. Koos had cited in our telephone conversation, was dynamite. In a country where profits of billions are made through the production of broiler chickens, this question is guaranteed to lead to hefty debates and plenty of uproar. In the document, the microbiologist listed a series of possible explanations for the rapid increase of ESBL. 'The reckless and excessive use of antibiotics is often cited as the main reason for the rise in resistance towards antibiotics. However it is noticeable that, despite the relatively low level of antibiotic use in human medicine in the Netherlands, the prevalence of ESBL[10] is similar to that of neighbouring countries'. On 13 March 2010, on the basis of Maurine Leverstein-van Hall's document to the ministers, NOS broadcast its first TV report on ESBL. One of the speakers in the broadcast was Roel Coutinho. 'The use of antibiotics in livestock farming must be reduced, whatever happens. This is a

---

[9]Professor Roel Coutinho was at the time director of the Centre for Infectious Disease Control of the RIVM.

[10]The term 'prevalence' refers to a figure used in the study of health and disease (epidemiology), and indicates how many people in a specific group (population) have contracted a particular disease.

serious problem. When we treat human beings we do everything we can to manage the use of antibiotics as carefully as possible, in order to avoid creating resistance for as long as possible. Absolutely the last thing we need is that the problem then gets served up to us via the back door. I'm referring to the use of antibiotics in the veterinary sector. We already had the problem of MRSA in pigs, and now we've got a similar problem in chickens as well. The use of antibiotics for animals must be reduced, since otherwise new problems will repeatedly be created'.

## Chicken as a Source

On 31 March 2010, a panel of experts on ESBL met at the RIVM in Bilthoven. The Director of the Centre for Infectious Disease Control (CIb) at the time, Roel Coutinho, had brought together these specialists in the field of ESBL. The agenda was as clear as it was complicated. As Coutinho said: 'There are signs that bacteria with ESBL are finding their way from chickens into the human organism. How certain is it that this is actually the case? And if it is the case, what must we then do?' On 8 April 2010, Coutinho sent a letter on behalf of the expert panel to the Secretaries General for Agriculture and Health, which both ministers forwarded to the Dutch parliament one day later (Verburg and Klink 2010a, b). 'There are strong indications that the increase in ESBL-producing bacteria in human medicine is not only being caused by the use of antibiotics for patients', he wrote, 'but in part can also be attributed to the creation of resistance in the veterinary sector. It should be pointed out that this problem is not confined to the Netherlands. Abroad, too—both within and outside the EU—there are reports of an increase in ESBL-producing bacteria in humans, animals and meat. There, too, the same strains are identified in humans and in meat products. The meat in Dutch shops partly originates from foreign countries'. Most of the EBSLs identified in humans differ from the types found in chickens. 'However, a considerable proportion of the ESBLs display similarities with those from broiler chickens, and a genetic similarity can be identified between the genes and plasmids of a limited number of isolates and those of isolates from humans and chickens from the Netherlands'. In their conclusions, the experts stress the role of the veterinary sector in the creation of the ESBL problem. 'An important factor for the emergence of resistance in bacteria is the use of antibiotics in humans and livestock. The experts unanimously agree that a more responsible and very restricted use of antibiotics is an important precondition for reducing the frequency with which resistances occur' (Coutinho 2010). The expert panel had some proposals for the ministers.

The first was an urgent recommendation that the veterinary sector should 'quickly and drastically reduce the use of antibiotics'. At the same time, initiatives should be introduced at an international and, in particular, European level to put the topic of ESBL on the agenda and to drastically reduce the use of antibiotics in livestock farming in other countries as well. The third recommendation concerned identifying gaps in knowledge and setting research priorities. The ministers wrote to parliament in the following terms: 'The recommendations of the expert panel give rise to concern, and it goes without saying that we take them very seriously'. Besides the 20% reduction that farmers were required to implement in 2011, farmers also had to ensure that antibiotic use would be reduced to half the level of 2009 by 2013. According to the figures published by the Diergeneesmiddelenautoriteit (veterinary medicine inspectorate), by the end of 2013, the use of antibiotics in cattle farming had been reduced by 57% (SDa 2014). By the end of 2019, the use of antibiotics in livestock had been reduced by almost 70% compared to 2009 (SDa 2020).

## A Classic Dilemma

By this time Wil Goessens, a microbiologist at the Erasmus University Medical Centre in Rotterdam, had already been involved in ESBL research for years. 'The ESBLs of today now also possess CTX-M genes.[11] These are very easily transferred from one bacterium to another, and also to other species of bacteria. In my view, this makes things scary'. Goessens was not exactly optimistic. 'Antibiotic resistance is becoming a real problem in healthcare across the world. Thanks to good policies, here in the Netherlands we've got off lightly so far. But believe me, MRSA is harmless compared to ESBL'. Patients with an ESBL infection can now only be treated with carbapenems. 'It's sometimes a real dilemma for doctors treating patients with severe infections caused by ESBL-positive bacteria', says Christina Vandenbroucke-Grauls, until October 2017 Head of the Department for Medical Microbiology at the VU University Medical Centre in Amsterdam. 'They know that such patients need carbapenems. But they also know only too well that the more you administer these medicines, the more probable it becomes that there will be bacteria which are resistant to it'. This is the classical contradiction between the needs of individual patients and the interests of public healthcare provision.

'In my opinion, the medical world is not equipped to react to this adequately', says Professor Vincent Jarlier, Head of the Department for Medical Microbiology at the Hôpital Universitaire Pitié-Salpêtrière in the south-east of Paris, one of the biggest hospitals in the city. 'We doctors try to cure patients, because that's what we've been trained to do. But we need help to see the bigger picture. Otherwise we will just carry on only doing what delivers short-term results. We must not just concentrate on the individual patient who has been infected by a resistant bacterium, but must also concern ourselves with the whole chain of cross-contamination[12] and selection pressure caused by the use of antibiotics. In hospitals we must continue to do everything humanly possible, but we must also become active beyond those four walls. We must convince politicians that people's state of hygiene at home and in schools must be improved, because at the moment only inadequate hygiene measures are in place, above all in the area of toilet hygiene, in other words

---

[11]The CTX-M gene is one of the genes that encodes bacteria fpr production of ESBLs.

[12]The term 'cross-contamination' is used when more than one patient is infected with an identical bacterium within the same period and at the same location.

everything connected with toilets. In schools the toilets are dirty, the children don't wash their hands, and often there's neither toilet paper nor sanitary towels. I can give you my guarantee that children spread their intestinal flora between one another there, and at home the situation is often no better. My former boss always used to say to me: "You know Jarlier, we all have the intestinal flora of the person cooking for us". There has been progress, which is why today we don't have typhus here anymore. But the resistances to antibiotics we're now seeing—the *E. coli* and Klebsiella with ESBL or carbapenemases—these are the faecal dangers of today. They are what typhus used to be.' Jarlier quotes the French statesman Clemenceau[13]: 'War is too serious a matter to be entrusted to the military'. In his view, this statement also applies to antibiotic resistance. 'Doctors and microbiologists cannot worry about whatever is getting into the sewer system or get involved in questions of general hygiene. They are not appropriately trained for this—at least, not in France. Doctors are not hygiene specialists. They care about their patients, they do everything for them. The most that one can expect of doctors is that they try to convince their patients of the benefits of vaccination, and also become vaccinated themselves. But we can't really expect them to acquire a comprehensive overview of this problem, which affects not only people, but also animals, plants, wastewater purification and nutrition', said Jarlier. 'The guidelines for using antibiotics that we have at present only refer to medicine, which includes a small proportion of veterinary medicine. The question of the environment doesn't feature in them at all. Various colleagues support me, and have said: "Are you actually aware what kinds of things are present in waste water?" There's a whole stack of publications about ESBL in hospital waste water. And about ESBL that's distributed over agricultural areas by the droppings of animals contaminated with it. But that doesn't mean that we don't have to do anything more about it. It's precisely because the situation is the way it is that we must look for solutions. Just as we also have to worry about the emissions of carbon dioxide, regardless of how complex the problem is. This exceeds the capacities of one single doctor. Until now, antibiotic resistance has almost always been a medical problem: an infection that can no longer be brought under control with the medicines prescribed for it. You had to reflect on how to deal with it. But now all that's changed. Here's an example: resistance of pneumococci[14] to beta-lactam antibiotics. We know that this resistance involves a connection between the use of antibiotics and children's contact with one another. This has led some colleagues to question whether we ought perhaps to organise child care differently.

---

[13]George Clemenceau, French doctor, politician, journalist and publicist. He was Prime Minister in the second half of the First World War and Minister of War (1917–1920).

[14]Every year worldwide around half a million children under five die from a pneumococcal infection. Thanks to sponsored vaccination programmes, a considerable reduction of pneumococcal infection deaths has been achieved in recent years (CDC 2018). Each year, about 10,000 people of all ages are admitted to hospital in the Netherlands with a pneumococcal disease of whom 6000 are aged 60 years and older. Of these people 900 die (RIVM 2020). In 2015, the member states of the EU reported more than 21,000 cases of confirmed invasive pneumococcal infections (ECDC 2019). In 2018, that number increased to nearly 25,000 (ECDC 2020c).

Should we not switch to a system with three or four children instead of big kindergartens? Paediatricians are aware of the problem. But it was absolutely impossible to speak with the responsible persons at the health ministry about the problem, because they were only interested in its medical aspects'.

One of the things investigated by the comprehensive European APRES study of the quality of antibiotic prescription in primary care was the disease burden caused by infectious diseases at kindergarten premises in the Netherlands. This study (Van Bijnen 2015) supports the comments about childcare made by Jarlier and his colleagues. Gastroenteritis and flu-like virus infections appear in children attending kindergarten almost twice as often as in children who do not. More than a third of the kindergartens stated that children did not always have to wash their hands before meals. Fifteen per cent could not always guarantee that children washed their hands after going to the toilet, and 17% of kindergartens stated that the kitchen and toilets were not cleaned every day.

## The Hot Topic: ESBL

'There is', says Jarlier, 'no means of preventing doctors in hospitals, or even outside them, from prescribing carbapenem antibiotics for a patient infected by a Gram-negative bacterium with ESBL. They have to treat the patient somehow or other! Doctors always decide in favour of the best treatment for their patients. And that's what they have to do—that is why they became doctors. Therefore, if we do nothing to stop the rise of ESBL, it's like continuing to row a leaky boat without sealing the hole through which water is pouring in. I can understand some doctors' reservations, because we don't just have to deal with the actual patients, who are still few in number, but also with the thousands of carriers of ESBL-positive bacteria and, above all, with the risk factors. Those who say this is impossible are in reality saying: "I give up". That's human—this is a complex problem, but it's like the debt crisis in Europe: we have no other choice. The task before us is to get the problem sufficiently under control for the risks to patients to remain acceptable. I fear that the true extent of the problem isn't yet clear. And I'm not alone in this assessment'.

A second French expert in the field of antibiotic resistance, Jean Carlet,[15] formerly Head of the ICU at the Hôpital Saint-Joseph in Paris' 14th arrondissement, says that many experts, including for example the scientist Patrice Nordmann, who is very highly respected internationally, regard the campaign against ESBL as already lost. 'Many people incline to accord central place to the role of carbapenemases. Journalists have indeed understood that resistance to carbapenems will lead to dramatic developments, since afterwards we really won't have anything anymore'. Above all else, Jarlier repeatedly draws attention to ESBL as the driving mechanism

---

[15]Jean Carlet is president of the World Alliance against Antibiotic Resistance (WAAR), founded in June 2012.

for the development of resistance to carbapenems. He is convinced that a lot more still needs to be done to prevent the further spread of ESBL.

When I spoke to Nordmann himself on the same day in December 2011, he seemed somewhat less rigid in his thinking than Carlet had described him. 'ESBLs are everywhere', he said. 'Many hens and a lot of chicken meat are contaminated with them, in the Netherlands as well. The import of hens from various European countries is one of the ways in which ESBL came to France. We must reduce the use of antibiotics, including their use in livestock farming. But nevertheless it will still be very difficult to control the spread of ESBL, since some of it is imported from other countries. The solutions are very difficult, even if the number of ESBL strains in the northern part of Europe is still manageable. In these countries, we see even fewer bacteria that have already overcome the next hurdle in their resistance towards carbapenems. But they will come, that's certain. We're approaching a situation where perhaps we'll no longer be in a position to treat several patients. The all-important thing is to screen patients as thoroughly as possible, above all patients at risk. Patients who carry highly resistant bacteria must be isolated. Perhaps in this way we can gain sufficient time while we're waiting for a new antibiotic. But there's absolutely no certainty of that', says Nordmann.

Carlet thinks that French hospitals have more or less reached the limits of their capacity to keep multiresistant bacteria under control. 'It would be unrealistic to imagine that a lot more could be done. We can't simply shut hospital departments down. The competition between hospitals is fierce. So if you announce a ban on admissions and have to treat the infected patients in cohorts, it's a disaster. Perhaps this is the reason why there's also a tendency to conceal outbreaks some- times—but not in the case of carbapenemases, as occurred at the Maasstad Hospital'. Carlet tells me that, alongside successful efforts to reduce MRSA cases in France, at the same time cases of *E. coli* and *Klebsiella* spp. with ESBL have increased.[16] 'The two curves have cancelled each other out. ESBLs are now public enemy number one. We occasionally have problems with carbapenemases as well, but they're still very limited'.[17]

---

[16]In 2002, less than 1% of all invasive *E. coli* and *Klebsiella pneumoniae* isolates in France produced ESBL. In 2010, the figures were 7.2% for *E. coli* and 17.8% for *K. pneumoniae,* and in 2015 they increased further, reaching 11% for *E. coli* and 30.5% for *K. pneumoniae*. In 2018, 30.8% of all invasive isolates of *K. pneumoniae* produced an ESBL and were resistant to third-generation cephalosporins. For *E. coli*, this figure was 9.6% (Pontiès et al. 2018, updated in 2019).

[17]From 2004 to 2009, there were between one and three episodes of enterobacteriaceae such as *E. coli* and *Klebsiella spp.* with carbapenemases in France every year. During each episode a number of linked cases of colonised or infected people occurred. From 2009 onwards the number of yearly episodes of CPE (Carbapenemase-Producing Enterobacteriaceae) were 10 episodes in 2009, 28 in 2010, 113 in 2011, 233 in 2012, 405 in 2013, 650 in 2014, 938 in 2015 and 1223 episodes in 2016. The cumulative number of cases in all episodes since 2004 was 5514. Almost half of all the episodes were imported from foreign countries, mostly from Northern Africa, by an index patient who was hospitalised there and then repatriated to a French hospital. Since 2009, the proportion of established import cases (an existing link to a foreign country is not always

It was not just in the Netherlands that 2010 was the year of ESBL. At the European Congress for Clinical Microbiology and Infectious Diseases in the same year, it was also the hottest topic. For four whole days, from 10 to 13 April, the item on the agenda at the Austria Center in Vienna was very often ESBL. A number of speakers related how ESBL was constantly multiplying across the continents and causing ever more problems.

The biggest outbreak of ESBL in the Netherlands affected the Zuiderziekenhuis site at the Maasstad Hospital in Rotterdam. It was there that, in 2009, *Klebsiella pneumoniae* with ESBL was diagnosed in four patients in the intensive care unit. Thirty-two patients were infected in 2010, and 39 in 2011. At some time in 2009 or 2010, the carbapenemase enzyme OXA-48 was also identified in certain Klebsiellas. This marked the beginning of the major outbreak of OXA-48-producing *Klebsiella pneumoniae,* whose inadequate management made the Maasstad Hospital in Rotterdam famous far beyond the borders of Holland.[18]

## Rotterdam on the Weser, Bremen on the Maas

At the beginning of November 2011, it became known that an outbreak of ESBL-producing *Klebsiella pneumoniae* had been going on for some time in the neonatal ward of the Bremen-Mitte Clinic. The story of the outbreak in Bremen bears similarities to the outbreak at the Maasstad Hospital in Rotterdam. At Bremen, too, the problem was hushed up for months, and the health authorities were informed too late. It was only after regional broadcaster Radio Bremen and the *Weser Kurier* newspaper reported that several babies at the Bremen-Mitte clinic had died that the hospital publicly disclosed the outbreak. 'The same story seems to have unfolded in Bremen as in Rotterdam', says Alex Friedrich, Head of the Department for Microbiology and Hospital Hygiene at UMC Groningen. 'The pattern is comparable to the events in Rotterdam: not recognising the problem, trying to solve it themselves for too long, not announcing the problem to the health authorities, not requesting any help from competent colleagues—with similarly grave consequences'. Friedrich made these comments in May 2012, in front of the parliamentary investigation committee set up by the Bremen city assembly. He had had the report on the Maasstad Hospital by the Lemstra Commission, *Oog voor het onzichtbare* ('An eye for the invisible') translated into German for the occasion (Lemstra 2012). Friedrich is German himself and has been working at the UMC Groningen since autumn 2010. 'I believe that the Lemstra Commission report contains an outstanding

---

reported) has decreased from 71% in 2010 to 42% in 2015, suggesting an increase in proliferation of CPE in French hospitals. Of the 2385 episodes of CPE reported in France up to 1 January 2016, more than half (58%) were caused by *Klebsiella pneumoniae* and more than a third (38%) by *E. coli*. The role of *E. coli* has been increasing over the past few years, from 24% in 2012 to 42% in 2015. OXA-48 (-like) is by far the most frequent carbapenemase encountered. It is responsible for 78% of all cases in France (Pontiès et al. 2018, updated in 2019).

[18]See Chap. 4, *Major outbreak at the Maasstad Hospital.*

reconstruction and analysis of the failures at the Maasstad Hospital, and I am convinced that those in Bremen could learn a lot from them'. At a press conference on 2 November 2011, the management of the Bremen hospital announced that three children—two boys and a girl—had died in the neonatal department of the hospital. The deaths occurred in connection with a hygiene problem involving *Klebsiella pneumoniae* producing ESBL, which had become resistant as a result. The first baby died in August, the other two in October 2011. During the same period, a further 12 babies became infected with the bacterium. Eight of them did not become sick as a result, but four did.

Thanks to the investigations of the media—including, particularly, those of Radio Bremen and the *Weser Kurier*—it emerged that the facts presented by the hospital did not quite correspond to the reality (Interdisziplinäre Hygiene-Aufklärung 2013). The ESBL-producing *Klebsiella* had already been identified in the neonatal ICU in April 2011. According to Radio Bremen, the hospital had even been battling against the bacterium as far back as 2009. The neonatal unit was reopened at the beginning of January 2012. Just 6 weeks later, the same ESBL-producing Klebsiella germ was diagnosed in two infant patients. On 29 February 2012, two babies died of blood poisoning caused by ESBL Klebsiella. In addition, a laboratory in Bochum testing older isolates demonstrated that the same bacteria strain had in fact already been present in the Bremen-Mitte Clinic in 2009.

After this, the neonatal ICU at the hospital Klinikum Bremen-Mitte was immediately closed permanently by the authorities. The health authorities decided that the neonatology department could only reopen again when the construction of new hospital buildings had been completed.

The cup of sorrows had yet to be drained to the dregs. In the middle of March, Klebsiellas were detected on a box of latex gloves. In mid-May 2012, the bacterium was found in a 10-week-old boy who had been admitted for a hernia operation. No bacteria had been detectable when he was admitted, but after the operation, he had them on his skin. The small boy became severely ill, but he survived. The number of infections rose to 23. On 22 May 2012, an assessment of cleaning activities by hygiene specialist Ludwig Weber, of the German Advice Centre for Hygiene, became known to the general public (Bremische Bürgerschaft 2012). Weber identified considerable failings that had been caused by ignorance and incapacity. The manual for the cleaning service was full of instructions that guaranteed unhygienic practices. Among others, Weber cited the following example: 'One pair of green gauntlets and one of red are used for all disinfection tasks in all wards or rooms. In this way the gloves and cleaning trolley can serve as vehicles for transferring any kind of pathogen from ward to ward and from room to room'. Weber's report is full of examples of such unhygienic methods.

For the parents of premature infants in the neonatal ICU at the Bremen-Mitte Clinic, the outbreak was sheer hell. 'When a mother learns that her helpless baby is lying there and turning blue, that itself is already heartrending', Beate Steffens told Radio Bremen 1 year after her son Niklas had been fighting for his life. Her husband Maik adds: 'Then the doctor took us aside and explained that he was in a really bad way, and that his chances of survival were only 30 to 70 per cent. A short while later he stopped breathing and was connected to the artificial respiration machine. The doctors told us that he was dying'.

For the sake of honesty, it must be said that there is always a high mortality rate in neonatal ICUs. 'This fact is all too often lost sight of when a bacterial outbreak occurs on a neonatal ward', thinks Jörg Hermann, Director of the Institute for Hospital Hygiene in Oldenburg. 'When premature babies become increasingly smaller and are born increasingly earlier, and they aren't actually capable of survival, then every infection can pose a problem. It's a shame that, in such cases, the media make a scandal out of something that possibly isn't a scandal at all. Because there's always a high risk of infection with these very young patients. It would make more sense to inform the public about those risks that already exist. And make it clear to them that everyone has the option of informing themselves beforehand and deciding: Which hospital shall I go to? Does it have the relevant hygiene experts? Does it have a microbiology department? Does it have orderly antibiotic therapy? Can I minimise my own personal risk by informing myself beforehand, and enter a hospital in which everything is being done to make risks as small as possible? This is really difficult when you're dealing with lethal pathogens. It then becomes very difficult to determine whether it was fate or whether mistakes really were made—we've seen this in Bremen as well. And it remains an open question whether it could have been prevented'. Hermann regularly travelled from Oldenburg to Bremen in order to help his colleagues there. 'The problem that nobody wants to hear about is that the children who died there only had a 50% chance of surviving to start with. If you look at the completed report on the events in Bremen you find criticism that the cleaning service was not ideal, and that the colleague who worked there was not a doctor, but a biologist, and he wasn't accredited either. Besides this, there's criticism that the health ministry wasn't sufficiently informed. But nobody has discovered how the infection was transmitted, and whether there was a lapse in hygiene somewhere or other. We can't just say: In Bremen they did the following things wrong, and that's why the children died there'.

Ranko Matijasevic and his wife knew very well that there were bacteria on the neonatal ward of the Bremen-Mitte Clinic when their twins Dana and Mila were born there on 27 October 2011. The babies weighed around 2 kilos each, and the duty paediatrician wanted to admit them for safety's sake. 'It was then that Dr. X[19] informed me that there were germs on the ward, but that I needn't worry about it', recalled Ranko Matijasevic during Gaby Mayr's radio documentary 'The trail of germs' (Mayr 2012). 'Some were wearing gloves, some not', he stated during the programme. 'They were playing with my children's lives. They were running the risk that something could happen. They were saying to themselves: I'll get through this, I'll manage it somehow. And then the whole thing backfired, and in the end even more children fell ill with the germ'. The attitude of repeatedly making hopeless attempts to bring the outbreak under control themselves, against their better

---

[19]The name of the doctor in question has been suppressed.

knowledge—as Ranko Matijasevic puts it—is exactly the same as what happened at the Maasstad Hospital in Rotterdam.

The reopening of the neonatal ward and intensive care unit closed by the health authorities was planned for 2015, at the same time as the opening of the new building of the hospital. But it was only in May 2019 that the new building was ready and that the neonatal ward and neonatal intensive care unit started functioning again.

## Patients in Danger

Bacterial outbreaks occur much more frequently on neonatal wards. This is to be expected, because the infant patients there are especially vulnerable to infections. Recent studies have shown that some tens of outbreaks of healthcare-associated infections are estimated to occur annually in neonatal intensive care units in Germany, and at least two patients fall ill with a severe infection (blood poisoning, pneumonia). According to the scientists' statements, the actual number of outbreaks is probably higher, since their calculations are based only on laboratory-confirmed infections in a subgroup of patients, premature babies with a very low birth weight (Schwab et al. 2014). At a lecture in Essen at the beginning of January 2013, Professor Walter Popp—Head of the Department of Hospital Hygiene at Essen University Hospital—also reported that neonatal wards are possibly affected more often than average by outbreaks of ESBL and MRSA.

Even after the clear breaches of regulations in Bremen, it could not be taken for granted that outbreaks that hospitals had a duty to report would be promptly announced. The Charité Hospital in Berlin, and the neighbouring German Heart Centre, were both given a reprimand for reporting an outbreak of *Serratia Marcescens* too late (Berliner Morgenpost 2012). According to the statements of the Berlin healthcare authorities, the bacterium was detected in the heart clinic in September 2012, but the outbreak was not reported until the latter half of October. The hospital disputes that it did anything wrong. For the Charité the case is particularly painful, because the hospital is the national reference centre for surveillance of nosocomial infections. The death of a baby who had developed a *Serratia* sepsis was attributed to the severe infection. Only after some time did it emerge that the baby had died of severe heart failure (Gastmeier 2014). At the 7th National Healthcare Quality Congress in Berlin, on 4 December 2013, the Medical Director of the Charité—Professor Ulrich Frei—reported on the events at his hospital. The negative coverage in the media had hit the hospital staff hard, he said. As a result of the closure of two neonatal wards for half a year and the negative reports in the press, the Charité had lost patients—and therefore income. It was not until 1 year after the outbreak that patient numbers reached their former level again. 'We have learned a great deal, and for example we have compiled a manual for crisis scenarios', Frei said. 'In addition, we know that the only way to take the wind out of the media's sails is to proceed proactively' (Gesundheitsstad Berlin 2013).

Just like in the Netherlands and in most other countries, the number of ESBLs is increasing significantly in Germany as well. 'The rates of ESBL-forming *E. coli* have been rising steadily over the past few years, and in German intensive care units now stand at almost 13 per cent', write the authors of an overview published in *Hygiene & Medizin* (Pfeiffer et al. 2013). 'Besides this, studies in Germany and the Netherlands show that an intestinal colonisation is present in between 4 and 8 per cent of the population. In Germany, too, ESBL is not a problem specific to hospitals', says Professor Markus Dettenkofer, at the time of our conversation Head of the Hospital Hygiene Section of the University Medical Centre Freiburg.

'We have not really succeeded in keeping these sources of ESBL in check. That must be clearly pointed out. In principle, we are now focusing more on the truly highly resistant Gram-negative pathogens. In the case of highly resistant 4MRGN and Acinetobacter and Klebsiella, as well as 3MRGN, we should definitely try to do this'.[20] Dettenkofer passes a harsh judgement on both the role of human medicine and that of intensive livestock farming and veterinary medicine. 'In the last analysis this is a self-cooked mess. You only have to consider how uncritically antibiotics have been used in the livestock sector. Certainly things are getting better, but people have acted very uncritically here. You could say that it's a criminal act, a big mistake. Microorganisms are sly. If we prescribe lots of antibiotics, then there'll be a lot of resistance. And in the last 10–15 years we haven't been doing our homework about antibiotic management, neither in the veterinary sector nor in human medicine' (Pfeiffer et al. 2013).

## Unsettling Figures

Many more topics relating to ESBL came up for discussion at EECMID 2010 in Vienna. For example, how easily it can be spread by tourists and other travellers. Or the fact that there's a virulent *E. coli* strain with ESBL that colonises people worldwide and is a frequent cause of urinary tract infections. Or that in the UK they have found the first *E. coli* that was not just ESBL-positive, but also possessed the NDM-1 enzyme that makes it resistant to carbapenems.

Another topic addressed was how easily ESBL can spread via the transfer of plasmids between different bacteria, and how difficult it is to bring this proliferation under control (Canton and Coque 2006). Jan Kluijtmans, from 2013 till December 2018 Director of the Dutch microbiologists' professional association NVMM, presented the findings of the studies of his group on the presence of ESBL in meat (Overdevest et al. 2011). Almost half of all the 249 meat products purchased for the study were contaminated with ESBL. Eighty-eight per cent of the chicken samples contained ESBL, and it could be detected in almost 19% of the samples of beef and pork. Fewer ESBLs could be found in organic meat, but the difference was not statistically significant. 'ESBLs are everywhere', Kluijtmans reported. 'Wherever we look, we'll find them. On meat, but also on vegetables, in water, in the soil, everywhere. However they occur much more frequently in developing countries, and

---

[20]For a definition of 4MRGN and 3 MRGN see Krinko (2013).

travellers can very easily become infected with them. Should we perhaps isolate and test all people who have been abroad and who, for that reason alone, have an approximately 40 per cent probability of being colonised by ESBL? It seems to me that we're already fighting a rearguard battle. We will have to concentrate on the management of risks, but it's an illusion to believe that we can still eliminate the problem'. Professor Georg Peeters, Head of the Institute for Medical Microbiology at the University of Münster, Westphalia, does not seem quite so pessimistic. 'With Gram-negative bacteria, ESBL and also carbapenemases, we can't yet say how things are going to develop. Many people act as though we aren't going to have any more antibiotics in ten years' time. Well yes, if we continue acting in this way and do nothing at all in the areas of prevention, new developments and new ideas, then it might indeed come to that 1 day. For some patients, unfortunately, it's already happening now. We have two or three patients suffering from total immunosuppression after bone marrow transplants, who have the misfortune of carrying a pseudomonas on which even colistin has no effect. But these infections do not spread, we can contain them'.

For both Kluijtmans and Christina Vandenbroucke-Grauls, there is only one possible solution left: we need new antibiotics that are effective against Gram-negative bacteria. 'And these must be so expensive', says Vandenbroucke-Grauls, 'that no farmer would even think of using them on their animals as a preventative measure. And no doctor would use them if it wasn't really necessary'.

## Suspicions Confirmed

At the autumn meeting of the Dutch Society for Medical Microbiology (NVMM) in 2010, the group headed by Christina Vandenbroucke-Grauls presented the findings of a study on the prevalence of ESBL in the Amsterdam population. For this study, they had examined the stools of 720 people who had visited their GP because of stomach pains. There is no known connection between stomach pains and antibiotic resistance. Ten per cent of all samples contained ESBL (Reuland et al. 2013). 'In the hospital we have six percent ESBL. Amongst the people in Amsterdam with ESBL, we found only a small number who had the same ESBL that we find in chickens.' In Tilburg, another Dutch town, ESBL was detected in 8 per cent of stool samples during a similar study in spring 2011. After their study of people who had visited the doctor with stomach pains, the research team at VU University Medical Centre Amsterdam began a new study of the population in general. More than 1700 people submitted their stool samples for analysis. 'ESBL-positive bacteria were found in 8.5 per cent of this group', recalled Vandenbroucke-Grauls at the beginning of November 2012. 'We even found an *E. coli* with OXA-48. When we found ESBL in ten per cent of patients with stomach pains, we still thought that many of these might have contracted these pains because of a trip on which they'd caught diarrhoea. But now that we've been able to identify ESBL amongst healthy people with almost exactly the same frequency, we must ask ourselves even more urgently: How do these people become infected with ESBL?'

The answers to this question were presented by Ascelijn Reuland, a clinical microbiologist at the VU University Medical Centre, as part of the symposium 'Antibiotic resistance—an ecological perspective' on 5 March 2013. Besides the use of antibiotics, travel behaviour is the most important explanation for the sharp increase in ESBL-carrier status among the general population. A stay in a foreign hospital remains by far the most important risk factor for infection with ESBL. But even without hospital treatment, travelling in places such as North Africa, the Middle and Far East, and even the United States increases the risk of colonisation by resistant bacteria by a factor of between two and four in comparison to people who do not undertake such trips.

In spring 2014, the research team at the VU University Amsterdam published an initial small study of EBSLs on vegetables (Reuland et al. 2014). As expected, they were also detected there. Amongst 119 vegetable samples, contamination with ESBL-producing bacteria was identified in 5%.[21] Before this, only one study of ESBL in vegetables had been carried out, in France (Ruimy et al. 2010). In this larger study, 13% of 399 fruit and vegetable samples were found to be contaminated. And there, too, organic products were affected.

The microbiologist Guido Werner, of the Robert Koch Institute in Wernigerode in Germany, thinks that in the case of some multiresistant Gram-negative bacteria, e.g. those producing ESBL, the species of the bacterium is a major factor. 'I'm always astonished by the fact that the proliferation is totally pathogen-specific, because the rates of multiresistant Gram-negative pathogens in Germany and the Netherlands are not very different—even though we follow quite different regimes and have quite different structures. I think that the pathogens and their epidemiology also play a decisive role. And we know from our studies of Gram-negative pathogens that the problem is not just limited to the sphere of healthcare institutions, but affects the general population as well. There are already many colonised patients amongst the general public, and naturally enough they then come to our hospitals. The rates are the same in Germany and the Netherlands. That means the starting basis is the same. If these persons enter a hospital environment, then the measures you take in response are certainly of decisive importance'.

That point was elegantly proven by the end of March 2019 in the thesis of Marjolein Kluijtmans-van den Bergh *Extended-Spectrum Beta-Lactamase-producing Enterobacteriaceae in Dutch hospitals* (Kluijtmans-van den Bergh 2019). She describes a study 'on the prevalence and acquisition of ESBL-positive *Enterobacteriaceae* in Dutch hospitals, given the application of contact precautions for known ESBL-E positive patients'. At admission of the patients, the prevalence of rectal carriage of ESBL-E varied from 6 to 7%, at discharge from 9 to 10%, numbers that were in line with the results of other studies in European hospitals. 'The absolute risk', writes Marjolein Kluijtmans-van den Bergh, 'of acquisition of ESBL-E rectal carriage ranged from 2% to 3% with an ESBL-E acquisition rate of 3 to 4 acquisitions

---

[21]The bacteria in question were a *Klebsiella pneumoniae*, a *Citrobacter freundii* and two *Enterobacter cloacae*.

per 1000 patients-days. Twenty-eight percent of acquisitions were attributable to patient-dependent transmission, and the per-admission reproduction number was 0.06'. These low numbers lead the author to the conclusion 'that is possible to control the nosocomial transmission of ESBL in a low-endemic, non-ICU setting where E. coli is the most prevalent ESBL-E and standard and contact precautions are applied for known ESBL-E positive patients'. In yet another chapter of her thesis, Marjolein Kluijtmans-van den Bergh studies the pros and cons of isolation in single-bed rooms. Some observational studies targeted at Gram-positive microbes like MRSA or VRE report that single-bed rooms may have a positive impact in limiting the spread of antimicrobial resistance. On the other hand, single-bed rooms are nowadays somewhat controversial due to the negative effects they may have on the quality of care in general. In a first randomised study, also published in *The Lancet Infectious Diseases*, Marjolein Kluijtmans-van den Bergh compared different isolation strategies of ESBL-E positive patients in non-ICU and non-haematology wards (Kluijtmans-van den Bergh et al. 2019). 'An isolation strategy of contact precautions in a multiple-bed room was non-inferior to a strategy of contact precautions in a single-bed room in terms of transmission of ESBL-E to wardmates (single-bed room 5% vs. multiple-bed room 6%)'. Older studies reported a risk for roommates of ESBL-E positive patients to acquire the ESBL-E. But these patients had unprotected exposure to their ESBL-E positive roommate and the studies did not compare the risk of acquisition of the ESBL-E by wardmates not sharing the patients room. According to Marjolein Kluijtmans-van den Bergh, these findings 'do provide evidence for the effectiveness of contact precautions in the control of ESBL-E'. Finally, the author comes with a warning. 'Without active surveillance, the vast majority of ESBL-E carriers go undetected during hospitalisation. This finding, together with the observed role of unprotected ESBL-E positive ward stay, warrants reconsideration of current control measures for ESBL-E. Infection control policies aimed at the prevention of nosocomial spread of ESBL-E should consider the endemic presence of ESBL-E rectal carriage in the community and thus in patients at hospital admission. Active surveillance at hospital admission in combination with pre-emptive isolation has been suggested, but its feasibility and cost-effectiveness are questionable. In light of the increasing variety of antimicrobial-resistant bacteria that require control measures in healthcare settings, possibilities to strengthen horizontal (general) control strategies should seriously be explored. Besides (re)-inforcement of compliance with current standard precautions guidelines and improvement of environmental cleaning practices, this should include identification of relevant gaps in current infection control strategies such as the availability of private sanitary (toilet and shower) for all patients, and hand hygiene for patients and visitors'.

The figures which the ECDC presents annually on 'European Antibiotic Awareness Day' in mid-November paint a picture that gives cause for concern, particularly regarding *Klebsiella pneumoniae* with ESBL. In 2013, more than 60% of all invasive isolates of *K. pneumoniae* in Greece, Bulgaria, Romania, Poland, Latvia and Slovakia were resistant to third-generation cephalosporins. The average amongst all EU-EEA countries was 30%. In 16 of 21 reporting countries, more than 80% of these isolates were ESBL-positive (ECDC 2014). By 2016, the European average of invasive *K. pneumoniae* isolates resistant to third-generation cephalosporins had increased to 31%. In Greece and Bulgaria, the percentage was more than 70%; in Romania, Poland and Slovakia more than 60%. The vast majority of these isolates—87%—were ESBL-positive (ECDC 2017). Things changed little since 2016. Those countries that had performed poorly continued to do so. In 2019 EU/EEA average rate of resistance to third-generation cephalosporines for *Klebsiella pneumoniae* isolates was still 31%. In Bulgaria, almost 76% of all invasive *Klebsiella pneumoniae* isolates were resistant to third-generation cephalosporins, in Greece and Romania far more than 60% and in Slovakia, Italy and Poland almost 60%. And just as in 2016, the vast majority of these isolates produced ESBLs (ECDC 2020a, b).

## Appeals for Clean Meat

The research team headed by Leverstein-van Hall of Utrecht[22] discovered that 20% of the ESBL present in humans was genetically identical with the ESBL that had been found in chicken meat. And almost exactly the same percentage of human ESBLs were genetically related to those in chicken. Ninety-four per cent of the chicken meat was contaminated with ESBL-producing *E. coli*. As the researchers noted in the journal *Clinical Microbiology and Infection* in June 2011: 'These results convey the impression that the transfer of ESBL-genes, plasmids and *E. coli* isolates from chickens to people tends to take place through the food chain' (Leverstein-van Hall et al. 2011). Other researchers at the University Medical Centre Utrecht (UMC), in collaboration with researchers and colleagues from China, Spain and Norway, arrived at different results in December 2014 (De Been et al. 2014). They described how humans and chickens carried related antibiotic resistance genes, and how the plasmids on which the genes are located in both people and humans are also closely related to one another. But according to the authors of this study, which appeared in *PLOS Genetics,* the ESBL-positive *E. coli* in humans and animals are different. They concluded that resistances against cephalosporins probably arise through the transfer of parts of the plasmids containing the genetic information.

It emerged from data presented by Leverstein during a meeting at the end of 2010—and referred to in an article in the NTvG (Dutch Journal of Medicine—that the number of hospital patients with resistant ESBL bacteria had increased by a half in less than 2 years (Kuijpers and van Dissel 2010). In GPs' surgeries, the number of patients with ESBL bacteria in blood cultures has even tripled. This is causing deep concern amongst clinical microbiologists. The bacteria can cause blood poisoning (sepsis). Then you have to act quickly, because sepsis is life-threatening. Often you only have a little time to test which bacteria are causing the sepsis. Potentially that

---

[22]She is now working at the Bronovo Hospital in The Hague.

may have grave consequences, because the antibiotic you administer may not be effective if the bacteria are resistant. This can waste precious time.

In an interview with NOS, Leverstein called on supermarkets to use their influence (NOS 2010). 'If the supermarkets only buy ESBL-free meat, then something will change'. Supermarkets initially reacted dismissively to Leverstein-van Hall's appeal, but a year later her moment of glory came. On paper, at least. On 2 September 2011, the Van Doorn Commission published the report *Sustainable Meat: the transition to a healthy, safe and respectful livestock industry by 2020* (Commissie Van Doorn 2011). Farmers, supermarkets, animal feed suppliers and meat processing enterprises jointly agreed that all meat in the Netherlands must be produced sustainably from 2020 onwards, using as few antibiotics as possible.

## Q Fever and Collisions of Interests

The supermarket sector's initial reaction to Leverstein-van Hall's appeal revealed the same conflict between the interests of public health and those of business as the Q fever affair of the time. The first indications of a possible health problem at the end of 2005 and beginning of 2006, which led to a proposal for an extensive research programme on Q fever in January 2007, did not result in any activity. In the summer of 2007, the health authorities demanded the addresses of the four farms where Q fever had occurred. However, these were not released, since this would have compromised the farmers' data protection. Shortly after this, the waiting room of the local GP's surgery in Herpen, a village in Brabant, was full of people with flu-like symptoms and respiratory tract problems.[23] Q fever was not classed as a disease requiring mandatory notification until 9 months later, after another 1000 people had become infected with it. All kinds of countermeasures were subject to long delays, and in the meantime, Q fever was spreading. Heart patients and pregnant women in the areas surrounding infected facilities were exposed to an increased risk of infection and miscarriage for 3 years, for the most part without knowing it. The people became sick. They came to the hospital with severe pneumonia. Several acquired chronic heart valve inflammations. Others died. And many of them became furious. It was not until 9 December 2009 that the interests of public health were finally accorded higher importance than those of economics. The ministers announcing the emergency slaughter of all pregnant goats and sheep in the facilities infected. Instead of the original four, there were by this time around hundreds of infected premises. And thousands of infected people, hundreds of

---

[23]In February 2014, work began on a major study of the incidence of Q fever in the population of Herpen. The preliminary findings were published at the end of May 2014, the final report in June 2015 (GGD Hart voor Brabant 2015). More than a third of the population of Herpen had fallen ill with Q fever at some time. A further 25% may possibly have been affected, although without further research this cannot be stated with certainty.

severely sick, and 25 deaths. By the end of 2018, the number of deaths caused by the Q fever outbreak had increased to 95.[24]

On 22 November 2010, the Q fever Commission founded in January 2010 presented its report *Van verwerping tot verheffing* ('From abortion to outbreak') (Evaluatiecommissie Q-koorts 2010). The commission's judgement was damning. During the Q fever outbreak, the minsters could have and indeed ought to have acted more boldly and more resolutely. Important information, such as the addresses of the infected farms, should not have been withheld from the health authorities for reasons of data protection. The commission also decided that the health ministry must assume control in cases of veterinary diseases dangerous to humans, which included the authority to make decisions even when other ministries affected did not agree with them. The commission decided that data protection considerations must not play any role in problems where public health is at stake and that the Dutch food safety authorities must become independent.

## One World: One Medicine—One Health

The Q fever outbreak was not only a complete surprise for the health authorities, but also for all the veterinary services. The competing interests—public health versus economic interests—did the rest. The authorities' reaction to the Q fever outbreak was a perfect example of the most important conclusion of the study *Emerging zoonoses: early warning and surveillance in the Netherlands* (Van der Giessen et al. 2010). The Netherlands is not well prepared for outbreaks of zoonoses, i.e. diseases that can be transferred from animals to people. The report recommended a drastic improvement in cooperation between human and veterinary medicine—of the kind also described in the concept 'One world—one medicine—one health' (Gyles 2016).

In November 2017, the WHO issued new recommendations to stop farmers and the food industry 'using antibiotics routinely to promote growth and prevent disease in healthy animals'. If these WHO-recommendations were followed, it would help 'preserve the effectiveness of antibiotics that are important for human medicine by reducing their unnecessary use in animals' (WHO 2017a, b).

In the Netherlands, work on the problem had already begun. Experts from human and veterinary medicine discussed matters with one another more often than before. The Dutch authority for veterinary medicine (Stichting Diergeneesmiddelen Autoriteit) is one example of this. It is addressing the issue of antibiotic use in intensive livestock farming under the guidance of a veterinary microbiologist, an epidemiologist and a medical microbiologist. Roel Coutinho, until August 2013 Director of the Centre for Infectious Disease Control (CIb) at the RIVM, has been

---

[24]These are confirmed cases. Roel Coutinho—at that time of the Q fever outbreak head of the Dutch Center of infectious diseases control—estimates that in reality about 50,000 people were infected with Q fever, and that moreover the number of deaths was two to three times greater than the official figures (RIVM 2018).

Professor of Life Sciences in the Faculty of Medicine and Veterinary Medicine at the University of Utrecht since 2011 and until the end of September 2018. He taught the epidemiology and prevention of zoonoses. In his inaugural lecture on 10 February 2012, Coutinho explained that there are reasons why everyone should urgently address the control of zoonoses (Coutinho 2012). 'In a recent study', Coutinho said, 'the new infectious diseases appearing during the period 1940–2004 were listed with the aid of articles in scientific journals (Jones et al. 2008). During the 65-year period investigated, 335 new infectious diseases were described. Over time, the number of newly appearing infectious diseases grew. The fact that there are now more scientific publications than before was taken into account here. Two thirds of the 335 newly occurring infectious diseases mentioned originated in animals. [...] If we look at the many new zoonoses, what is striking is that it is particularly ecological and social changes that contribute to the increasing speed with which they appear'. In his speech, Coutinho spoke against the abolition of intensive livestock farming and romantic ideas of small-scale agriculture. 'We can't go back to the past and we don't want to either, because all these changes in society have formed the foundation of our affluence.

An affluence that other parts of the world are slowly attaining as well. "Back to the past " isn't possible. It is never a solution. And neither is it a solution now'. Between 2006 and 2010, as part of the study *Emerging zoonoses: early warning and surveillance in the Netherlands,* a list was compiled of the microorganisms occurring in animals that posed the greatest risks for humans (Van der Giessen et al. 2010). 'A sensible exercise', Coutinho said in his inaugural speech. 'But recent history teaches us that new infectious diseases have appeared of which we had no idea. It is important that we have strong structures for the control of infectious diseases in place, which cooperate well with one another'.

## Ecological Changes

It is equally important to have a good surveillance system, in order to be able to identify outbreaks of old or new zoonoses as quickly as possible. Such surveillance should primarily be carried out in those areas where the risk of zoonoses occurring is at its greatest. 'But', says Coutinho, 'we must also extend our surveillance globally to include those areas where major ecological and social changes are taking place. Where woods are being deforested, where agriculture is becoming more intensive, or where major social changes are being brought about by wars. Where more wild animals are being hunted and traded than before. Or where you can buy antibiotics without a prescription: antibiotics that, for us, are a last resort to treat serious infections. That sounds like "a tale of faraway lands". But in our country as well, surveillance of infectious diseases in animals is of great importance. In intensive livestock farming, the excessive use of antibiotics leads to the creation of resistant microorganisms that pose a new danger for humans. And as a result of the presence of a large number of genetically similar animals, the risk of new pathogens spreading quickly is increasing. Close collaboration with the veterinary sector, and also with farmers, is therefore indispensable. Thanks to the report on the Q fever epidemic, an important step in this direction has been taken. But things could be better. There is still a lack of transparency, and of willingness to report new diseases in animals immediately. But even in this field, considerable progress has been made in recent years'. The rich countries have the resources and expertise to set up surveillance systems for themselves. Developing countries cannot do this without extensive technical support from industrialised countries, said Coutinho in his inaugural speech. 'Our society is changing constantly and with ever greater rapidity. What I would like to draw your attention to is the fact that social and ecological changes result in our having to deal with newly emerging zoonoses more often than previously. The HIV epidemic—a zoonosis—has shown us that the consequences can be very far-reaching'.

At the end of February 2016, seven Dutch universities and university hospitals responded to the ever more frequent international appeals for a 'one health' approach and founded the Netherlands Centre for One Health. 'The 4 NCOH strategic research themes are complementary and interactive', according to the organisation's website. 'They focus on studying the interactions and connections between human, veterinary, wildlife, and environmental health in pursuit of durable solutions to grand societal challenges requiring a One Health approach'. The key points of NCOH research are the prevention and control of outbreaks of infectious diseases; prevention of antibiotic resistance; and the development of new medicines and new treatments. 'As the causes and possible solutions also include components of healthy farming and healthy wildlife and ecosystems, a One Health approach is required to solve these major societal challenges'. In June 2019 the new institute received a considerable grant of 10 million euros from taxpayers money to study how to better prepare for outbreaks of vector-borne infectious diseases that are reckoned to come about more often in the future due to climate change, growth of the world population and increase in international travel and trade (NCOH 2019).

In September 2016, 4 years after his inaugural lecture, Roel Coutinho gave an interview for the TV news magazine Zembla, during which he was asked whether he was confident that human health would now become the no. 1 priority in a zoonosis-related crisis like the Q fever outbreak. 'I would not be so rash as to say that we have organised things properly now', Mr. Coutinho said. 'Our structures are better organised, but I cannot say that this is a guarantee'. According to Mr. Coutinho, the cooperation between all the players involved has evolved in the right direction, but the conflict between economic and public health interests has not changed at all. That means it remains to be seen whether public health interests come first in the next zoonosis-related crisis. Mr. Coutinho fears that they will not (Zembla 2016).

## Meat Safety Under the Spotlight

If there is one area where the 'One World—One Health' approach proposed by Coutinho in his inaugural lecture is important, then it is food safety. The meat that goes on sale in shops in the Netherlands, as we have already seen, is full of ESBL-producing bacteria, and this applies quite especially to chicken. Things are no different on the farms: ESBL was detected at all the Dutch chicken farms investigated (Dierikx 2012). The same applies to more than 40% of pig farms (Dohmen 2012) and more than half the veal calves tested. This is an international problem. The findings of the research teams led by Kluijtmans and Leverstein-van Hall have all been extensively confirmed. For example, in 2012, a Canadian research team in Montreal identified genetic similarities between *E. coli* that caused urinary tract infections in humans and *E. coli* taken from the intestines of animals from abattoirs. More than 70% of the strains that caused urinary tract infections came from chickens (Bergeron et al. 2012). Pathogenic *E. coli* cause more than 80% of all urinary tract infections in humans (Lee et al. 2018). In the USA, between 6 and 8 million urinary tract infections are diagnosed every year. Around the world, there are between 130 and 175 million cases annually. In the USA, urinary tract infections give rise to costs of between 1 and 2 billion dollars per year (Russo and Johnson 2003). The percentage of ESBL-positive *Klebsiella pneumoniae* is very high in many Asian countries: in India, Pakistan and Jordan it is 70%, in Saudi Arabia 55%, in South Korea 29%, in Taiwan 26% and in Kuwait 24% (Wertheim 2011). At the beginning of January 2015, researchers from Japan, Vietnam and Thailand published a study in *Infection and Drugs Resistance*. According to their research, ESBL-producing *E. coli* are endemic amongst the general population in the Indo-Chinese countries Thailand, Laos and Vietnam. Of all the *E. coli* isolates studied, 47% were ESBL-positive in Vietnam, 66% in Thailand and as many as 70% in Laos (Nakayama et al. 2014).

These figures give few grounds for optimism, but it still seems that appropriate interventions can have a significant impact. This, at least, is what is suggested by the findings of the research team led by Jan Kluijtmans. They repeated the study that had originally revealed how a lot of the meat sold in Dutch shops—above all chicken—contains ESBL-producing microbes. At the end of 2014, Kluijtmans and his team once again bought meat in supermarkets and subjected it to selective culturing in the microbiological laboratory. They identified a considerable decrease of ESBL-producing bacteria in the chicken they tested. 'It was so big we didn't trust the results', Mr. Kluijtmans told me in December 2015. 'In summer 2015 we started all over again with freshly purchased meat and confirmed the results. 47% of the chicken contained ESBLs, compared with 84% in 2013 and 81% in 2009'. Mr. Kluijtmans thinks that, where the chicken is of Dutch origin, the decrease is linked to the significant reduction of antibiotic use in livestock farming. This amounted to 69.6% by the end of 2019 versus the reference year 2009 (SDA 2020). The authors of a study on the effects of the drastic decrease in the use of veterinary antibiotics in the Netherlands identified a minor effect on resistance in broilers. In the study, published in September 2016 in the *Journal of Antimicrobial Chemotherapy*, they write that 'recent Dutch policies reducing the total veterinary use of antimicrobials, and restricting the use of critically important antimicrobials, appear to have reduced (and are projected to further curb) *E. coli* resistance levels in veal calves and slaughter pigs. The impact on dairy cattle and broilers was, however, minor' (Dorado-Garcia et al. 2016). In February 2018, the ESBLAT (ESBL attribution analysis) research group, composed of researchers from various institutes—mostly, but not exclusively, veterinary institutes—published their report (Mevius et al. 2018). Their main conclusions were that ESBLs are everywhere: in the intestines of animals (pets and livestock), in human intestines and in the environment. Around 5% of the total human population is colonised by ESBL-carrying bacteria. The highest prevalence of ESBL-producing bacteria—over 60%—was found in sewage, broiler chickens and chicken meat. The researchers found that ESBL-producing microbes in the intestines of healthy colonised people are very similar to the ESBLs causing infections in others that are hard to treat. They concluded that humans themselves are an important source of transmission of ESBL-positive bacteria, and that transmission between animals or meat, especially chicken, plays a less significant role. Nevertheless, depending on the level of detail of genetic analysis, between 10 and 30% of the ESBLs found in humans might originate from livestock reservoirs, mainly chicken. People working in sectors involving close contact with animals run a greater risk of being colonised by ESBL-positive microbes. Farmers are colonised by ESBLs very similar to those of their livestock.

## A Garden That Needs Looking After

Until the end of 2016, Jan van Wijngaarden was Chief Inspector for Public Health at the Dutch Health Care Inspectorate (Inspectie voor de Gezondheidszorg—IGZ). Infectious diseases, and how to prevent and deal with them, are second nature to him. He is very concerned about the rapid spread of ESBL, both inside and outside hospitals. 'We don't exactly know where they are coming from. Certainly from abroad, but not exclusively so. Outside hospitals, I don't think we can control them. In hospitals there are sick and vulnerable people, who are becoming increasingly older and more severely ill, and invasive interventions take place there.[25] You're therefore dealing with a population for whom resistant bacteria pose a risk. With ESBL, it's no different from MRSA. The main challenge, therefore, is to try and keep hospitals as free from these germs as possible. But how are we going to bring that about? Already at present, between 5 and 10 per cent of people who enter hospital bring ESBL along with them. If people become infected as a result of an ESBL-producing bacterium, then nothing has changed. You have to discover which bacterium is causing the infection, which resistances it is carrying, and then administer the right antibiotic. When you act preventatively, you must also learn which resistances are to be expected. This is the usual way of proceeding. But how do you determine that such and such an ESBL is spreading in the hospital, infecting new patients and thus becoming a problem for all the patients throughout the entire building—and, of course, for other hospitals, nursing homes and retirement homes? You must first notice that you have a germ in the building which, apparently,

---

[25] 'Invasive' in the sense that an instrument is introduced into the human body.

spreads easily from one patient to another'. Clinical microbiologists can then use molecular diagnostics to determine whether the ESBL bacteria of two or more patients are identical. 'But', says Van Wijngaarden, 'that is expensive, complicated and time-consuming'. The alternative is to use an algorithm, i.e. a mathematical model. 'If you have a specific number of infected patients on a ward during a defined timeframe, then you probably have a problem'.

Van Wijngaarden has a very clear conception of the prevention and control of infectious diseases. 'We must make maximum efforts to keep multiresistant bacteria out of the hospital as far as is possible. That includes VRE, which are perhaps not so dangerous for patients. The health ministry thinks that controlling these germs continues to be worthwhile, and I trust their opinion. Moreover, this has a major additional benefit: it enables us to keep a good infrastructure for preventing infection in working order. This makes it easier for us to react to new problems quickly. This well-functioning infrastructure is an important factor in the present situation. Thanks to this, we have a good chance of getting the problems that are now surfacing under control as well. The investments that we have made in the area of MRSA control are now paying off. For example, we know that multiresistant tuberculosis (MR TB) is being diagnosed more and more frequently. We have constructed a system for keeping this problem under control—a kind of flood warning system—that functions very well. But this is a problem we're aware of. We know much less about ESBL and carbapenemases. It is therefore all the more important that we keep our structures intact. Infection prevention is like a garden that needs to be properly looked after. You must never neglect it, because otherwise weeds will immediately shoot up all over it.'

# References

Beemer, F., Van Velzen, G., Van den Berg, C., et al. (2010). *Wat zijn de effecten van het ontkoppelen van voorschrijven en verhandelen van diergeneesmiddelen door de dierenarts?* (In Dutch). Accessed November 1, 2020, from https://edepot.wur.nl/133692

Bergeron, C., Prussing, C., Boerlin, P., et al. (2012). Chicken as Reservoir for Extraintestinal Pathogenic *Escherichia coli* in Humans, Canada. *Emerging Infectious Diseases, 18*(3), 415–421. https://doi.org/10.3201/eid1803.111099. Accessed from https://wwwnc.cdc.gov/eid/article/18/3/11-1099_article

Berliner Morgenpost. (2012). *In German.* Accessed November 2, 2020, from https://bit.ly/2Lummv6

Bremische Bürgerschaft. (2012). *Landtag, 18e Wahlperiode, 18/677.* In German. (Amongst others pages 170–175). Accessed November 2, 2020, from https://bit.ly/38kN8ig

Canton, R., & Coque, T. M. (2006). The CTX-M β-lactamase pandemic. *Current Opinion in Microbiology, 9*(5), 466–475. https://doi.org/10.1016/j.mib.2006.08.011.

CDC (Centers for Disease Control and Prevention). (2018). *Global pneumococcal disease and vaccine.* Accessed November 1, 2020, from https://www.cdc.gov/pneumococcal/global.html

Commissie Van Doorn. (2011). *Al het vlees duurzaam De doorbraak naar een gezonde, veilige en gewaardeerde veehouderij in 2020 (Sustainable Meat: the transition to a healthy, safe and respectful livestock industry by 2020).* Accessed November 9, 2020, from https://edepot.wur.nl/176874

Coutinho, R. A. (2010). *Advies met betrekking tot ESBL's in Nederland*. In Dutch. Accessed November 1, 2020, from (see second part of the document) https://bit.ly/3hYOD9i

Coutinho, R. A. (2012). *Van dier naar mens: Zoönosen in een wereld in verandering*. Accessed from https://dspace.library.uu.nl/handle/1874/251744

De Been, M., Lanza, V. F., de Toro, M., et al. (2014). Dissemination of cephalosporin resistance genes between *Escherichia coli* strains from farm animals and humans by specific plasmid lineages. *PLoS Genetics*. https://doi.org/10.1371/journal.pgen.1004776.

Dierikx, C. (2012). *ESBLs in de vleeskuiken productiekolom. Oral presentation at the seminar Vóórkomen van ESBLs in de voedselketen en bij de mens in Utrecht*. In Dutch. Accessed November 9, 2020, from https://bit.ly/3kbdrKx

Dohmen, W. (*2012*). *ESBLs in de varkenshouderij Transmissie van dier naar mens. Oral presentation at the seminar Vóórkomen van ESBLs in de voedselketen en bij de mens in Utrecht*. In Dutch. Accessed November 9, 2020, from https://bit.ly/36efrgc

Dorado-Garcia, A., Mevius, D. J., Jacobs, J. J. H., et al. (2016). Quantitative assessment of antimicrobial resistance in livestock during the course of a nationwide antimicrobial use reduction in the Netherlands. *Journal of Antimicrobial Chemotherapy, 71*(12), 3607–3619. https://doi.org/10.1093/jac/dkw308.

ECDC (European Centre for Disease Prevention and Control). (2014). *Antimicrobial resistance surveillance in Europe 2013. Annual Report of the European Antimicrobial Resistance Surveillance Network (EARS-Net)*. https://doi.org/10.2900/39777. Accessed November 9, 2020, from https://bit.ly/39bwyRm

ECDC (European Centre for Disease Prevention and Control). (2017). *Surveillance of antimicrobial resistance in Europe 2016. Annual Report of the European Antimicrobial Resistance Surveillance Network (EARS-Net)*. https://doi.org/10.2900/296939. Accessed November 9, 2020, from https://bit.ly/35jIHCz

ECDC (European Centre for Disease Prevention and Control). (2019). *Invasive pneumococcal disease. Annual epidemiological report for 2017*. Accessed November 1, 2020, from https://bit.ly/3hTnrZe

ECDC (European Centre for Disease Prevention and Control). (2020a). *Additional tables EU/EEA population weighted mean 2019*. Accessed January 7, 2021, from https://bit.ly/35jUHEa

ECDC (European Centre for Disease Prevention and Control). (2020b). *Antimicrobial resistance in the EU/EEA (EARS-Net) – Annual Epidemiological Report for 2019*. Accessed January 7, 2021, from https://bit.ly/3ntksIw

ECDC (European Centre for Disease Prevention and Control). (2020c). *Invasive pneumococcal disease. Annual epidemiological report for 2018*. Accessed November 1, 2020, from https://bit.ly/2Xm8J3L

Evaluatiecommissie Q koorts. (2010). *Van verwerping tot verheffing* ('From abortion to outbreak'). In Dutch. Accessed November 9, 2020, from https://edepot.wur.nl/156218

Gastmeier, P. (2014). *Serratia marcescens*: An outbreak experience. *Frontiers in Microbiology, 5*, 81. https://doi.org/10.3389/fmicb.2014.00081.

Gesundheitsstad Berlin. (2013). *Bei Infektionsausbrüchen pro-aktiv vorgehen*. In German. Accessed November 2, 2020, from https://bit.ly/3f5KRt6

GGD Hart voor Brabant. (2015). *Rapportage uitkomsten Q-koorts Herpen II onderzoek*. In Dutch. Accessed November 9, 2020, from https://bit.ly/3nssWQn

Gyles, C. (2016). One medicine, one health, one world. *Canadian Veterinary Journal, 57*(4), 345–346. Accessed from https://bit.ly/2XiWc0V

Interdisziplinäre Hygiene-Aufklärung. (2013). *Medien-Chronik des Frühchen-Skandals in Bremen*. In German. Accessed November 2, 2020, from https://bit.ly/2Uw0IYH

Jones, K. E., Patel, N. G., Levy, M. A., et al. (2008). Global trends in emerging infectious diseases. *Nature, 451*(7181), 990–993. https://doi.org/10.1038/nature06536.

Klink, A. (2010). 29683 Dierziektebeleid. Accessed November 1, 2020, from https://zoek.officielebekendmakingen.nl/kst-29683-52.html. In Dutch (This link leads to a letter of the Ministers on the ESBL-problem. It contains a link to Coutinho R (2010), the scientific advice, signed by Professor Roel Coutinho, on how to deal with ESBLs that is a largely based on the document written by Maureen Leverstein-van Hall I am referring to. Unfortunately it does not link to it).

Kluijtmans-van den Bergh, M. F. Q. (2019). *Extended-spectrum beta-lactamase-producing enterobacteriaceae in Dutch hospitals.* Accessed from https://bit.ly/3nbdt7f

Kluijtmans-van den Bergh, M. F. Q., Bruijning-Verhagen, P. C. J., Vandenbroucke-Grauls, C. M. J. E., et al. (2019). Contact precautions in single-bed or multiple-bed rooms for patients with extended-spectrum β-lactamase-producing Enterobacteriaceae in Dutch hospitals: A cluster-randomised, crossover, non-inferiority study. *The Lancet Infectious Diseases, 19*(10), 1069–1079. https://doi.org/10.1016/S1473-3099(19)30262-2.

KRINKO - Kommission für Krankenhaushygiene und Infektions prävention. (2013). Praktische Umsetzung sowie krankenhaushygienische und infektionspräventive Konsequenzen des mikrobiellen Kolonisationsscreenings bei intensivmedizinisch behandelten Früh- und Neugeborenen. *Epidemiologisches Bulletin,* (42). Accessed November 8, 2020, from https://bit.ly/3nnNUiW

Kuijpers, E. J., & van Dissel, J. T. (2010). *Opmars van resistente gramnegatieve bacteriën.* 154: A2868. In Dutch. Accessed from https://bit.ly/3pVOuWO. English abstract: The rise of resistant gram-negative bacteria. Accessed from https://bit.ly/3bhGOdx

Lee, D. S., Lee, S. J., & Choe, H. S. (2018). Community-acquired urinary tract infection by *Escherichia coli* in the era of antibiotic resistance. *Biomed Research International.* https://doi.org/10.1155/2018/7656752.

Lemstra, W. (2012). *Oog voor het onzichtbare (An eye for the invisible).* Accessed November 16, 2020 in Dutch https://bit.ly/3hQF9g8 or in German https://bit.ly/3pYYIG4

Leverstein-van Hall, M. A., Dierikx, C. M., Cohen Stuart, J., et al. (2011). Dutch patients, retail chicken meat and poultry share the same ESBL genes, plasmids and strains. *Clinical Microbiology and Infection, 17*(6), 873–880. https://doi.org/10.1111/j.1469-0691.2011.03497.x.

Mayr, G. (2012). Die Spur der Keime. In German. Accessed November 2, 2020, from https://bit.ly/3bgUGo9

Mevius, D. J., Heederik, D., & Van Duijkeren, E. (2018). *Summary ESBL-Attribution-analysis (ESBLAT) searching for the sources of antimicrobial resistance in humans.* Accessed November 9, 2020, from https://bit.ly/2IjwW6Q

Nakayama, T., Ueda, S., Uong, B., et al. (2014). Wide dissemination of extended-spectrum β-lactamase-producing *Escherichia coli* in community residents in the Indochinese peninsula. *Infection and Drug Resistance, 2015*(8), 1–5. https://doi.org/10.2147/IDR.S74934.

NCOH. (2019). *Netherlands Centre for One Health. 10 million for One Health research in the Netherlands.* Accessed November 9, 2020, from https://bit.ly/2XkeZco

NOS. (2010). *Eerste dode door ESBL-bacterie.* Accessed November 9, 2020, from https://nos.nl/artikel/187040-eerste-dode-door-esbl-bacterie.html

Overdevest, I., Willemsen, I., Rijnsburger, M., et al. (2011). Extended-spectrum β-lactamase genes of *Escherichia coli* in chicken meat and humans, the Netherlands. *Emerging Infectious Diseases, 17*(7), 1216–1222. https://doi.org/10.3201/eid1707.110209.

Pfeiffer, Y., Eller, C., Leistner, R., et al. (2013). ESBL-Bildner als Infektionserreger beim Menschen und die Frage nach dem zoonotischen Reservoir. *Hygiene & Medizin, 38*(7/8): 294–299. In German, with English summary. Accessed November 2, 2020, from https://bit.ly/3s3f4z5

Pontiès, V., Savitch, Y., Soing-Altrach, S., et al. (2018). *Episodes impliquant des EPC en France.* Situation épidémiologique du 31 décembre 2016. Updated 12 May 2019. In French. Accessed November 2, 2020, from https://bit.ly/3mMW6sW

Reuland, E. A., Overdevest, I. T. M. A., Al Naiemi, N., et al. (2013). High prevalence of ESBL-producing Enterobacteriaceae carriage in Dutch community patients with gastrointestinal complaints. *Clinical Microbiology and Infection, 19*(6), 542–549. https://doi.org/10.1111/j.1469-0691.2012.03947.x.

Reuland, E. A., Al Naiemi, N., Raadsen, S. A., et al. (2014). Prevalence of ESBL-producing Enterobacteriaceae in raw vegetables. *European Journal of Clinical Microbiology and Infectious Diseases, 33*, 1843–1846. https://doi.org/10.1007/s10096-014-2142-7.

RIVM. (2018). *Q koorts*. In Dutch. Accessed November 9, 2020, from https://www.rivm.nl/q-koorts

RIVM. (2020). *Pneumococcal disease*. Accessed November 1, 2020, from https://bit.ly/3nm3yv9

Ruimy, R., Brisabois, A., Bernede, C., et al. (2010). Organic and conventional fruits and vegetables contain equivalent counts of Gram-negative bacteria expressing resistance to antibacterial agents. *Environmental Microbiology, 12*(3), 608–615. https://doi.org/10.1111/j.1462-2920. 2009.02100.x.

Russo, T. A., & Johnson, J. R. (2003). Medical and economic impact of extraintestinal infections due to *Escherichia coli*: Focus on an increasingly important endemic problem. *Microbes and Infection, 5*(5), 449–456. https://doi.org/10.1016/S1286-4579(03)00049-2.

Schwab, F., Geffers, C., Piening, B., et al. (2014). How many outbreaks of nosocomial infections occur in German neonatal intensive care units annually? *Infection, 42*, 73–78. https://doi.org/10. 1007/s15010-013-0516-x.

SDa. (2014). *The Netherlands Veterinary Medicines Authority. Usage of antibiotics in agricultural livestock in the Netherlands in 2013 trends and benchmarking of livestock farms and veterinarians SDa/1145/201*. Accessed November 1, 2020, from https://bit.ly/3n8frVT

SDa. (2020). *The Netherlands Veterinary Medicines Institute. Usage of antibiotics in agricultural livestock in the Netherlands in 2019. Trends and benchmarking of livestock farms and veterinarians*. Accessed November 1, 2020, from https://bit.ly/38t0xpc

Van Bijnen, E. M. E. (2015). *Antibiotic treatment and commensal Staphylococcus aureus resistance in primary care in Europe. A nine-country study*. Accessed November 2, 2020, from https://bit.ly/35i2ulZ

Van der Giessen, J. W. B., van de Giessen, A. W., & Braks, M. A. H. (2010). *Emerging zoonoses: Early warning and surveillance in the Netherlands*. RIVM-rapport 330214002. Accessed November 9, 2020, from https://www.rivm.nl/bibliotheek/rapporten/330214002.pdf

Verburg, G., & Klink, A. (2010a). *29683 Dierziektebeleid*. In Dutch. Accessed Nov 1, 2020, from https://zoek.officielebekendmakingen.nl/kst-29683-52.html (This link leads to a letter of the Ministers on the ESBL-problem. It contains a link to Coutinho R (2010), the scientific advice, signed by Professor Roel Coutinho, on how to deal with ESBLs that is a largely based on the document written by Maureen Leverstein-van Hall I am referring to. Unfortunately it does not link to it).

Verburg, G., & Klink, A. (2010b). *Deskundigenberaad RIVM en reductie antibioticumgebruik*. In Dutch. Accessed November 1, 2020, from https://bit.ly/35dK71N (see first part of the document).

Wertheim, H. F. L. (2011). *Inappropriate antibiotic use and resistance in Asia and its global impact; a delicate balance of antibiotic accessibility*. Oral presentation at the spring meeting of the NVMM (Dutch Society for Medical Microbiology), Arnhem 18–20 Apr 2011. See pages S39 and S40, abstract Oo60. Accessed November 9, 2020, from https://bit.ly/3k9Z3SJ

WHO. (2017a). *WHO guidelines on use of medically important antimicrobials in food-producing animals*. Accessed November 9, 2020, from https://bit.ly/2LtxW9E

WHO. (2017b). *Stop using antibiotics in healthy animals to prevent the spread of antibiotic resistance*. Factsheet. Accessed November 9, 2020, from https://bit.ly/3opUR4e

Zembla. (2016). *Volksgezondheid niet op 1 bij uitbraak dierziekte*, Zembla 28 Sept 2016. Accessed January 7, 2021, from https://bit.ly/3pXT1b9

# The End in Sight?

## 7

Medical tourism to India is becoming ever more important. More important for the Indian economy, but also—in a negative sense—more important for the spread of highly resistant microorganisms. Take, for example, the first three NDM-1 cases identified by the Center for Disease Control (CDC) in the United States in 2010 (CDC 2010). All three cases involved NDM-1-producing Enterobacteriaceae.[1] All three bacteria were detected in patients who had recently undergone medical treatment in India. Often this consists of acute treatment for people on holiday or business travellers. But it may also mean that the patients had gone to India as medical tourists, for example in order to undergo plastic surgery there. Substantial numbers of Indians and Pakistanis in the USA and—above all—the United Kingdom do likewise. But many patients also come from Middle East countries. Every year several hundred thousands of patients visit India in order to have an operation. The revenue this generated during 2015 is estimated at 3 billion US dollars. The value of the Indian medical tourism market is expected to grow to 8 billion dollars by 2020 (The Economic Times 2015).

In May 2011, a woman from the United States travelled back to her homeland, Cambodia. She became sick and was informed that she had a tumour on her spine. In order to be treated, she had to go to the neighbouring country of Vietnam, where she was admitted to a hospital in Ho Chi Minh City in December 2011. There a catheter was inserted into her body, and she received two kinds of antibiotics as a prophylactic measure. On 6 January 2012, the woman returned to America, where she was immediately admitted to hospital again. One month later, two different strains of *Klebsiella pneumoniae* with NDM-1 were identified in the patient. Antibiotic resistance is a major problem in Vietnam, but reliable data concerning this are hard to

---

[1] These were: a *Klebsiella pneumoniae,* an *Escherichia coli* and an *Enterobacter cloacae.*

© The Author(s), under exclusive license to Springer Nature Switzerland AG 2021     125
R. van den Brink, *The End of an Antibiotic Era*,
https://doi.org/10.1007/978-3-030-70723-1_7

come by.[2] There is a national working group of the Global Antibiotic Resistance Partnership (GARP) in Vietnam. GARP is an initiative of the US Center for Disease Dynamics, Economics and Policy. Until mid-2015, the Dutch clinical microbiologist Heiman Wertheim was the Supervisor of GARP in Vietnam. In October 2010, the GARP working group in Vietnam published its report *Situation analysis: Antibiotic use and Resistance in Vietnam* (GARP 2010). In his foreword, Nguyen Van Kinh, Director of the Vietnamese GARP working group, writes: 'The global problem of antimicrobial resistance is particularly pressing in developing countries, where the infectious disease burden is high and cost constrains the replacement of older antibiotics with newer, more expensive ones. Gastrointestinal, respiratory, sexually transmitted, and nosocomial infections are leading causes of disease and death in the developing world, and management of all these conditions has been critically compromised by the appearance and rapid spread of resistance'. Kinh believes that too little attention is being devoted to this problem. 'Antibiotic resistance does not currently top any list of national problems. Strategies to control antibiotic resistance should not drain resources from more pressing concerns. Correctly carried out, antibiotic resistance control should be either cost-neutral or, in fact, one of the few health interventions that actually save money'.

On the basis of the limited data available and interviews with experts, the report reaches some harsh conclusions. Multiple resistance occurs frequently in Vietnam[3]—in the case of some bacteria, more frequently than in other south-east Asian countries.[4] Until now Vietnam has been struggling to control a black market in medicines, in which many antibiotics are also offered for sale (KI-Media 2008; VietnamNet Bridge 2017).[5] In April 2010 and again in January 2018, the WHO warned of a flourishing black market for medicines, above all in Asia and Africa (WHO 2010, 2018). Often these illegally supplied medicines consist of poor imitation products with much too little active ingredient. In the case of antibiotics, the efficacy of the medicines is too low to contribute to effective treatment, while at the same time they promote the development of resistance. 'Or they don't contain any active ingredient at all', says Wertheim, 'and then they don't contribute to resistance either'.

---

[2]In 2012, Jan Kluijtmans told me that he had heard from some colleagues in Asia that they were not allowed to publish anything about resistance problems any more. At the same time people were becoming more aware of the link between antibiotics use and resistance, for example in India and China.

[3]In 2000 and 2001, *Streptococcus pneumoniae* was resistant to penicillin in 71% of cases, and in 92% of cases resistant to erythromycin (GARP 2010).

[4]Forty-two per cent of Gram-negative *Enterobacteriaceae* were resistant to ceftazidime, 63% to gentamicin and 74% to nalidixic acid. Ceftazidime is a third-generation cephalosporin. Gentamicin is an aminoglycoside antibiotic and nalidixic acid is one of the (fluoro)quinolones (GARP 2010).

[5]According to the GARP report on Vietnam, 25 types of antibiotics were withdrawn from the market in 2008 because of their poor quality. These included both medicines produced in Vietnam and imported ones. Antibiotics make up roughly a quarter of all illegal medicines taken off the market (GARP 2010).

## Everybody Is a Pharmacist

At the 2011 spring meeting of the Dutch Society for Medical Microbiology, Heiman Wertheim gave a presentation about the report mentioned above and a survey of pharmacists (Wertheim 2011). More than 90% of all antibiotics sold in Vietnam are purchased without prescription, even though this is prescribed by law. A quarter of all medicines sold in Vietnam is antibiotics.

Vietnam has a population of almost 90 million, and around 57,000 pharmacies (Viêt Nam News 2010). That equals 6.5 pharmacies per 10,000 inhabitants. Even kiosks and stalls where medicines can be obtained are counted as pharmacies. According to the GARP report, the country has 39,000 official pharmacies. This would still amount to 4.3 per 10,000 inhabitants. By way of comparison, in the Netherlands, there were exactly 2.000 pharmacies for a population of 17.4 million people as of 1 January 2020 (SFK 2020; CBS Statline 2020). That's almost 1.2 pharmacies per 10,000.

Vietnamese people who feel sick prefer to go to a pharmacy rather than a clinic or hospital. This saves time and money, according to the authors of the GARP report on the country. By not going to the doctor first, these people avoid the need to pay their own contribution to basic medical care.[6] 'The high out-of-pocket expenditures encourage people to bypass providers and purchase drugs—including antibiotics—directly, without proper diagnosis. [...] Even though prescriptions are legally required, antibiotics (and a wide range of other drugs) can be purchased directly by consumers at pharmacies or drug outlets. Self-diagnosis is not very accurate, but self-treatment is very common. In a community-based study undertaken in 2007, 78 per cent of antibiotics taken by the study participants were purchased in private pharmacies without prescription. Buying drugs directly is cheaper and faster than going to a practitioner' (GARP 2010). According to Vietnamese regulations, only pharmacists with 5 years' experience may own a pharmacy. However, the reality is otherwise. Practically anyone with the licence of an authorised pharmacist can open a pharmacy. The patients explain what is wrong with them to the pharmacy staff, who usually have only little medical training or none at all. Pharmacies naturally have a commercial interest in selling antibiotics. The GARP report for Vietnam announced that, in 2006, there were 230 full-time inspectors with 1000 staff dealing with antibiotics prices and preventing corruption. Moreover, this is said to be a major problem, which in addition to fraudulent pharmacist licensing also includes payments from pharma firms to doctors. And then, of course, there are also the patients who want antibiotics at all costs because they believe they are effective

---

[6]Every worker or employee must contribute to the compulsory health insurance scheme. Insurance is free for pensioners and the poor. The insurance covers the costs of basic care, but also requires a patient contribution of around 20%. Since 2005, all medical treatment for children under six has been free.

against everything. This must naturally lead to a high use of antibiotics and, therefore, to the formation of resistance.[7]

Wertheim told me that Vietnamese children under five receive five treatments with antibiotics annually. Dutch GPs prescribe on average considerably less than one treatment per year for children under five (Otters et al. 2004).[8] Little is known about antibiotic resistance in Vietnam. Wertheim said that 58 Vietnamese studies of infectious diseases were published in international medical journals between 2000 and 2010. Only one of these dealt with antibiotic resistance in Vietnamese intensive care units. A few were concerned with postoperative infections, and the rest with infections picked up outside hospitals. In the meantime, the first cases of NDM-1 were reported (Nguyen et al. 2013). Wertheim described another case that was as remarkable as it was tragic. A patient was lying in a Vietnamese intensive care unit with pneumonia they had contracted in the hospital, caused by multiresistant Gram-negative bacteria. The patient had to be treated with colistin, which is not available for human use in Vietnam. It is, however, most certainly available for use with animals. In the veterinary sector, colistin is used in vast quantities. The patient in question died. Wertheim showed his audience an ominous slide on which a long series of antibiotics was listed, all of which are used as growth promoters in livestock feed. In Vietnam, there is hardly any livestock feed without antibiotics. Moreover, important medicines from all classes of antibiotics are used (Wertheim 2011). In neighbouring China, half of all antibiotics are used in the veterinary sector. The equivalent figures for antibiotics use in the veterinary sector in Vietnam are not known. But the data that are known speak volumes. Seventy per cent of all medicines given to animals are antibiotics. In Vietnam, large quantities of antibiotics are also used in fish farming. The GARP report refers to a Dutch study by the food safety authorities from 2009, in which the antibiotics use in Vietnamese fish farming is estimated at 700 grammes per tonne of fish. In Norway and Sweden, approximately 2 grammes of antibiotics are used per tonne of fish, in the UK 10–20 grammes, and in Canada 157. Only in a third of cases is a veterinarian involved in the use of antibiotics in livestock or fish farming (GARP 2010; Wakker Dier 2014). A study of other researchers estimates the use of antibiotics in the aquaculture of panga at 93 grammes per tonne (Rico et al. 2013). In a 2020 study, a research group estimated the global antibiotic use in the fast-growing aquaculture industry at 10,259 tonnes. They foresee an estimated increase of 33% to 13,600 tonnes in 2030. The usage in aquaculture in the Asia-Pacific region represents almost 94% of the global use, with China representing 58% of it. The antibiotic use in aquaculture has the highest intensity per kilogram of biomass, write the authors of the study. The total

---

[7]Vietnam and India still use much fewer antibiotics per capita than the United States or southern European countries. Many Indian and Vietnamese people have very limited access to medical care, or none at all. They often buy antibiotics for a short period. That leads to underdosing, which considerably encourages the formation of resistance.

[8]In the Netherlands, the consumption of antibiotics in the community was 9.5 DDD per 1000 inhabitants per day in 2019. The EU average was 19.4 DDD per 1000 inhabitants per day (ECDC 2020a).

global use of antimicrobials by humans, in food-producing animals and in aquaculture is estimated at 236,757 tonnes in 2030. Humans will by then use 48,608 tonnes and food-producing animals 174,549 tonnes (Schar et al. 2020).

Meanwhile, Wertheim and his team have been concentrating on developing a surveillance project to monitor the use of antibiotics and the emergence of resistance. 'That's working pretty well', he told me in summer 2012. The project has to be carried out in 20 hospitals in collaboration with the health ministry, and an annual report must be published. It is also intended to set up something similar for the veterinary sector (Wertheim et al. 2013). Professor Jan Kluijtmans welcomes the creation of the surveillance structures but warns of unrealistic expectations. 'Measurement is only the beginning', he says. 'It's really about the actions that follow'. In 2013 the Vietnamese Ministry of Health presented a national action plan for combatting drug resistance in the period from 2013 to 2020. As the scientists taking part write in *The Lancet Global Health* of November 2016, a working group from the Oxford University Clinical Research Unit and the Vietnamese Ministry of Health developed 'evidence-informed quality standards for appropriate antibiotic prescribing for community-acquired pneumonia and acute exacerbation of COPD' (Li et al. 2016). In June 2016 the draft standards were shared at a meeting with officials from the Ministry of Health and 'over 40 managers, physicians, pharmacists and microbiologists from central and provincial hospitals across Vietnam'. All those present at this meeting recognised 'that international standards need local adaptation. [. . .] However, in an environment with high prevalence of antimicrobial resistance, patients self-medicating with over-the-counter antibiotics before presenting themselves at hospitals, and absence of national surveillance, determining appropriate first-line therapy was more challenging than establishing the standards for thorough clinical diagnostic assessment. Further collection and analysis of susceptibility data from the Vietnam resistance network of 16 hospitals will allow formal standards to be recommended' (Li et al. 2016). At the beginning of August 2017, Vietnam launched a 'National Action Plan for management of antibiotic use and control of antibiotic resistance in livestock production and aquaculture 2017–2020'. This plan is intended to complement the National Action Plan launched by the Ministry of Health in June 2013 (FAO 2017).

## Microorganisms with Itchy Feet

Up to a few years ago, there were no microorganisms in Europe that were resistant to carbapenem antibiotics. However, that quickly changed, and travel played a decisive role in spreading them. Akke van der Bij, who works now at the Diakonessenhuis Hospital in Utrecht, and her Canadian colleague Johann Pitout, from the University of Calgary, wrote an article about this in the *Journal of Antimicrobial Chemotherapy* (Van der Bij and Pitout 2012). 'Not just international tourism, but also the refugee migrations caused by war result in a situation where more people are on the move than ever before. As a result, a large number of antibiotic-resistant bacteria are given a chance to move from one geographical location to another. Germs from the

Enterobacteriaceae group are one of the most important causes of severe healthcare-associated and community-acquired infections in human beings, and antibiotic-resistant strains of these bacteria have become an increasingly serious problem. As a result of international travel and tourism, there is a risk that people can become infected with antibiotic-resistant Enterobacteria, particularly CTX-M-producing[9] *Escherichia coli*, or spread them. In developed countries, links can be identified between infections and Enterobacteria producing KPC, VIM, OXA-48 and NDM[10] and hospital visits or admissions in regions where they are endemic[11]—e.g. the United States, Greece and Israel (KPC), Greece (VIM), Turkey (OXA-48)[12] and the Indian subcontinent (NDM)'.

A Swedish study of travel as a source of infection with multiresistant bacteria, carried out by the University of Linköping, shows this quite clearly. Before leaving for Africa, Asia and Latin America, ESBL was identified in 4% of travellers. After they came back, 32% were positive (Ostholm-Balkhed et al. 2013). Hundred Swedish people making trips to destinations outside Europe took part in another study for the University of Uppsala. ESBL-producing *E. coli* bacteria could be identified in 24 of the 100 participants after they returned from their trip. Eighty-eight per cent of those who travelled to India were colonised[13] when they returned. Amongst those travellers in the study who visited other countries in Asia and the Middle East, ESBL-producing *E. coli* strains could be identified in 32 and 29%, respectively (Tängdén et al. 2010). A French study confirmed the findings of the Swedish one. The researchers described how three healthy French people who travelled to India were colonised over there by carbapenemase-producing Enterobacteriaceae. In one case this was NDM-1, and in the other two, it was OXA-181. It took a month before the bacteria disappeared from the French travellers' intestines (Ruppé et al. 2014). In 2016, a study by a group of researchers at the VU University Medical Centre in Amsterdam confirmed the hypothesis that travel outside Europe is a major risk factor for faecal colonisation with ESBL-producing Enterobacteriaceae. The risk was also heightened by travel to the USA (Reuland et al. 2016).

Of the first nine Dutch patients with carbapenem-resistant bacteria to be identified, five had become infected by the bacteria in the intensive care unit of a Greek hospital, three on trips to India, and one in the Netherlands. All nine patients were infected with *Klebsiella pneumoniae*. The enzymes causing the resistance were

---

[9]CTX-M is the name of a group of plasmids that are closely related to one another. The latter are sections of DNA which are found loose in bacteria.

[10]*Klebsiella pneumoniae* carbapenemase (KPC), Verona integron-coded metallo-beta-lactamase (VIM), OXA-48 (oxacillinase) und New Delhi metallo-beta-lactamase (NDM) are all carbapenemases—enzymes that make bacteria resistant to carbapenems.

[11]A bacterium is endemic somewhere if it can be identified there by standard procedures.

[12]At ECCMID 2012 it emerged that this was already out of date, since OXA-48 was by then already endemic in Turkey, Morocco, Tunisia and India. For more on the spread of OXA-48 in Europe see for example Albiger et al. (2015) and for the global spread, see e.g. Fursova et al. (2015).

[13]If someone is colonised by bacteria they become a carrier. The bacteria multiply, but without causing disease symptoms.

identified as KPC in five cases, NDM-1 in two, and OXA-48 and VIM in one case each. In 2008–2009, for the first time in the Netherlands, there was an outbreak of *Pseudomonas aeruginosa* that the VIM-2 enzyme had made resistant to the carbapenem antibiotic imipenem. The outbreak affected the intensive care unit and ten general wards at the Erasmus University Medical Centre in Rotterdam (Van der Bij et al. 2011). Not long afterwards a second outbreak occurred, this time at the centre for severe burns injuries at the Red Cross Hospital in Beverwijk. In February 2011, a particularly resistant pseudomonas strain was identified in two patients there in quick succession. In the same period, a patient at the hospital's general intensive care unit became infected by this bacterium, which was resistant to all antibiotics except colistin. Tests revealed that the bacteria involved were genetically identical. Two of the three patients developed a sepsis. A retrospective study carried out afterwards revealed that between 2006 and 2011, a total of 14 patients had become colonised with these VIM bacteria at the centre for severe burns injuries of the Red Cross Hospital, and seven more in the general intensive care unit. The bacterium had, therefore, already been present in the hospital for 5 years before the outbreak was noticed. According to clinical microbiologist Bram Diederen, at that time working at the regional healthcare laboratory in Haarlem, this oversight had been possible 'because there was no temporal or spatial coincidence of cases'. Since it had not affected the patients simultaneously and surfaced in different wards, the outbreak only became apparent when two cases occurred in the severe burns centre simultaneously (Diederen et al. 2012). Because of the highly pathogenic nature of VIM-2 *Pseudomonas aeruginosa,* a study was carried out immediately after the outbreak at the Red Cross Hospital, in order to investigate how often VIM-producing *Pseudomonas aeruginosa* strains appear in the Netherlands. The study was able to identify VIM-2-producing bacteria in eight Dutch hospitals, two burn wound centres and a long-term care facility between 2010 and 2011. Eighty-five per cent of the VIM-2 bacteria strains found were genetically identical. 'Since isolates producing metallo-beta-lactamase cause severe infections that are difficult to treat', the researchers wrote, 'the discovery of isolates of the same clone in several hospitals in the Netherlands must be regarded as a significant national problem' (Van der Bij et al. 2012). A recent meta-analysis shows that there are two important risk factors for the occurrence of carbapenem-resistant *Pseudomonas aeruginosa:* the use of carbapenems, and the deployment of medical devices such as catheters and infusion systems (Voor in 't Holt et al. 2014).

## The First Carbapenemases in Germany

During the period in which the first outbreaks of carbapenemase-producing bacteria occurred in Dutch hospitals, the same thing happened in Germany. In an article that appeared in the *European Journal of Clinical Microbiology and Infectious Diseases* in March 2010, scientists and doctors from Heidelberg described the first verified case of KPC in Germany. In January 2008 a *Klebsiella pneumoniae* was identified in the wound fluid of an intensive care patient at the University Hospital Heidelberg, which was resistant to ertapenem and a number of other antibiotics. Since the bacterium was still susceptible to meropenem and imipenem, the staff did not immediately think of KPC. But when identical Klebsiella isolates were isolated from the respiratory tracts of two other patients in the same department, it was confirmed that they were dealing with KPC-2. The isolation measures introduced, and the training given to medical staff on KPC and how to deal with it, were not able to prevent five more patients from becoming infected by June 2008. All eight colonised patients became severely ill. Three developed a critical infection and died of it. At the end of 2008, 5 months after the last patient to be affected by the outbreak, a KPC-producing *Klebsiella pneumoniae* was once again isolated in another patient. The patient had previously received cancer treatment in Greece. 'During determination of the type', the authors wrote, 'it emerged that these isolates were indistinguishable from those associated with the outbreak'. In November 2007, this patient had been treated in the same intensive care unit as the index patient of the KPC outbreak. 'The KPC *Klebsiella pneumoniae* had possibly been introduced into Germany from Greece, and it is probable that it has been carried to other treatment facilities' (Wendt et al. 2010).

In response to questions in parliament, the German federal government presented an overview of all known reports of carbapenemase-producing bacteria from hospitals during the period 2008 to the end of August 2013. The report showed all resistances to meropenem and imipenem separately. The absolute figures are low, but the trend is nevertheless clear. A constant increase in the number of reports of carbapenemase-producing bacteria can be identified from 2008 onwards (Widmann-Mauz 2013). This trend has not changed since then. In June 2017, the German national reference laboratory NRZ published its annual report on carbapenemase in Germany. The number of isolates submitted increased by 12% between 2015 and 2016. Of the 5878 isolates with reduced susceptibility to carbapenems, half of these were either a *Pseudomanas aeruginosa* or a *Klebsiella pneumoniae*. Two thousand, two hundred and sixty-two of the suspect isolates actually carried a carbapenemase. Among those *Enterobacteriaceae* tested, OXA-48 was by far the most frequent carbapenemase, followed by VIM-1, KPC-2 and NDM-1. In *Pseudomonas aeruginosa,* VIM-2 is mainly predominant. Finally, in *Acinetobacter baumannii* OXA-23 was as predominant as in previous years. Nevertheless, the diversity of the carbapenemase genes found by the NRZ increased sharply, from 24 in 2015 to 38 in 2016 (Pfennigwerth 2017). In 2017, 6481 isolates with reduced susceptibility to carbapenems were submitted to the NRZ. *Pseudomonas aeruginosa* (1532) and *Klebsiella pneumoniae* (1412) were the most frequent isolates. Among the suspect isolates, 2533 carried a carbapenemase. Almost all 500 isolates of *Acinetobacter baumannii* submitted were resistant to carbapenems. For *E. coli* and *K. pneumoniae* more than half were and for *P. aeruginosa* a little more than a quarter. OXA-48 was by far the most predominant carbepenase, followed by VIM-1, NDM-1 and KPC-2 (Pfennigwerth 2018). In 2018, the number of carbapenemase-producing *Enterobacteriaceae* isolates increased further, as did the number of isolates carrying more than one carbapenemase gene. OXA-48 overall remained the most frequent found carbapenemase, but in *Pseudomonas aeruginosa* VIM-2 was predominant, as was OXA-23 in *Acinetobacter baumannii* (Pfennigwerth 2019). The picture did not change in 2019. A slight increase of the number of isolates carrying a carbapenemase, in total 2.843, and the same types of carbapenmase remained predominant (Pfennigwerth 2020).

Matthias Pulz is President of the Lower Saxony Regional Health Authority in Hannover. 'All of us treat 4MRGN[14] and, above all, carbapenemase-producing bacteria with great respect, since we have almost nothing left to treat them with. If the germs spread, then we have an enormous problem. We now have some new recommendations on how to handle them, but at present I would not venture to make any prognoses about these. I hope that we'll succeed in recognising these outbreaks in the early stages and keeping the problem contained. In retrospect, we in Germany have waited too long before tightening up our strategies where MRSA is concerned. We thought we could somehow keep things contained, and then suddenly we were faced with over 20 per cent. We certainly still have methodological problems with these Gram-negative germs as well. In contrast to MRSA these form a colourful array of quite different pathogens, and it isn't so easy to determine everything immediately by running a test. Once the germ is there, the people remain colonised. Unlike with MRSA, we can't try to counteract the colonisation by decolonisation. That means the basic conditions tend to be even less favourable than with MRSA. You just have to live with that'.

## No.1: But on the Wrong Lists

Greece is the no. 1 user of antibiotics in Europe. The Greeks use more than one and a half times the European average, and as much as three and a half times the usage in the Netherlands, which is the lowest in Europe (ECDC 2020a). In March 2018, the *Proceedings of the National Academy of Sciences* (PNAS) published a major study on the 'global increase and geographic convergence in antibiotic consumption between 2000 and 2015'. Carried out by an international team of researchers, the study analysed trends in antibiotic consumption in 76 countries, making it the largest study of its kind ever attempted. Between 2000 and 2015, the overall global usage of antibiotics in human medicine increased by 39%, from 11.3 defined daily doses (DDDs) per 1000 of population per day to 15.7. The total human consumption increased by 65%, from an estimated 21.1 billion DDDs to an estimated 34.8 billion. The rise in total usage is higher than the increase in DDDs per 1000 of the population per day due to the increase in the world population. The increase in antibiotic consumption is driven by low- and middle-income countries, where the rate of antibiotic consumption 'is rapidly converging to rates similar to high-income countries'. In low- to middle-income countries, the researchers found there was 'a significant positive association between gross domestic product per capita and

---

[14]4MRGN, multiresistant Gram-negative pathogens (bacilli) with resistance to four antibiotic groups (penicillins, cephalosporins, quinolones, carbapenems).

changes in the antibiotic consumption rate'. The consumption of broad-spectrum penicillins increased by 36% worldwide between 2000 and 2015. The usage of last-resort antibiotics increased in both high-income and low- to middle-income countries (Klein et al. 2018).

Back to Greece. The resistance rates in Greece for most bacteria under surveillance were the highest in the EU for years, and this still applies to several types, such as carbapenem resistance in *Klebsiella pneumoniae* or *Acinetobacter* spp. Naturally, therefore, Greece is often cited as the source of the outbreaks that doctors in other countries have to control. The 2019 ECDC data on the number of invasive isolates of *Acinetobacter Sp.* with resistance to carbapenems, as reported in the ECDC Surveillance Atlas of Infectious Diseases, show a mean value of 32.6% for the 27 EU/EEA countries contributing data. In Greece and Croatia, 92% of all invasive Acinetobacter isolates are resistant to carbapenems, in Romania, Lithuania and Latvia far more than 80% and in Italy almost 80%. The best-performing countries are Denmark, Norway, Finland and the Netherlands with a value close to zero or zero (ECDC 2020b).

Olympia Zarkotou is a microbiologist at the Tzaneio Hospital in Piraeus. The work that she and her colleagues perform could very aptly be described by such terms as 'labours of Hercules' or 'Sisyphean tasks'. 'In the hospital we are, of course, confronted by all these infections with highly resistant bacteria which in the Netherlands, for example, don't exist. This is one factor that partly explains the high use of antibiotics, but naturally the question also arises: what was there first, the chicken or the egg? Did the frequent use of antibiotics come first, or the resistant bacteria? The use of antibiotics is also high outside hospitals. We haven't succeeded in reducing use, for example by restraining from treating viral infections with antibiotics. Even though they don't help at all in such cases, doctors still prescribe them because of patient pressure. In the patients' eyes, a doctor who doesn't prescribe antibiotics isn't a good doctor. The frequent use of antibiotics leads to resistance, which makes it necessary to use even more effective antibiotics, which in turn leads to more resistance, and so on. We're caught in a vicious circle'.

In Greece, many antibiotics are obtained without a prescription. 'There are several other countries in which this happens', says Dominique Monnet, Expert and Coordinator of the Department for Antibiotic Resistance and Nosocomial Infections at the European Centre for Disease Prevention and Control (ECDC). 'Selling antibiotics without a prescription is illegal in all member states of the European Union. And this abuse is certainly a partial explanation for the problem'. Olympia Zarkotou stresses that not all antibiotics are available without a prescription, and then goes on to describe the role of pharmacists in Greece. 'Of course, no antibiotics at all should be sold without a prescription, but the pharmacists in Greece play a special role. Every district has its own pharmacy, and everyone knows their pharmacist. They're a neighbour, a kind of friend you have your morning coffee with in the café. And this 'friend' naturally doesn't refuse to sell you an antibiotic if you want one'. Anna-Pelagia Magiorakos, one of Monnet's colleagues at the ECDC, is Greek and has very precise knowledge of the situation in her homeland. 'In reality this still happens, but recently a lot has been done to ensure that no medicines are being handed out without a prescription any more. For example, doctors must now write their prescriptions electronically. This makes it much more difficult to sell without a prescription or copy a prescription, which also occurred. These changes were certainly introduced for economic reasons, but in part they're also political decisions'.

The Greek health ministry has also carried out several information campaigns to explain to the population that the unnecessary use of large quantities of antibiotics is a bad thing. 'But paediatricians, for example, find themselves in a very difficult situation. Parents are often very frightened of fever and exercise considerable pressure on them. Greek children take large quantities of macrolides.[15] And of course, what's the result? The streptococci become very resistant to antibiotics. But this massive use of antibiotics is only one of the problems. Another, completely different problem is what to do about the high percentage of multiresistant bacteria in hospitals'.

Since 2010, the health ministry and the HCDCP,[16] the Greek equivalent of the CDC in the US, have had an action plan. 'The most important aims of the plan are surveillance—in order to be able to form a reliable picture of the situation—and a mandatory obligation to report infections by multiresistant bacteria. But for this, serious surveillance and honest reporting are required. Apart from the information from the EARS-net[17] we have no insight into what's going on in Greece. How many patients are carrying a multiresistant bacterium, how many have fallen sick because of an infection, and how many patients die of an infection? We don't know. And it's also very important that the plan includes centrally agreed recommendations for identifying multiresistant bacteria and about measures for preventing and treating infections. If you don't know precisely how and where to look for multiresistant bacteria, then you have a problem with infection prevention'. Roughly a month after my conversation with Zarkotou, the HCDCP published the first results of Action Plan Procrustes.[18] Up to this point, out of a total of 133 Greek hospitals, 64 public and military hospitals had taken part in this surveillance network. As part of a major cost-cutting exercise, the government plans to reduce the number of hospitals to approximately 80. This would reduce the number of hospital beds to approximately 30,000, compared with more than 54,000 in 2009. To put it differently, this equals

---

[15]A group of antibiotics that are principally effective against Gram-positive bacteria such as streptococci and pneumococci. The best-known are erythromycin und clarithromycin.

[16]Hellenic Centre for Disease Control and Prevention.

[17]The European Antibiotic Resistance Surveillance Network is coordinated by the ECDC in Stockholm. Over 900 laboratories from EU countries supply data. They work for 1400 hospitals, which are responsible for approx. 100 million people.

[18]Procrustes is a character from Greek mythology. He was an innkeeper who offered his guests food and drink. When they went to bed, he checked that they fitted the bed exactly. If they did not, they were forcibly stretched. However, if there were too long, he cut them down to the correct size by hacking off their limbs. According to Olympia Zartokou, Procrustes' lack of scruples is a metaphor for the strict measures that are necessary to restrict antibiotics use and antibiotic resistance to an acceptable level once again.

480 hospital beds per 100,000 inhabitants in 2009, and 273 per 100,000 after the reduction. By the end of December 2018, Greece had 45,045 hospital beds left, that is 427 beds per 100,000 (Statista 2020a). By way of comparison, according to Dutch data, there were 39,900 hospital beds in the Netherlands at the end of 2018, which equals 231 hospital beds per 100,000 of the population (De Staat van Volksgezondheid en Zorg 2020). According to data from the German Hospital Federation, at the end of 2018, there were still 498,000 hospital beds in Germany for 82.8 million people, which equals 600 beds per 100,000 inhabitants. Still, the number of hospital beds sharply reduced compared to the 666,000 beds in 1991 (D-Statis 2020).

## India, Where All the Plagues of Egypt Come From

India is possibly linked even more so with any kinds of 'superbugs' that keep cropping up than Greece. This term refers to highly resistant pathogens, which can cause infections that can hardly be treated any more, or cannot be treated at all. With regard to this matter, the Indian health ministry speaks of 'malicious propaganda'. It has been suggested in the Indian parliament that a conspiracy of multinational companies is involved. In India, the pharmaceutical industry and medical tourism are booming businesses (BBC 2010). Just like Vietnam, there is also a GARP report about India which was published in March 2011 (GARP 2011). Of course, it is easy to say things on paper, but without a group of pioneers who want to limit the excessive use of antibiotics, improve the inadequate access to medicines of a large part of the population, and remedy the dire lack of sanitary facilities in India, nothing will change. And this is not just a problem for India's 1.2 billion people, but also for the rest of the world. It is a gigantic problem. The British professor Timothy Walsh estimates that around 100 million Indians are carrying intestinal bacteria with NDM-1. Walsh has also investigated drinking water and surface water samples from New Delhi for NDM-1. Four per cent of the drinking water samples and 30% of the surface water samples were contaminated with NDM-1 bacteria (Walsh et al. 2011). After this second article was published in *The Lancet Infectious Diseases,* the Indian government once again reacted critically to Walsh and his co-authors—although less so than after the publication of his first article on NDM on 12 August 2010 (Kumarasamy et al. 2010). At that time, considerable pressure was exerted on Walsh's Indian co-authors in particular. The Indian scientists were even instructed not to concern themselves with NDM-1 any longer. They were also informed that it is illegal to send bacterial strains abroad. But in the same month that Walsh's second article appeared, the Indian government made financial resources available for research into NDM-1. Christina Vandenbroucke-Grauls, Professor and, until October 2017, Head of the Department of Medical Microbiology at the VU University Medical Centre in Amsterdam, visited India in October 2011 to take part in a conference. 'The Indians now seem to becoming proactive themselves. They are beginning to understand that they themselves have to do something to stop all bacteria from becoming resistant to all the medicines that are still available to us. This makes one feel somewhat more positive again. While over there I noticed, despite all the problems, there are doctors who have the courage to tackle these vast problems with infection prevention and further training of colleagues. I was in a state-run hospital in Mumbai that was incredibly old, dirty and overcrowded. But the microbiologist there was an impressive woman, who tried to do everything that was possible'. The GARP report on India hits the nail on the head. 'The infectious disease burden in India is among the highest in the world. A large amount of antibiotics are consumed in fighting infections, some of them saving lives, but every use adding to antibiotic resistance in bacteria' (GARP 2011).

Between 2005 and 2010, the profits from carbapenem antibiotics in Indian pharmacies more or less quadrupled (CCDEP 2011). The trend was similar in Pakistan. In many cases, no doctor was consulted nor any prescription issued, which suggests that we are often looking at unnecessary use. At the same time, many Indians have no access to antibiotics, and certainly none at all to the relatively expensive carbapenems. Around 8% of all deaths in India are the result of diarrhoeal diseases, and a further 6% are caused by infections of the respiratory tracts. More than 5 million children under five contract pneumonia or a sepsis ever year. In 2005 and 2006, only 13% of children with pneumonia received antibiotics, and only a third of children with pneumonia symptoms were taken to a doctor. And this is a problem of poverty. Besides the lack of money other factors also play a role, such as the low level of education and the lack of hospitals, clinics and doctors in some parts of the country. At the same time, there is considerable misuse of antibiotics. This is linked to the lack of knowledge about how to manage antibiotics correctly on the part of doctors and the general public—and not just in India. Patients' expectations also play a role, as well as, of course, the desires of pharmacists—and some doctors—to earn money from the sale of medicines. At the time the report appeared, 20% of all antibiotics in New Delhi were sold over the counter without a prescription. Between 2005 and 2009, the registered turnover in antibiotics outside hospitals in India almost doubled. In 1995, 3% of India's GDP went on healthcare expenses; in 2017 the figure was 3.53% (World Bank 2020a). According to World Bank data, in 2017 almost 63% of all healthcare expenditure in India came out of people's own pockets—one of the highest out-of-pocket rates in the world. In many Western countries, the ratio is the precise opposite (World Bank 2020b). State expenditure on healthcare has increased in recent years, and more people have been given access to healthcare provision. But in such a vast country as India, with its enormous population, the situation is improving only very slowly.

In India, there are not really any reliable data on the occurrence of resistance, because there is no national system of surveillance. There are also hardly any data on the use of antibiotics for animals. However, scientists addressing the use of antibiotics and resistance to them in cattle, poultry and seafood have found high rates of resistance to a number of antibiotics (Singh 2009).

## The Scoping Report

For the CCDEP, who published the 2011 GARP report on India, the fact that our knowledge of antibiotic resistance rates in India continues to contain several gaps was the spur to undertake a new study, commissioned by a branch of the Indian government. *The Scoping report on antimicrobial resistance in India* was published in November 2017 (Gandra et al. 2017). 'AMR is a global public health threat, but nowhere it is as stark as in India', the authors write in the summary of their report. 'India has some of the highest resistance rates among bacteria that commonly cause infections in community and healthcare facilities. Resistance to broad-spectrum antibiotics, fluoroquinolones and third-generation cephalosporin was more than 70% in *Acinetobacter baumannii*, *Eschericia coli*, and *Klebsiella pneumoniae*, and more than 50% in *Pseudomonas aeruginosa*'. Not surprisingly this leads to high usage, and thus high rates of resistance to last-resort carbapenems. 'The highest level of carbapenems resistance was observed in *A. baumannii* (either 67.3% or 70.9%, depending on the study), followed by *K. pneumoniae* (56.6% or 56.6%), *P. aeruginosa* (46.8% or 41.8%) and *E. coli* (11.5% or 16.2%)'. The authors also note the appearance of colistin resistance in Gram-negative bacteria, a logical consequence of the increase in the use of colistin to treat carbapenem-resistant bacterial infections. 'However, known plasmid-mediated colistin resistance genes *mcr-1* and *mcr-2* were not detected frequently'. They stress the important role antibiotic usage in livestock farming plays in human health, 'since antibiotic-resistant bacteria can be transmitted between humans and animals through contact, food, and from the environment'. The researchers quote a series of studies reporting isolates of ESBL-producing *E. coli* in poultry and pigs, Gram-negative bacteria producing NDM-1 and ESBL in milk and, in one study, VRSA (vancomycin-resistant *S. Aureus*) in milk from cows with mastitis. In aquaculture the findings were similar. *The 2017 Scoping report on antimicrobial resistance in India* states that 'a limited number of published studies on the environment indicate high levels of antibiotic-resistant bacteria and antibiotic-resistance genes (ARGs) in various bodies of water' (Gandra et al. 2017). Hospital wastewater contains high levels of bacteria resistant to antibiotics, for example third-generation cephalosporins, as do some major Indian rivers. Antibiotic resistance genes that make bacteria resistant were in fact also found in major rivers in India, including genes that confer resistance to last-resort antibiotics. The authors quote studies that detected the genes CTX-M, NDM-1 and *mcr-1* in rivers. Sources for drinking water and recreational water also contain microbes with high levels of resistance to broad-spectrum antibiotics, especially third-generation cephalosporins. 'And a study involving four tap water samples, one borehole water sample and 23 environmental water samples in the Hyderabad area found that among 23 environmental samples, 22 had Enterobacteriaceae and other gram-negative bacteria, 100% of them were ESBL-producing, and more than 95% were producing blaOXA-48 producers'. Interestingly enough, some important pharmaceutical factories are located in Hyderabad. The pharmaceutical industry is big in India. According to the GARP study, there are at least 40 companies in India that produce active pharmaceutical ingredients for antibiotics, and 250 factories that produce at least one antibiotic for human use. Although India has established standards for pharmaceutical wastewater, there are no such standards for residues of antibiotics in wastewater. Antibiotic pollution by wastewater is only one of the many drivers of antibiotic resistance in India that the authors mention. These also include (high) consumption of antibiotics in humans and animals, high consumption of broad-spectrum antibiotics, heavy prescription of fixed-dose combinations of two antibiotics, poor infection control practices in hospitals, and social factors such as self-medication, over-the-counter sales of antibiotics without prescription, lack of knowledge of the proper use of antibiotics, mass bathing as part of religious gatherings and, of course, the sanitation situation in India, which is still very poor.

## Killing Rather Than Curing

On 14 March 2012, Margaret Chan—until July 2017—General Director of the World Health Organisation (WHO)[19]—spoke at the opening ceremony of the 'Combatting Antimicrobial Resistance' conference, which was organised by the Danish Presidency of the EU in Copenhagen. Chan issued a warning: 'The antibiotic threat is easily described. It has an irrefutable logic. Antimicrobial resistance is on the rise in Europe, and elsewhere in the world. We are losing our first-line antimicrobials. Replacement treatments are more costly, more toxic, have much longer duration, and may require treatment in intensive care units'. Later in her speech the head of the WHO made an almost apocalyptic prediction. 'Hospitals have become hotbeds for highly resistant pathogens such as MRSA, ESBL, and CPE—increasing the risk that hospitalisation kills instead of cures. [...] If current trends continue unabated, the future is easy to predict. Some experts say we are moving back to the pre-antibiotic era. No. This will be a post-antibiotic era'. Chan also specified what that would mean. 'A post-antibiotic era means, in effect, an end to modern medicine as we know it. Things as common as strep throat or a child's scratched knee could once again kill. Some sophisticated interventions, like hip replacements, organ transplants, cancer chemotherapy and care of preterm infants, would become far more difficult or even too dangerous to undertake. At a time of multiple calamities in the world, we cannot allow the loss of essential antimicrobials, essential cures for many millions of people, to become the next global crisis' (Chan 2012).

Chan continued her offensive in May 2014, at the 67th World Health Assembly in Geneva, where representatives of civil society organisations from all six continents founded an Antibiotic Resistance Coalition (ARC). At the same time, the coalition adopted a resolution on antibiotic resistance, in which the delegates called on governments to increase their national efforts and develop international cooperation.

---

[19]Chan was succeeded on the 23th of May 2017 by Dr. Tedros Adhanom Ghebreyesus from Ethiopia as Director General of the WHO.

According to the declaration, this requires an exchange of information on the extent of resistance development and the use of antibiotics in humans and animals. It is also a question of improving the sensitivity of healthcare professionals and the general public towards the threat from resistance, the need for a responsible use of antibiotics, and the importance of good hand hygiene and other infection prevention measures (ARC 2014). At the same time, the 67th World Health Assembly adopted a declaration that was entirely in accord with the ARC's resolution on antibiotic resistance. Among other things, in the declaration the WHO member states were urged to improve their medicine management systems, promote research into the way the usability of the presently available antibiotics could be extended, and support the development of new diagnostic methods and treatment options (WHO 2014).

Professor Martin Mielke, Head of the Department for Infectious Diseases at the Robert Koch Institute in Berlin, welcomed the WHO declaration. 'However, we can see that in many countries resources are needed. Think of Africa or India, for example. China is actually supposed to have sufficient resources, and yet the antibiotic resistance problem there is grave. Or take South America—where, in places, very few laboratories have taken part in the surveys. Basically this is also a very important aspect—everyone around the world laying the relevant cards on the table, so as to inject some dynamism into the issue of perceiving the problem. And we must do some capacity building, and transport everything that we've established here over there. Development aid is, I think, a good task for the G8[20] to become actively involved with. It's always about countries with a problematic social structure, or crisis countries. That's comparable to the way it was in Europe at the end of the 19th century. In those days there were similar relationships here, and the greatest changes came about through improving the social structure: clean water, toilets, higher incomes, better living conditions. These are laws that can't be by-passed. There's little sense in just installing PCR[21] machines if you don't also install toilets at the same time'.

In June 2014, the World Alliance Against Antibiotic Resistance, an organisation comprising hundreds of doctors, pharmacists, nurses, microbiologists, veterinarians, biologists and patient representatives from 55 countries, published an emphatic appeal. According to the WAAAR we need a worldwide crusade in order to continue having effective antibiotics available for patients with infections. The appeal underscores the necessity for increased education of the general public and medical specialists. WAAAR also suggests that antibiotics could be included in the UNESCO world heritage list. Moreover, the group also demands that antibiotics should be made available worldwide, even for people in poor countries, and that

---

[20]The G8 (Group of Eight) is comprised of the eight richest industrial nations. It was founded in 1975 by the USA, Germany, the UK, France, Italy and Japan as the G6. As a result of Canada's entry in 1976, it became the G7. Since 1998, Russia has also been taking part, as a result of which it has become the G8. In March 2014, Russia's membership was suspended during the Crimean crisis.

[21]The polymerase chain reaction (PCR) is a test in which very small quantities of genetic material are sufficient to identify a germ quickly.

surveillance systems should be developed in all countries in order to promote and monitor the proper use of antibiotics (WAAAR 2014).

## 'This Announcement Could Have Been Made Earlier'

Problems in a neonatal department are always good for eye-catching headlines. When babies or children are involved, emotions quickly run high. The outbreak in Bremen[22] received far more attention in the media than another outbreak that occurred almost simultaneously, and which in the end proved to be much worse. This was also in Germany, but this time at the University of Leipzig Medical Centre (UKL). And here, too, the hospital did not immediately report the outbreak to the authorities. And here too it took a long time before they asked for help from outside specialists. On 9 July 2010, the hospital admitted a patient from the Leipzig area who had been on holiday on Rhodes and was in hospital there. A Klebsiella germ that produced the KPC enzyme was discovered in the man. This made the bacterium resistant to almost all antibiotics. The man was immediately isolated, hygiene measures were heightened, and the patients who had had contact with the patient, as well as the room he had stayed in, were examined. No further infections were found. Somewhat time-delayed, however, they then appeared.

In autumn 2010, an outbreak of this Klebsiella germ occurred on several wards of the hospital. Between the start of the outbreak and February 2011, when it ended, 30 patients were infected. Until January 2011, the University Medical Centre saw no reason to inform the local health authority. 'From a present-day perspective, this announcement could have been made sooner', said Medical Director Wolfgang Fleig during the press conference in which the hospital announced the outbreak. This was on 24 May 2012, more than a year later (UKL 2012). Nor was the press conference itself set up until journalists from the Mitteldeutscher Rundfunk radio station (MDR) discovered that the hospital was struggling with KPC, and questions were asked. By then the number of patients with KPC-producing Klebsiellas had already risen to 58. In almost all the cases it affected patients with severe underlying diseases. 'Obviously there is a long latency period between infection and possible detection of the germ', explained Fleig. Colonised patients who did not know that they were carrying the bacteria could therefore transfer them to other patients without being aware of it. That could explain the outbreak in autumn 2010, said Fleig at the press conference. 'The outbreak at the University of Leipzig Medical Centre could certainly have been contained by introducing additional preventative measures, but the chain of transmission could not have been definitively broken. To achieve that, people outside the UKL carrying KPC would have to be identified'.

Matthias Pulz, President of the Lower Saxony Regional Health Authority, stressed the importance of openness. 'We cannot screen every patient for KPC. That's simply not on. Therefore it's very important to tell people openly where

---

[22]See Chap. 6 The beginning of the end.

there's a problem in the region. This can prepare other hospitals for it. If a patient who is positive is transferred, then I assume that this will be communicated. I was amazed that all I ever heard was "we successfully controlled the KPC outbreak". People always like to say that. But if it isn't the case, then you have to warn others. Communication is one of the key points. You have to put your cards on the table'.

Marcus Dettenkofer, until Summer 2014 Head of the section for hospital hygiene at the University Medical Centre Freiburg and now working at the Clinic in Constance, regrets that his colleagues in Leipzig waited so long. 'It was also intriguing for us to follow this development: to see that in only the past three years in Saxony, with the University of Leipzig Medical Centre as its epicentre, there has actually been a KPC outbreak which has now been made public (Lübbert and Rodloff 2014). The staff have disclosed the data and no longer kept quiet about it. But the fact that it took a while before the significance of the outbreak was really taken seriously was naturally dramatic. Action should have been taken earlier. But now the staff have really told it like it is. And that also fits in with the idea of screening risk patients for these multiresistant gram-negative pathogens relatively consistently in large centres'.

The outbreak at the University of Leipzig Medical Centre is the biggest outbreak of such pathogenic intestinal bacteria ever identified in Germany. On 24 June 2013, the hospital published a press release announcing that the KPC outbreak was over (UKL 2013). The definitive figures appeared in the spring. Christoph Lübbert writes that between June 2010 and April 2013 a total of 103 patients were colonised with a KPC-2-producing *Klebsiella pneumoniae*, 43 patients developed an infection. 'The mean duration of hospital stay for all the 103 patients affected by KPC-2-KP was 44 days. Hospital mortality amounted to 41 per cent (42/103). The deaths of seven patients could be traced directly back to a KPC-2 infection, and in the case of 11 other patients most likely to polymicrobial infections including KPC-2' (Lübbert et al. 2014).

In spring 2014, Christoph Lübbert published yet another paper on the KPC outbreak entitled 'What can we learn from the Leipzig KPC outbreak?' (Lübbert 2014). Lübbert is in a suitable position to present speculations on this topic. From July 2012 to June 2013 he headed the internal task force of the University of Leipzig Medical Centre, in order to bring the KPC-2 outbreak under control. His most important observations are:

- 'The experience gained from the Leipzig KPC outbreak shows that separate cohorting of KPC-positive patients and KPC contact patients in inpatient areas specially set up for them, with associated demarcation of staff (i.e. deployment of nursing staff who care exclusively for KPC-positive patients or KPC contact patients) is a very important measure for the successful management of outbreaks'.
- 'In the light of the Leipzig experience, a systematic screening programme is not just an integral component of a concept for management of KPC outbreaks, but also an indispensable tool for identifying new cases entering the clinic. Here regional prevalence data should be the decisive determinant of the intensity of

screening. In a manner analogous to the already widely established MRSA screening process, therefore, a superordinate screening for carbapenem-resistant Enterobacteria (CRE) and/or 4MRGN will probably be necessary, particularly when patients are admitted to intensive care units, in order to enable at-risk populations of hospitalised patients to be effectively protected from CRE transmission'.

The ease with which the KPC-2 spread in the hospital is astonishing. 'The outbreak occurred after a 66-year-old man was admitted as an inpatient. He was suffering from a nosocomial pneumonia, and had been transferred to the University of Leipzig Medical Centre from a hospital in Rhodes, Greece, where KPC-producing Klebsiella strains are highly endemic (Munoz-Price et al. 2013). The patient was initially admitted to the hospital intensive care unit needing respiration. After the patient had been moved to a general ward—at which time the exact microbiological type of pathogen he had brought from Greece was still unknown—a fatal chain of infections began. One single night in a multi-bed room, which was occupied by a patient who later tested positive for KPC, was enough to transfer the pathogen to other patients'.

It is only when you look at the 2010 figures for all the cases of *Klebsiella pneumoniae* resistant to carbapenem antibiotics identified in Germany that the full extent of the outbreak becomes clear (Kaase 2011). The total was 113, and that included not just KPC, but all resistance mechanisms taken together. KPC was identifiable in 53 cases, in other words almost half the total. The University of Leipzig Medical Centre was responsible for half of all these cases. Even for a teaching hospital that admits severely ill patients and exchanges many patients with other hospitals, this is an excessively high percentage. In a press release dated 24 June 2013, the hospital announced: 'The analyses show that KPC can obviously survive in hospitals for a very long period. At the same time it has emerged that early isolation and long-term, intensive surveillance of pathogenic status are necessary where KPC carriers are concerned' (UKL 2013).

In May 2013, the NRZ data for 2012 were published in the *Epidemiological Bulletin* of the RKI. They show that from a total of 151 KPC-2 isolates, 59 came from Saxony, and this does not include the outbreak at the University of Leipzig Medical Centre. In their analysis, the scientists do not mince their words. 'The data collected by the NRZ make it clear that carbapenemases have not only arrived in *P. aeruginosa* and *A. baumannii,* but also in *K. pneumoniae* and other Enterobacteriaceae in Germany. In this respect the epidemiology of the carbapenemases obviously differs from that in other countries. While KPC are the most frequently occurring carbapenemases in Enterobacteriaceae in South America, the USA, China, Israel, Italy and—alongside type VIM metallo beta lactamases—Greece, the NRZ data to date indicate that there is a great diversity of carbapenemase-producing Enterobacteriaceae in Germany. (...) At present Germany is still in the initial phase of a worrying spread of carbapenem-resistant Gram-negative pathogens. (...) Since it is impossible to prevent carbapenemase-producing Gram-negative bacteria from entering hospitals via appropriate carriers, it is all the more important to identify the patients affected and avoid the spread of multiresistant pathogens within the hospital and the occurrence of severe infection through suitable measures.' The most important risk factor remains contact with the healthcare systems of other countries. 'It goes without saying that patients who were in a German hospital where they might have had contact with infected or colonised patients should be screened as well. Therefore, an exchange of information between hospitals on the appearance of 4MRGN (MRGN = multiresistant, gram-negative bacilli) is necessary, and the established regional networks could provide a suitable platform for this' (Kaase 2013). The NRZ data up till 2019 show an increasing rise in the number of carbapenemases found in Enterobacteriaceae over the years, most of all in *Klebsiella pneumoniae*. But in 2019, for the first time in 10 years, this increase was limited. OXA-48 is by far the most predominant carbapenemase, followed by VIM-1 and KPC-2 (Pfennigwerth 2020).

## Combination Therapy with Colistin

Since colistin is now used frequently to combat infections with carbapenem-resistant bacteria, resistances to colistin are increasingly being formed. Combination therapy with colistin may be a better solution. At the end of January 2015, researchers from Pennsylvania published a study of 20 patients who were connected to respiratory devices and who had contracted pneumonia as a result. Nineteen of them were treated with colistin, in order to control their infection by a carbapenem-resistant but colistin-susceptible *Acinetobacter baumannii*. After 30 days, the mortality rate was 30%. For patients who were treated with a combination of colistin, a carbapenem and ampicillin-sulbactam, the mortality rate was lowest (Qureshi et al. 2015. Researchers from the General Hospital of the Chinese People's Liberation Army in Beijing also came to the conclusion that combination therapy with colistin delivers better success rates in the treatment of carbapenem-resistant Enterobacteriaceae than monotherapy with colistin (Ni et al. 2015).

## Food Chain

Carbapenemases are the bogeyman of modern medicine, the superlative form of antibiotic resistance. It is hard to imagine what might happen if they found their way into the food chain. And yet that has already happened—for example in India, but also in Europe. In January 2014, the Federal Institute for Risk Assessment in Berlin published an unsettling newsletter. For the first time, the institute had found carbapenemase-producing bacteria in samples from livestock. These consisted of three salmonella isolates from fattened pigs and one from broiler chickens. One of the pigs was also carrying an *E. coli* with a carbapenemase gene. In all cases, the gene in question was VIM-1. As well as this, salmonella with NDM-1 was also found in a migratory bird. Similar results to the 2011 findings originally reported in 2014 were obtained in 2015 and 2016, according to an updated version of the newsletter published in December 2016 (BfR 2016). The national reference centre for Gram-negative hospital pathogens is concerned about this discovery of carbapenemases in intensive livestock farming. 'These findings too show that molecular surveillance of resistance mechanisms from clinical samples in Germany is of crucial importance' (Kaase 2013). There are not many studies on carbapenemase in livestock. A review article published in *EFSA Journal* on 17 December 2013 provides some more examples from three other countries: OXA-23-producing Acinetobacter in isolates from cattle and horses in France and Belgium and NDM-producing Acinetobacter isolates from pigs and poultry in China (EFSA 2013). In a study from January 2016 carried out on the faeces of dairy cattle on the High Plains in the American mid-West, a limited number of carbapenemase genes were detected. In an article published in *Science* in November 2017, the authors argue that much remains unclear on the extent to which livestock contribute to the spread of antimicrobial resistance (genes) in humans. 'Overall', they conclude, 'events leading to the occurrence of ESBL/AmpC- and carbapenemase-encoding genes in animals seem very much multifactorial. The impact of animal reservoirs on human health still remains debatable and unclear; nonetheless, there are some examples of direct links that have been identified' (Webb et al. 2017).

In 2018, a group of German and Dutch scientists introduced a paper that systematically reviewed topic-relevant articles from the PubMed database, published between 1980 and 2017. 'We identified 68 articles describing CRE among pigs, poultry, cattle, seafood, dogs, cats, horses, pet birds, swallows, wild boars, wild stork, gulls, and black kites in Africa, America, Asia, Australia, and Europe. The following carbapenemases have been detected (predominantly affecting the genera *Escherichia* and *Klebsiella*): VIM, KPC, NDM, OXA, and IMP. Two studies found that 33–67% of exposed humans on poultry farms carried carbapenemase-producing CRE closely related to isolates from the farm environment. Twenty-seven studies selectively screened samples for CRE and found a prevalence of <1% among livestock and companion animals in Europe, 2–26% in Africa, and 1–15% in Asia. Wildlife (gulls) in Australia and Europe carried CRE in 16–19%'. And they conclude: 'The occurrence of CRE in livestock, seafood, wildlife, pets, and directly exposed humans poses a risk for public health. Prospective prevalence studies using molecular and cultural microbiological methods are needed to better define the scope and transmission of CRE' (Köck et al. 2018).

An article in the Italian Journal of Food Safety reiterates this warning. The authors also stress the possible role of migratory birds in the spread of carbapenemases. 'Despite the use of carbapenems in food-producing animals is banned in Europe and other countries, detection of CP[23] microorganisms in livestock has been reported in EU as well as non-EU countries. Selection pressure exerted by β-lactams antimicrobial treatments in farm animals, as well as CP bacteria transmission from human sources, are considered responsible for the occurrence of CP microorganisms in livestock. Likely, meat and milk might become a source of CP

---

[23]CP, carbapenemase producing.

bacteria for the consumers, with the worst scenario to be displayed in countries with high prevalence of CP bacterial infections in humans. In this context, the role of hospital sewage and WWTPs in the environmental distribution of human CP bacteria has been effectively assessed. Furthermore, human activities on natural habitats, as the use of manure to amend soil in agricultural practises, strongly contribute to the diffusion and maintenance of resistance bacteria and their transferable genetic elements in the terrestrial and aquatic environments. In this scenario, wild animals, and especially migratory birds, may amplify both maintenance and long-distance distribution of CP microorganisms' (Bonardi and Pitino 2019).

## KPC on the American East Coast

KPC was identified for the first time in 1996 in the US state of North Carolina. The first scientific paper addressing this was published some 20 years ago (Yigit et al. 2001). Up until 2005 eight types of KPC had appeared, which are all very closely related. The dominant types are KPC-2 and KPC-3. KPC appears most frequently in the north-east of the United States. In New York, there have been regular outbreaks since 2003. In autumn 2004, a quarter of all the *Klebsiella pneumoniae* in the hospitals of Brooklyn contained the KPC enzyme (Bratu et al. 2005). According to data from the Center for Disease Control in the USA, in 2007, 8% of all *Klebsiella pneumoniae* investigated were producing KPC (CDC 2009). In the same year, KPC also reached Chicago.

Researchers described a 2008 outbreak in four neighbouring counties in Illinois and Indiana. Centered around one acute care hospital but affecting none less than 26 health care institutions. The patients were frequently transferred between hospitals and long-time care facilities, making it easy for resistant bacteria to spread. Intensive contact between hospitals within a region also played an important role (Won et al. 2011).

This same phenomenon is shown very neatly by a study carried out in Orange County, California, in which all the 32 hospitals located there took part. Of the 173,000 patients admitted to hospitals in Orange County in 2005, approximately 30% were admitted at least twice. On average, these readmissions took place within 53 days of being discharged from the hospital. In all the total number of hospital admissions was 320,000, and three-quarters of the group who stayed in the hospital multiple times (approx. 35,000 patients) were admitted to more than one hospital. The researchers calculated that within a 6-month period, 6 of the 32 hospitals in Orange County shared patients with more than half the other hospitals in the county. After a year the number of hospitals that shared patients with more than half the hospitals in the region was 17. They shared at least one patient with the other hospitals but in average 28. These figures included both patients with and without an infection (Huang et al. 2010).

On New Year's Eve 2013, the CDC published an alarming graph depicting the 'Threat from a nightmare bacterium'. In 2001, KPC was identified in one hospital in one American state. By 2013 KPC had spread to healthcare facilities in

46 states (CDC 2013a). In New York, New Jersey and Chicago the bacterium was already endemic. This rapid proliferation must certainly have been one of the factors contributing to the publication of the report *Antibiotic Resistance Threats in the United States 2013* by the Center for Disease Control in September 2013. The report describes the status of antibiotic resistance in the USA very precisely: more than 2 million cases of illness, 23,000 deaths and tens of billion dollars in additional treatment expenses and social costs (CDC 2013b). By 2017, there were at least 18 variants of KPC known (Stoesser et al. 2017).

At the end of 2013, the US Food and Drug Administration (FDA) published a plan for reducing antibiotic resistance. This included measures that had to be implemented voluntarily by the pharma industry, veterinary surgeons and farmers. In this way, the FDA hopes to ensure that no antibiotics that are important for humans are used in livestock farming, that no more animal feed containing these substances is manufactured, and that the use of antibiotics by veterinarians without a prescription is curtailed. In the USA three quarters of all for human beings important antibiotics are used 'in an unjudicious manner' for intensive livestock farming (FDA 2013). The FDA has been severely criticised for this plan. The National Resources Defense Council (NRDC) expressed itself in very negative terms: 'The FDA's policy is an early holiday gift to industry. It is a hollow gesture that does little to tackle a widely recognised threat to human health. The FDA has essentially followed a voluntary approach for more than 35 years, but use of these drugs to raise animals has increased. There's no reason why voluntary recommendations will make a difference now, especially when the FDA's policy covers only some of the many uses of antibiotics on animals that are not sick. The FDA is failing the American people' (NRDC 2013). The Pew Charitable Trusts were less severe in their reaction. This important lobby group welcomed the initiative. 'There's a lot more that must still be done, but this is a very promising start, particularly after decades of stagnation', said Laura Rogers, Director of the PEW Human Health and Farming campaign (PEW 2013).

## Mega-Outbreak in Israel

Professor Yehuda Carmeli is Head of the Department for Epidemiology and Preventative Medicine at the Tel Aviv Medical Centre. I had a conversation with him during the ECCMID 2012 European congress of microbiologists in London. 'Up to 2005, we in Israel had never actually seen a Klebsiella with KPC', said Carmeli. 'But in the course of 2006, that changed at lightning speed'. At the end of 2005, someone from the USA brought KPC to Israel. A patient with KPC was admitted to one of the Israelian hospitals. Even though they had received a kidney transplant in Miami shortly before, they were placed in the intensive care unit without isolation. 'The patient had brought a letter from the US with them, stating that he was colonised with KPC, but the surgeon who admitted him didn't know what that was', says Carmeli. 'Nine other patients in the intensive care unit promptly became colonised with KPC. Some of them died'.

The Klebsiellas with KPC caused an unprecedented outbreak that spread throughout the whole of Israel (Schwaber et al. 2011). 'On the day after admission, a urine culture of the patient was ordered', explained Carmeli. 'One day later it was suspected that he had antibiotic resistance to carbapenems. While this was being confirmed a technical problem arose, and then came the weekend'. Carmeli relates this with a sense of shame, shaking his head. After the weekend, the patient was confirmed as having KPC, and it was possible to start contact tests of his fellow patients. 'That's the story of the outbreak in one of the hospitals', he said. The KPC spread like wildfire across the whole country. In the first 6 months of 2006, the number of patients in Israel rose by 40 new cases per month, and in the second half of the same year by 89 KPC patients per month. In the first quarter of 2007, there were on average 143 new patients per month. In March, it was as many as 185 new patients. On 31 March 2007, there were 1275 patients in 27 different hospitals that had been infected by a KPC bacterium. In 92% of cases, this was *Klebsiella pneumoniae*. Eight per cent involved other bacteria to which KPC had migrated.

'By the beginning of 2006 it was clear to me almost at once that it was not possible to stop the outbreak. And what applies in my hospital naturally applies to the other hospitals as well. It was then that we decided to tackle the outbreak nationwide'. The health ministry published guidelines on isolating carriers of KPC. They had to be strictly isolated in single rooms or treated by cohort care in one room together. Additionally, a system was introduced in which nursing staff caring for KPC-positive patients were forbidden from caring for any non-infected patients during the same shift. That is important, because bacteria are often spread by the nursing staff. On top of this, a task force for antibiotic resistance and infection prevention was set up. These specialists visited all the hospitals, in order to ensure that the campaign against the outbreak could be coordinated. Between May and September 2007, the number of new infections fell to 57 per month. In October, there was a renewed sharp increase to 87 new patients, but then a downward trend appeared. In May 2008, there were still 45 reports of new patients infected by a KPC-producing bacterium. Up to the present day, Israel has still been unable to completely resolve its KPC problem. The outbreak was accompanied by a significantly increased mortality rate. Of all the patients in Israel who contracted an infection caused by a KPC-producing bacterium, almost half died (44%). Other countries with high rates of KPC cases, such as Greece and the USA, reported similar mortality rates. Carmeli thinks that the number of deaths actually caused by the KPC infections is somewhat lower than the high mortality rate of 44% might suggest. 'Based on previous findings, the corrected figure for mortality caused by these bacteria can be estimated at around 35 per cent', he says in one of his many articles on the Israeli outbreak (Schwaber and Carmeli 2008). Four thousand to six thousand patients die annually in Israel from all healthcare-associated infections taken together, as was revealed during a debate in the Knesset, the Israeli parliament on 1 January 2014. Carmeli was one of the experts who had been invited to the Knesset as a speaker (Jerusalem Post 2014). In a meta-analysis of the relevant studies published before 9 April 2012, Greek researchers established that patient mortality resulting from infection with carbapenem-resistant Enterobacteriaceae—which, in almost all cases, means *Klebsiella pneumoniae*—fluctuates between 26 and 44%. The researchers also found that the mortality resulting from infections by a carbapenem-resistant Enterobacter is twice as high as the mortality caused by infections with *Enterobacteriaceae* that are susceptible to carbapenems (Falagas et al. 2014).

Meanwhile, KPC has spread over the entire world. During one session at ECCMID 2012, reports of large and small KPC outbreaks in a whole series of countries in Asia, North America, Latin America and Europe followed one after the other. In the Netherlands, too, the number of carbapenemases has already been increasing for several years. The absolute figures are not very high, but the upward trend gives experts cause for concern. In 2011, a total of 169 Gram-negative bacteria strains with carbapenemases were discovered. Most of these came from the 117 patients from the Maasstad outbreak of OXA-48-producing *Klebsiella pneumoniae* known at that time. Similar bacteria were found in 30 patients from other Dutch hospitals (RIVM 2012). In 2012, 68 carbapenemases were identified, two-thirds of which were found in *Klebsiella pneumoniae*. In over half these cases (36), the resistance mechanism was OXA-48 (RIVM 2013). In 2013, the number of carbapenemases rose to 91. In over half the cases this was OXA-48. In 60% of the cases the bacteria were Klebsiella pneumoniae, and in 30% *Eschericia coli* (RIVM 2014). In 2014 there was a decrease in the number of carbapenemase genes detected: 66. Roughly half of these were OXA-48. *K. pneumoniae* was involved in almost two-thirds of all cases (RIVM 2015). In 2015, there was an increase in the number of carbapenemase-producing isolates detected by the Dutch national reference laboratory at the RIVM. A total of 130 unique isolates were found, originating from 124 people. Almost 40% carried OXA-48, and 35% NDM (Nethmap/Maran 2016). The upward trend continued in 2016 as the RIVM detected 165 unique carbapenemase-producing *Enterobacteriaceae* isolates obtained from 151 different persons. Eighty-three of the isolates carried an OXA-48 gene, and 49 an NDMgene (Nethmap/Maran 2017). In 2017, 235 unique carbapenemase-producing *Enterobacteriaceae* isolates were obtained from 201 different persons (Nethmap/ Maran 2018) and that number increased further in 2018 to 306 unique carbapenemase-producing *Enterobacteriaceae* isolates from 266 persons (Nethmap/Maran 2019). The most frequently identified genes encoding for carbapenemases were like in 2017: OXA-48, NDM, VIM and KPC. In 2019, a total of 363 unique carbapenemase-producing *Enterobacteriaceae* isolates—most of the time *Klebsiella pneumoniae* and *Eschericia coli*—were obtained from 316 persons, again a relatively big increase in the number of collected carbapenenmase genes, predominantly OXA-48, NDM-5 and NDM-1 (Nethmap/ Maran 2020).

In 2017, there were three outbreaks with carbapenemase-producing *Enterobacteriaceae*, in 2018 four, among which one bigger in the Zaans MC, a general hospital in Zaandam, a town north of Amsterdam. That outbreak continued until fall 2019. Since February 2018 in total 39 patients were detected as carrying an NDM-1positive *Citrobacter freundii*. One patient died of an infection by this microbe. In 2019, two new outbreaks of carbapenemase-producing *Enterobacteriaceae* occurred.

## KPC-Outbreak

In 2013, the first KPC outbreak occurred in the Netherlands. It was actually a double outbreak, but a limited one. In August 2013, the Amphia Hospital in Breda admitted a patient who had spent 5 weeks in an intensive care unit in Greece. The woman was KPC-positive. She was treated under isolation, but nevertheless, the bacterium was transferred to a second patient. The woman who had been infected in Greece was transferred to a nursing home and isolated according to all the necessary procedures. Two months later, KPC was identified in a patient from the same section of the nursing home. Despite heightened hygiene and infection prevention measures, three more patients in the nursing home became infected with the KPC. They were transferred to a separate section of the nursing home, where they were looked after by staff who never came into contact with other patients. Two of the patients died in December. One of these deaths involved a KPC infection. The KPC isolates were not only resistant to carbapenem antibiotics, but also to colistin (Weterings et al. 2015).

In October 2017, a group of Dutch researchers published a study on what they called 'the unnoticed spread to different regions' of carbapenemase-producing *Enterobacteriaceae*. They found that 8 isolates of NDM-1-producing *Klebsiella pneumoniae*, originating from 8 patients in 4 different hospitals and a long-term care facility, were closely related genetically to isolates from 26 patients collected during a hospital outbreak in the southern part of the Netherlands. Since the authors found no indications of shared exposure or contact between the outbreak patients and the others, they concluded that CPE is quietly spreading throughout the Netherlands. Healthcare institutions seem to play a role in the spread of this NDM-1-producing *K. pneumoniae*. 'These unexpected findings underline the importance of national surveillance of CPE and the use of NGS' (next-generation sequencing, a method for establishing the complete genetic code of a microorganism) (Leenstra et al. 2017).

## Sint-Niklaas and Duffel

In Belgium, the first Gram-negative bacterium resistant to carbapenems was identified in 2008. The case involved five different patients in three Brussels hospitals, who were all colonised by VIM-producing *Klebsiella pneumoniae*. Two patients came from two different Greek hospitals, where they had been treated after a serious car accident. In the middle of 2010, Klebsiellas with NDM-1 also appeared. Patients who had been in Pakistan and the Balkans brought the bacteria back to Belgium with them. In a statement, the Health Council of Belgium wrote that 'in the first ten months of 2011, epidemics were identified in three hospitals and sporadic cases of CPE were found in a dozen institutions. Most of the patients affected had not previously visited any country where CPE was endemic' (Hoge Gezondheidsraad

2011). In response to this, a national surveillance system for CPE was introduced from 1 January 2012. 'Where carbapenemases are concerned, we reacted pretty quickly', says Professor Youri Glupczynski, Head of the Department for Medical Microbiology at the UCL University Clinic Mont Godinne of the Catholic University of Leuven. Among other things, Glupczynski's laboratory at the Mont Godinne hospital is also the national reference lab for carbapenemases. Two of the outbreaks that occurred in 2011 were major: one at Duffel near Mechelen, and the other at the Nikolaas general hospital in Sint Niklaas, near Antwerp. In both outbreaks it was predominantly *Klebsiella pneumoniae* with OXA-48 that was involved.

On 1 July 2012, precisely 100 patients in the Sint-Niklaas hospital were colonised by OXA-48-producing bacteria. In most cases, these consisted of *Klebsiella pneumoniae*. By the end, more than 180 patients had become infected by OXA-48. It was not until the second half of 2013 that the outbreak showed signs of slowly abating—although according to Bart Galloway, the Clinical Microbiologist of the Antwerp hospital network, even by the end of February 2014 it was still not completely over.[24] In the Sint-Maarten Hospital in Duffel, the outbreak was under control much sooner. On 1 July 2012, there were 13 patients, one of whom developed a severe infection. After this, a few more infections with the outbreak germ occurred sporadically at the Duffel hospital.

In 2012, a total of 478 carbapenemase-producing bacteria (CPEs) were identified in Belgium, 469 CPEs were detected in 2013, and 276 in the first half of 2014. In 2012 three quarters of these cases involved *Klebsiella pneumoniae,* and in 2014 the figure was still a little less than 60% of cases. The resistance mechanism was OXA-48 in 89% of cases in 2012, while in the first half of 2014 that figure was 73% of cases. Roughly half of the patients had been in a Belgian treatment facility shortly before CPE was identified. A third had not had contact with healthcare facilities in the previous year. Only 11% had been a healthcare facility abroad in the year before CPE was identified. Screening of each patient who has stayed in a hospital abroad remains necessary during admission, but this measure alone will not be adequate, because the majority of current cases are of domestic origin (Jans et al. 2014). Of all Belgian blood isolates of *Klebsiella pneumoniae*, 0.5% were resistant to carbapenems in 2014, just like in 2015. After a peak at 2.4% in 2016, 2017 showed a decrease to 1.1% and in 2018 an increase to 1.4% of all *Klebsiella pneumoniae* blood isolates being resistant to carbapenems (Catteau and Mertens 2020).

Glupczynski is very satisfied with the way the hospital in Sint-Niklaas has been tackling its problems in 2011, 2012 and 2013. 'They're open, they send us bacteria strains, they've requested specialist help, they follow the guidelines—they're really doing very well'.[25] And yet it has not been possible to bring the outbreak in Sint-

---

[24]Personal message from Bart Galloway to the author, 21 February 2014.

[25]However, the 'openness' of the Nikolaas General Hospital praised by Glupczynski was limited to its openness towards colleagues. There is nothing about the outbreak of bacteria on the hospitals' website, and the annual reports for 2011 and 2012 do not mention it either.

Niklaas under control. In Glupczynski's opinion, this has undoubtedly got to do with certain specific circumstances. 'The hospital in Sint-Niklaas comprises five sites. They treat many older patients, who stay for long periods and, as a result, are often transferred within the hospital. Also, the older patients are often readmitted to the hospital before long. That enables the germs to spread'. In Belgium, almost a third of all hospitalisation cases involve elderly people. A large proportion of older patients are transferred back and forth between elderly care facilities, nursing homes and hospitals more or less regularly.[26] 'It is a great pity that at the end of 2011, when we were working out our recommendations on how to proceed against carbapenemases, we didn't take sufficient account of the role of elderly care and nursing homes. Now we must quickly investigate how often these bacteria appear in elderly people. Even amongst patients who visit their GP. At the moment we have no information about this. There are already elderly care facilities and nursing homes that decline to accept patients with OXA-48. There's no justification for this, but they do it anyway, because they don't know enough about it'. In elderly care facilities, data collection on antibiotic resistance is often hampered by the low frequency of testing to establish the susceptibility of isolates for different antibiotics.

Glupczynski is convinced that major educational efforts are needed to inform doctors, laboratories, nursing staff and the general public about bacteria, antibiotic resistance and the importance of hygienic measures. 'But you hardly find any course content relating to the hygiene of doctors and nursing staff, or patients and hospitals, in the curricula of universities and teaching institutions. There is no training in this subject area', he says.

Professor Glupczynski observes a striking similarity between the hospitals that have to deal with CPE: almost all of them were affected by outbreaks of *Klebsiella pneumoniae* with ESBL in the past. But this does not apply to the hospital in Sint-Niklaas. 'We are now looking at the old ESBL strains again, in order to compare them with the current OXA-48 bacterial strains. It may be that we're dealing with one and the same strain, which was initially ESBL-positive and later became OXA-48-positive as well—as happened at the Maasstad Hospital in Rotterdam'.

## Hidden Reservoir

Glupczynski thinks that a reservoir of carbapenemases has developed in the Belgian population without being noticed. 'It's a result of trips to countries where these bacteria occur frequently, for example North Africa and particularly Morocco, where OXA-48 appears often. Migrants who return to their country of origin for a holiday can bring it from there to Belgium'. In this connection, he points to the slowly

---

[26]In September 2012, there was also an outbreak of multiresistant Klebsiellas, in which the transfer of patients to the UMC Groningen Beatrixoord rehabilitation centre played a role. The bacterium was introduced into the ward for spinal injuries at the Beatrixoord rehabilitation centre via a patient from the hospital. At both sites, a total of 11 carriers of the bacterium were identified.

changing population of elderly care facilities and nursing homes. 'More and more first-generation migrants are living there. At the end of 2011 we had the first patients who had never been admitted to hospital and never undertaken any travels, and who were nevertheless colonised with carbapenemase-producing germs'. Recently a whole series of cases in which patients were colonised by a KPC-positive bacterium was reported near Liège.[27] 'In Liège and the surrounding area there is a large Italian community. KPCs occur frequently in Italy. Perhaps one thing explains the other. I am sure that there is a hidden system of transfer within the general population. More than any other germ, *Klebsiella pneumoniae* feels at home both inside and outside hospitals. This germ functions as a kind of link between hospitals and the general public. This isn't quite as true for *E. coli*. There is a lot more of it, and it's much more easily transferred too, but it's less pathogenic than *Klebsiella*. Transfer to the general population is very easy, especially if there's a lack of personal hygiene or food hygiene. And you tend to find that more often in elderly people'. In the Franco-Belgian border region, there is also a specific factor at work, says Glupczynski. 'French health insurance allows elderly people from France to live in an elderly care home in Belgium if they wish to. They're happy to do this, because the homes in Belgium offer better care, and they can find a place more quickly there than in France. In the Belgian town of Tournai, for example, 80 per cent of all residents of elderly care homes have French citizenship. However, if these people need to go to hospital, because of their health insurance they have to be admitted to a French hospital. That creates risks of spreading resistant bacteria that no-one has thought about'. The few available Dutch figures seem to support Glupczynski's plea to pay more attention to antibiotic resistance in long-term care facilities. More and more multiresistant bacteria are being identified in the residents of Dutch elderly care and nursing homes. MRSA, *E. coli* with ESBL and *Klebsiella pneumoniae* with ESBL occur there more frequently than in hospitals, outpatient clinics or GPs' surgeries.

Peter Bergen is a hygiene specialist for the Lower Saxony Regional Health Authority. He is investigating the most significant differences between hospitals and elderly care or nursing homes. 'In a nursing home or elderly care home the residents have private living spaces. The presence of multiresistant pathogens does not change this is any way. It's a different situation from that in a hospital, where the length of stay is limited. People live in elderly care and nursing homes. So if someone there catches such germs, it often tends to be the case that they remain colonised for the rest of their life. However, the question is whether other residents are infected inside the home, or whether it is just a reservoir for what has happened in clinics'.

According to Bergen, all these factors make it difficult to compare hospitals with nursing homes and elderly care homes. 'Both are healthcare institutions, but no elderly care home is a medical facility—at least in Germany. And—what's much

---

[27]In 2012, seven hospitals in the province of Liege were affected by KPC. There were outbreaks in three hospitals in which a total of 26 patients were colonised by KPC. Only in one case did a patient bring in the KPC from abroad (Jans et al. 2014).

more important—there aren't any in-house medics. Patients are cared for by the residents' GPs. This is a disadvantage where a holistic approach to hygiene is concerned, because no-one in elderly care homes has any medical skills. People are quick to suppose that the high incidence of multiresistant pathogens in an elderly care home is the result of a lack of hygiene. But they forget that it's impossible to carry out the same measures there as in a hospital, even for purely legal reasons. They can't, for example, seriously think of isolating a resident of an elderly care home who's carrying multiresistant pathogens in a separate space. At least, not for an unlimited period. You very quickly get the impression that people in an elderly care home are working unhygienically, because they do things differently there than in a hospital. But very often there's a reason for that. Infection prophylaxis is only one slice of the pie, not the whole. The second point is that patients with dementia have infectiological problems that they simply can't solve. They can rest assured that their surrounding will be smeared with faeces and secretions or excretions of every kind. You can't rely on any rules. This means that you find yourself in a kind of tolerance zone—in other words, an unsatisfactory situation that ultimately, however, you can't get rid of'.

## Harbingers of Doom?

Professor Glupczynski confirms that Belgium is facing a 'rapid rise' in the number of carbapenemases. But he isn't one of those medical microbiologists who see the resistance mechanisms spreading quickly around the world as harbingers of doom. 'There are colleagues who say that NDM stands for "Apocalypse Now". It's a big problem, but we can end it if we have the will. And therefore—apart from hygiene, hygiene and more hygiene—it mainly comes down to what I've just said about elderly care. But in India you're fighting a losing battle'. Glupczynski's Parisian colleague Patrice Nordmann doesn't expect much from India either. '650 million Indians don't have a toilet. Several hundred million have no access to medical provision of any kind. What we need to do over here is track down these resistant bacteria and isolate their carriers. And, more than anywhere else, this applies to the United Kingdom. This is because you find NDM wherever there are links to the Indian subcontinent. It's primarily a Commonwealth problem'.

In November 2011, the European Centre for Disease Prevention and Control (ECDC) published an overview of the confirmed cases of NDM-producing Enterobacteriaceae in the EU up to that time (ECDC 2011). Up to then, 68 patients had been recorded in the UK. Two-thirds of these cases involved *Klebsiella pneumoniae*. Of the 40 British patients whose travel behaviour was known, 20 had been in India shortly before, 5 in Pakistan and 1 in Spain. Fourteen had not travelled. In the rest of the European Union, only 38 patients had been reported up to November 2011, more than half of them carrying *Klebsiella pneumoniae*. Fifteen of these had developed an infection. Twenty-five of the patients had stayed in a hospital abroad within a month before they were identified as having NDM: 13 in India, 3 in Pakistan, 6 in one of the countries of former Yugoslavia, and 2 in Iraq.

One of the colonised patients had lived for some time in India. In June 2019, ECDC published a so called *Rapid risk assessment* on a large regional outbreak of NDM-producing carbapenem resistant Enterobacteriaceae that took place in the Italian region of Tuscany. 'Between November 2018 and May 2019, seven Tuscan hospitals notified a total of 350 cases. Due to its size and the resulting change in the epidemiology of CRE, the reported outbreak is a significant event, despite previous endemicity of *Klebsiella pneumoniae* carbapenamase (KPC)-producing CRE in this geographic area. The change in the type of carbapenemase further reduces treatment options because NDM-producing CRE are not susceptible to some of the new beta-lactam/beta-lactamase inhibitor combinations such as ceftazidime-avibactam and meropenem-vaborbactam. Numerous reported outbreaks and examples of cross-border transmission of NDM-producing CRE in the European Union/European Economic Area (EU/EEA) demonstrate the transmission potential of NDM-producing CRE in European healthcare systems. Outbreaks such as the one in Tuscany present a risk for cross-border transmission and further spread to other EU/EEA countries, especially since the affected area is a major tourist destination. Given the previous rapid establishment of KPC-producing CRE in Italy (which resulted in an endemic situation), the risk for further spread of NDM-producing CRE from the current outbreak is considered to be high for Italy and moderate for cross-border spread to other EU/EEA countries. Sporadic cases of community acquisition of NDM-producing CRE have also been described for other European countries. However, the introduction and dissemination of these bacteria have mainly been associated with healthcare settings. Therefore, the risk of acquisition of NDM-producing CRE related to this outbreak is likely restricted to persons with recent healthcare contact. (. . .) After the initial report of NDM-1 from Sweden in 2008, Public Health England, concerned with the rapid increase in the number of human cases with NDM-1-producing CRE in hospitals across the UK, issued a national alert in July 2009. By November 2010, a survey distributed among 29 European countries showed that 13 had already identified and reported NDM-producing CRE cases. The first reported outbreak in Europe occurred in a hospital in Bologna in northern Italy in 2011. In 2012, a large interregional outbreak of NDM-producing *K. pneumoniae* was reported in Poland, only a few months after a first case of NDM-1-producing *K. pneumoniae* was detected in a patient with previous travel history to Africa. Most of the early cases with known travel history were shown to be associated with previous hospitalisation in the Indian subcontinent or in the Balkans. In 2015, EuSCAPE (the European survey on carbapenem-producing Enterobacteriaceae) confirmed that NDM-producing CRE were spreading in the Balkan region, with large numbers of isolates collected in Montenegro, Serbia, and Greece. In 2015, NDM was the third most frequent carbapenemase detected in the EU/EEA. A national expert assessment indicated that a number of EU countries were facing outbreaks of NDM-producing CRE in hospitals located either in the same or different regions, suggesting autochthonous interinstitutional transmission' (ECDC 2019; Albiger et al. 2015).

The first Dutch patient with NDM-1 to be identified was a 66-year-old woman who was admitted to a Belgrade hospital after a brain haemorrhage. From there she was transferred to the neurology department of the Medisch Spectrum Twente in Enschede on 27 August 2008. It was known that the woman was carrying an MRSA, so she was isolated as soon as she was admitted. A *Klebsiella pneumoniae* with ESBL was also found in the patient. The woman was discharged from the hospital on 15 October 2008 and transferred to a nursing home, where further isolation measures were taken. On 10 October 2008, a 73-year-old woman was admitted to the pulmonary disease ward of the same hospital in Enschede. At the end of October, a Klebsiella with ESBL was identified in a culture taken from this second patient. On 8 November, she was discharged from the hospital. On 25 June 2010, she was readmitted with severe lung problems. She died on 18 July. The first patient also died. A Klebsiella with ESBL and enzymes that made it resistant to carbapenems was found in both patients by the Laboratory for Microbiology in Twente and Gelderland (Labmicta) in Enschede. Among these enzymes was NDM-1 (Halaby et al. 2012).

In summer 2013, the University Medical Centre Groningen was confronted by a quite special case of imported carbapenemases. The patient involved had been admitted to a private clinic in Egypt with severe stomach pains. There she was given two types of antibiotics by infusion for 13 days. Four days after she returned to the Netherlands, she was admitted to the University Medical Centre Groningen with fever and severe stomach pains. Of course, she was isolated. The woman was infected by a *Klebsiella pneumoniae* with NDM-1 and OXA-48. Moreover, she was colonised by an *E. coli* with OXA-48 and an *E. coli* with two different ESBLs. Her husband and two children, who had visited her in the clinic in Egypt were also colonised by multiresistant bacteria. In the case of her husband, it was *E. coli* with two different ESBLs. Two different *E. coli* with ESBL were identified in her elder child, while a germ with KPC was found in the younger one. In the opinion of the authors of an article on this case, 'in countries where resistant Enterobacteria rarely appear, the guidelines for infection control should perhaps be extended to include screening the increasing number of international travellers, including the family members who have visited a patient abroad' (Bathoorn et al. 2013).

'We can't meddle with India', said Nordmann. We were sitting in his small office at the Hôpital Bicêtre near Paris. 'By contrast, we can set something in motion in countries that are members of the European Union, for example Greece. The excessive use of antibiotics there—although not just there—must come to an end'. Nordmann abides by the maxim that, in order to improve the world, you have to start with yourself. 'For me, it is the patients over here with a higher risk of infection that are important. In their case, we can stop them being colonised by these kinds of multiresistant bacteria. That is our mission. We must screen "at-risk" patients on hospital wards and then implement the necessary measures. Up to now this has still been easy.[28] And you in the Netherlands can achieve even more. Let's look at the

---

[28]The French data show still very low numbers of *Enterobacteriaceae* resistant to carbapenems. In 2017, the number was 0.65% for all *Enterobacteriaceae*, but 1, 56% for *Klebsiella pneumoniae*. (Santé Publique France 2018).

example of MRSA in the Netherlands. This problem has been under control for 30 years thanks to the guidelines applied there, and the incidence is very low'. As Nordmann says: 'I don't think that patients who have been transferred to European hospitals from abroad are always identifiable as such. We must find that out on the day the patient is admitted. And we also need to get our house in order here in Europe first. What is happening in Italy? What's going on in Greece? How is it that the rate of resistance to antibiotics in hospitals there is so high?' Nordmann gives the answer to this question at once: 'Three things are responsible for this: too many antibiotics are prescribed, hygiene regulations are not observed, and they don't search for multiresistant bacteria. This has got to do with cultural habits. In general, in Europe there's a correlation between the incidence of antibiotic resistance in a country and the size of its debts. It has everything to do with the degree of social organisation. In north European countries such as Sweden, Denmark, the Netherlands and also Germany, antibiotic resistance is much rarer than in south Europe, because society is less organised there. A stay in Greece is an important risk factor for colonisation by multiresistant bacteria. And members of the European Parliament do not talk about this very often. Just as, 20 years ago, they said nothing about the deficits and debts of a particular country. They lack the courage for this'. The Greek statistics support Nordmann's view. In the second half of 2015—the Greek publish data every 6 months—on average more than 80% of the *Klebsiella pneumoniae* isolates from blood cultures on intensive care units of Greek hospitals were resistant to imipenem and meropenem. On surgical wards, the resistance rate was 60%, and on general wards more than 40%. One year later, in the second half of 2016, the resistance rates of blood isolates of *Klebsiella pneumoniae* to meropenem and imipenem were around 84% on ICUs, 55% on surgical wards and 50% on general wards. In the second semester of 2017, the resistance rates on Greek ICUs were lower but still around 80%, on surgical wards about 55%, and on general wards still above 50%. Over the period July–December 2018, things did not really change. Resistance to carbapenems on the ICUs was still around 90%, on surgical wards almost 60% and on medical wards around 45%. In the second semester of 2019 finally, a decrease was registered in the number of *Klebsiella pneumoniae* blood isolates resistant to carbapenems. In the ICUs of Greek hospitals, 80% were resistant to carbapenems, on surgical wards 60% and in medical wards around 40%. In the first six months of 2020 the figures went up again: 86% of all Klebsiella pneumoniae blood isolates on the ICUs were resistant to carbepenems, on surgical wards 57%—a slight decrease—and on medical wards 52% (WHONET 2021).

Professor Evelina Tacconelli, Full Professor of Infectious Diseases at the University Hospital in Verona and Medical Director of the Department for Internal Medicine at the University Hospital Tübingen and a specialist in healthcare-associated infections supports her French colleague's statements.[29] Tacconelli was educated in her homeland of Italy and, before coming to Tübingen, was at the Harvard Medical

---

[29]In 2004, Professor Tacconelli was awarded the ESCMID Prize for the nosocomial infections field by the European Society of Clinical Microbiology and Infectious Diseases.

School in Boston. 'It now looks as though there's a problem in southern Europe, even though nobody's made any mistakes. I have worked in south Europe. The problem isn't there because it somehow just happened. It's there because every time we requested an isolation room, we were told: "No, that's not necessary." It's there because there's no education and training in antibiotics. It's there for several reasons, but above all because of the defective structures in south Europe. It's time to stand up and say: "These things don't just happen." One fine day there was KPC in Rome, and now we have 300 cases in Modena or some other place as well. If we don't stand up and say that something's not right, then a day will come when it's impossible even for a country like Sweden to keep this type of bacteria at bay. Because not just in south Europe, but also in Sweden or the Netherlands, the budgets for infection prevention and control of healthcare-associated infections are under pressure. In most southern European countries there are enough infectious disease specialists or microbiologists. But then why isn't it working? It's not just a matter of money. In Italy the situation for infectious disease specialists, in contrast to nursing staff, is similar to that in the Netherlands. And yet despite this there's a big problem. It's not a matter of what the machine looks like, but of how it works'.

## Rowing with Rudders That Are Too Short

In Piraeus, Olympia Zarkotou tries to do everything that is possible. She is not angered by all the criticism that rains down on Greece. 'It's the truth', she says, 'we're the worst students in the class'. At the Tzaneio Hospital, where she works, at-risk patients are screened on admission to see if they are carrying carbapenem-resistant bacteria. 'Just like with MRSA in the Netherlands. We have to know what the patients are bringing with them. We therefore screen patients who have been transferred from a nursing home or another Greek or foreign hospital. In this way we've been able to reduce the number of infections with Klebsiellas and Acinetobacter that are resistant to carbapenems. In 2010 the number of infections in the intensive care unit fell by around a half. We achieved this through screening, isolation of infected patients and better compliance with hygiene regulations. Everyone is paying more attention now'. At the Tzaneio Hospital, there are also antibiotics advisers, who coordinate compliance with the antibiotics guidelines. 'For example, they advise alternating the use of antibiotics. Three months of one medicine, and then three months of an alternative medicine. In this way, fewer resistances are created. Up to date this procedure has produced very good results'. These cautious initial attempts to reduce antibiotic resistance in Greece—or at least, to stop it increasing—are under great pressure as a result of the commercial and financial crisis that has befallen the country (EUobserver 2011). One of the biggest problems facing the prevention and control of infectious diseases, according to Zarkotou, is the lack of nursing staff. 'We have enough doctors, but too few nursing staff. This makes infection prevention almost impossible. If a nurse has to look after too many patients, then hygiene fails to come up to scratch. Even the nursing staff complain about it. If you have to work under stress, because you're responsible for too many patients, then sometimes you can just forget to wash your hands and put new gloves on when moving from one patient to another. And I haven't even mentioned the fact that we need more rooms than we have now, in order to be able to isolate patients'. Zarkotou believes that antibiotics advisers and specialist hygiene staff are important in order to reduce the use of antibiotics or, if they are nevertheless necessary, to ensure that they are used properly. 'We have them in my clinic and in several other hospitals in Athens too, but outside the city there are no specialist hygiene staff and hardly any microbiologists. The HCDCP[30] is trying to change this situation, but it has far too little money. Working groups of microbiologists, hygiene specialists, doctors and nursing staff have been formed. They've been meeting at least three times a year in different hospitals to provide help and make recommendations. This has worked well. But instead of more money to develop the programme, there's now less. So all these activities are carried out less frequently, or no longer carried out at all. Fortunately a lot has happened since 2010. All hospitals have received written instructions. Since November 2010, there have been training events in many towns. Surveillance is up and running. The most important things—and, I believe, the most expensive—are being carried out'.

At the beginning of June 2014, I met Olympia Zarkotou again. 'Greek hospitals are battling with several problems, because they get less money and employ fewer staff. But I believe the main problem is that there's no culture of infection prevention in the healthcare sector, and that Greek patients are not sufficiently well informed to insist on their rights with regard to patient safety'. But Zarkotou also has some good news. In February 2014 a new law was passed, setting out a general framework for combatting antibiotic resistance. The role of infection prevention committees in hospitals was enhanced, and it was stipulated that a commission for antibiotics advice must be set up. The frequency with which infections with multiresistant bacteria occurred had to be documented, as did the number of bacteria with antibiotic resistance and the level of compliance with hand hygiene. Reference measurements to determine baseline values had to be carried out in order to determine the prevalence of healthcare-associated infections or antibiotics use. In addition, all hospitals had to introduce a surveillance system to monitor the use of antibacterial medicines and isolation or cohort care of patients. The results of these measurements are used to assess hospitals. According to the new law, the hospital director is responsible for effectively reducing the number of healthcare-associated infections.[31] 'Sensible use of the available financial resources is another challenge for our healthcare system', says Flora Kontopidou.[32] She is Head of the Office for Antibiotic Resistance at the Hellenic Centre for Disease Control and Prevention (HCDCP). 'The hospitals must tell the health ministry what annual budget they need for infection prevention and control, and they must provide evidence of the means they use to combat healthcare-associated infections'. Procrustes has worked, in

---

[30]Hellenic Centre for Disease Control and Prevention.

[31]E-mail message from Olympia Zarkotou to the author on 6 June 2014.

[32]Flora Kontopidou in an e-mail to the author on 4 July 2014.

Kontopidou's opinion. 'The number of hospitals that have voluntarily taken part in the action plan has reached a surprisingly high level—85 per cent of public hospitals and the largest military and private hospitals. In 2013, the continuing increase in cases of sepsis caused by carbapenem-resistant bacteria was halted for the first time'. The overriding aim of the Procrustes programme, according to Kontopidou, is 'to control the spread of multiresistant bacteria in hospitals with the resources we have at our disposal. The HCDCP has played a key role in this, because it has encouraged the departments for infection prevention and control of healthcare-associated infections to make use of the new law to improve the quality of treatment. In the HCDCP's view, introducing fixed structures and procedures in Greek hospitals is the most suitable method of dealing effectively with problems in the healthcare system—for example antibiotic resistance—which are not just serious threats for Greece, but also for the rest of the world'. The somewhat optimistic statements by Olympia Zarkotou and Flora Kontopidou concerning Greek efforts to stop the increase of antibiotic resistance cannot allay all the concerns about healthcare provision in this country, which has been hit hard by the financial crisis. Resistance rates have remained high up to today (WHONET 2021). In an interview with the Reuters news agency, Marc Sprenger—then Director of the ECDC[33]—sounded a warning about the situation in Greece (Reuters 2012). After visiting the country, he warned that basic medical provision in Greece is threatened by the ongoing financial cuts. These were introduced by the Greek government in order to obtain European financial aid. On 12 May 2013, the *New York Times* reported that healthcare expenditure had been cut by 40% since 2008. Because of the lack of resources, some hospitals could no longer even buy gloves, bandaging materials or catheters. Approximately 35,000 doctors and nursing staff had lost their jobs (The New York Times 2013). The workload of the remaining medical staff is therefore very high (Reuters 2012). Moreover, a year after losing their job, unemployed people also lose their health insurance. In 2012, more than 24% of Greeks were unemployed. In 2013, that increased to even more than 27%. Now, in 2020 the unemployment rate is considerably lower at 15.5% but is still the highest in the European Union (Statista 2020b). The salaries of those who still have work have fallen considerably. As a result of this, many Greeks no longer have any access to medical care, which has resulted in a sharp rise in infant mortality and a considerable increase in HIV infections (Kentikelenis et al. 2014). But there was also some positive news in that dark period. Greek doctors and nurses have set up outpatient clinics where non-insured patients can get free treatment. The clinics are financed by donations from companies and private individuals (BBC 2013).

---

[33]Sprenger, at the time director general of ECDC, joined the World Health Organisation in July 2015. He has been Director of the WHO's Antimicrobial Resistance Secretariat until 2021 and is now Special Envoy Covid-19 Vaccination for the Dutch Carribean.

## Cynical Examples

On the other side of Europe, Karin Tegmark-Wisell is preoccupied with precisely the same topics as Olympia Zarkotou—but from a quite different, and more favourable, perspective. Tegmark-Wisell is Head of the Department of Antibiotic Resistance and Infection Prevention at the Smittskyddsinstitutet (SMI), the Swedish centre for disease control, which is situated in Solna, right next to the famous Karolinska University Hospital and the ECDC central office. Antibiotic resistance is not a big problem in Sweden. Relatively few antibiotics are used, and the infection prevention system works. 'Compared with many other countries Sweden seems to be in good shape, but even we can see that the threat will assume alarming proportions in future if things continue as they are. At the moment we've still got a more or less firm grip on the situation. But even in Sweden, individual patients are affected by antibiotic resistance. Up to now, we haven't had to ask ourselves whether it would be better not to replace a hip, or no longer transplant an organ, because of possible infections that we can't treat any more. But we do address such questions, in order to keep politicians and the general public informed. Because even we have to deal with the import of resistant bacteria, and nowadays we're seeing more outbreaks than we used to'. Tegmark-Wisell cites an example from Germany. 'In Essen, some transplant patients in an intensive care unit contracted severe infections by a Klebsiella with KPC, which had presumably been brought in by a patient from Greece. Five of the patients died.[34] What I'm now going to say will sound very cynical, because it's tragic that people have died. But clear, concrete examples that we can use to illustrate the importance of infection prevention help us to give weight to our demands. And that's necessary, because here too in the healthcare sector savings are being made, which weakens our position. We've also used the outbreak at the Maasstad Hospital in Rotterdam as an example in talks with Swedish politicians. If such outbreaks occur in India or Greece, then it's difficult for us in Sweden to identify with them. We're good at infection prevention, we have all sorts of quality assurance systems, and our microbiological laboratories do first-rate work. But if it emerges that something like this can also happen in a country that's similar to ours, then from an educational point of view that's a very useful example'.

In Sweden too, hospitals compete for patients. There are public and private hospitals. 'For hospitals, of course, transplantation patients also mean business. You never want to lose them. Therefore there might possibly be an incentive to hush up the fact that you've got resistant bacteria in the building. So, now and then, hospital directors perhaps suppress data. The result is that their hospitals possibly don't take the best countermeasures'. Swedish hospitals have an obligation to report bacterial outbreaks. Hospitals that report them honestly run the risk of looking bad

---

[34] At Essen University Hospital, five transplant patients and two cancer patients became infected with the same *Klebsiella pneumoniae* with KPC-2 and VIM-1 between July 2010 and January 2011. Five patients developed a severe infection as a result of the bacterium and died. In four cases, the bacterium was the cause. One of the patients who died had been in a Greek hospital shortly before they were first admitted to Essen (Steinmann et al. 2011).

by comparison with hospitals that withhold these data. 'You have to report them and then ask the authorities to investigate the outbreak. Some hospitals decline to do this, because they prefer to conceal the fact that something's gone wrong. Hospitals that do report their cases are therefore particularly conspicuous—but I'm convinced that in the long run they'll be the winners'.

'What applies to the SMI in Sweden also applies to the ECDC, except that here it's on a European level. We show the EU member states the figures in the form of a rankings list', said in 2012 then ECDC-director Marc Sprenger, with whom I was sitting in his office in Solna's former institute for the blind. 'And then we hope that national governments will grasp that they might possibly have to do something'. The ECDC is trying to give individual help to Greece—the country which, according to Sprenger, is battling with these problems the most. 'We're approaching this in a quite structured way. We're trying to provide them with a kind of custom-fit support. I was positively surprised that the Greeks requested this from us'.

## References

Albiger, B., Glasner, C., Struelens, M. J., et al. (2015). Carbapenemase-producing *Enterobacteriaceae* in Europe: Assessment by national experts from 38 countries, May 2015. *Eurosurveillance, 20*(45). https://doi.org/10.2807/1560-7917.ES.2015.20.45.30062.

ARC - Antibiotic Resistance Coalition. (2014). *Declaration on antibiotic resistance.* Accessed November 26, 2020, from https://bit.ly/2MHskJv

Bathoorn, E., Friedrich, A. W., Zhou, K., et al. (2013). Latent introduction to the Netherlands of multiple antibiotic resistance including NDM-1 after hospitalisation in Egypt. *Eurosurveillance, 18*(42). https://doi.org/10.2807/1560-7917.ES2013.18.42.20610.

BBC. (2010). *India rejects UK scientists' 'superbug' claim.* Accessed November 24, 2020, from https://www.bbc.com/news/world-south-asia-10954890

BBC. (2013). *Greece's life-saving austerity medics.* Accessed from https://www.bbc.com/news/magazine-23247914

BfR. (2016). *Bundesinstitut für Risikobewertung. Antibiotikaresistenz: Carbapenemase-bildende Keime in Nutztierbeständen.* In German. Accessed November 26, 2020, from https://bit.ly/33h30iW

Bonardi, S., & Pitino, R. (2019). Carbapenemase-producing bacteria in food-producing animals, wildlife and environment: A challenge for human health. *Italian Journal of Food Safety, 8*(2), 7956. https://doi.org/10.4081/ijfs.2019.7956.

Bratu, S., Mooti, M., Nichani, S., et al. (2005). Emergence of KPC-possessing *Klebsiella pneumoniae* in Brooklyn, New York: Epidemiology and recommendations for detection. *Antimicrobial Agents and Chemotherapy, 49*(7), 3018–3020. https://doi.org/10.1128/AAC.49.7.3018-3020.2005.

Catteau, L., & Mertens, K. (2020). *European antimicrobial resistance surveillance for Belgium (EARS-BE) - Report 2018.* Accessed November 28, 2020, from https://bit.ly/35mzKIG

CBS Statline. (2020). *Bevolking op 1 januari en gemiddeld; geslacht, leeftijd en regio. Population statistics.* Accessed November 16, 2020, from https://bit.ly/3s5EPi9

CCDEP (The Center For Disease Dynamics, Economics & Policy). (2011). *Retail sales of carbapenem antibiotics to treat gram-negative bacteria are increasing rapidly in India and Pakistan.* Accessed November 24, 2020, from https://bit.ly/3799RvW

CDC (Centers for Disease Control and Prevention). (2009). Guidance for control of infections with Carbapenem-resistant or Carbapenemase-producing *Enterobacteriaceae* in acute care facilities.

*Morbidity and Mortality Weekly Report (MMWR), 58*(10), 256–260. Accessed November 25, 2020, from https://bit.ly/3orsVNx

CDC (Centers for Disease Control and Prevention). (2010). Detection of *Enterobacteriaceae* isolates carrying metallo-beta-lactamase—United States. *Morbidity and Mortality Weekly Report (MMWR), 59*(24), 750. Accessed November 26, 2020, from https://bit.ly/3q6jWln

CDC (Centers for Disease Control and Prevention). (2013a). *Antibiotic resistance threats in the United States 2013.* Accessed November 26, 2020, from https://bit.ly/2Ld0V1L

CDC (Centers for Disease Control and Prevention). (2013b). *"Nightmare bacteria" threat.* Accessed November 26, 2020, from https://bit.ly/2LvcelG

Chan, M. (2012). *Antimicrobial resistance in the European Union and the world.* Accessed November 25, 2020, from https://bit.ly/3np2JBW

De Staat van Volksgezondheid en Zorg. (2020). *Ziekenhuisbedden.* In Dutch. Accessed November 23, 2020, from https://bit.ly/3oqyAn6

Diederen, B. M. W, Hattink-Malipaard, C. J. R., Vloemans, A. F. P. M., et al. (2012). *A prolonged outbreak with Metallo-beta-lactamase producing* Pseudomonas aeruginosa *(PA) in a Burn Centre and Intensive Care unitlinked to an environmental reservoir.* Oral Presentation at the spring conference of the Dutch Society of Medical Microbiology (NVMM), Arnhem 17–18 April 2012. Nederlands Tijdschrift voor Medische Microbiologie 20 (Supplement). See page S96, P029. Accessed November 20, 2020, from https://bit.ly/394pt6y

D-Statis – Statistisches Bundesamt. (2020). *Zahl der Intensivbetten in Deutschland von 1991 bis 2018 um 36% gestiegen.* In German. Accessed November 24, 2020, from https://bit.ly/3bhBsip

ECDC (European Centre for Disease Prevention and Control). (2011). *Updated risk assessment on the spread of NDM and its variants within Europe.* https://doi.org/10.2900/14890. https://bit.ly/3nmU3f7

ECDC (European Centre for Disease Prevention and Control). (2019). *Regional outbreak of New Delhi metallo-beta-lactamase producing carbapenem-resistant Enterobacteriaceae, Italy, 2018–2019.* Accessed November 24, 2020, from https://bit.ly/3bfIILE

ECDC (European Centre for Disease Prevention and Control). (2020a). *Antimicrobial consumption in the EU/EEA – Annual Epidemiological Report 2019.* Accessed November 23, 2020, from https://bit.ly/2Lh2SdB

ECDC (European Centre for Disease Prevention and Control). (2020b). *Surveillance atlas of infectious diseases. Updated every year.* Accessed November 23, 2020, from https://bit.ly/2JX07NX

EFSA (European Food Safety Authority). (2013). Scientific opinion on carbapenem resistance in food animal ecosystems. *EFSA Journal, 11*(12). Accessed from https://bit.ly/3nt8Epk

EUobserver. (2011). *Ordinary Greeks turning to NGOs as health system hit by austerity.* Accessed 29 Nov 2020 https://euobserver.com/social/113841

Falagas, M. E., Tansarli, G. S., Karageorgopoulos, D. E., et al. (2014). Deaths attributable to Carbapenem-resistant *Enterobacteriaceae* infections. *Emerging Infectious Diseases, 20*(7), 1170–1175. https://doi.org/10.3201/eid2007.121004.

FAO (Food and Agricultural Organization of the United Nations). (2017). *Together and stronger against antimicrobial resistance in Viet Nam: National Action Plan launched today.* Accessed November 20, 2020, from https://bit.ly/3i2zzaI

FDA (Food and Drug Administration). (2013). *Guidance for industry new animal drugs and new animal drug combination products administered in or on medicated feed or drinking water of food producing animals: Recommendations for Drug sponsors for voluntarily aligning product use conditions with GFI #209.* Accessed November 26, 2020, from https://www.fda.gov/media/83488/download

Fursova, N. K., Astashkin, E. I., Knyazeva, A. I., et al. (2015). The spread of $bla_{OXA-48}$ and $bla_{OXA-244}$ carbapenemase genes among *Klebsiella pneumoniae, Proteus mirabilis* and *Enterobacter* spp. isolated in Moscow, Russia. *Annals of Clinical Microbiology and Antimicrobials, 14*(46). https://doi.org/10.1186/s12941-015-0108-y.

Gandra, S., Joshi, J., Trett, A., et al. (2017). *Scoping report on antimicrobial resistance in India.* Accessed November 25, 2020, from https://bit.ly/38qiXX6

GARP. (2010). *Global antibiotic resistance partnership. Situation analysis. Antibiotic use and resistance in Vietnam.* Accessed from https://bit.ly/3nvrZX4

GARP. (2011). *Global antibiotic resistance partnership. Situation analysis: Antibiotic use and resistance in India.* Accessed November 24, 2020, from https://bit.ly/2MM9Yao

Halaby, T., Reuland, A. E., Al Naiemi, N., et al. (2012). A case of New Delhi Metallo-β-lactamase 1 (NDM-1)-producing *Klebsiella pneumoniae* with putative secondary transmission from the Balkan region in the Netherlands. *Antimicrobial Agents and Chemotherapy, 56*(5), 2790–2791. https://doi.org/10.1128/AAC.00111-12. Accessed from https://aac.asm.org/content/aac/56/5/2790.full.pdf

Hoge Gezondheidsraad - Belgian Health Council. (2011). *Advies van de Hoge Gezondheidsraad nr. 8791 Maatregelen te nemen naar aanleiding van de toename van carbapenemase producerende enterobacteriën (CPE) in België.* In Dutch. Accessed November 28, 2020, from https://bit.ly/3q8i3oS

Huang, S. S., Avery, T. R., Song, Y., et al. (2010). Quantifying interhospital patient sharing as a mechanism for infectious disease spread. *Infection Control and Hospital Epidemiology, 31*(11), 1160–1169. Accessed from https://bit.ly/2JV7JQT

Jans, B., Catry, B., & Glupczynski, Y. (2014). *Microbiologische- en epidemiologische surveillance van carbapenemase producerende Enterobacteriaceae in België januari 2012 - juni 2014.* In Dutch. Accessed November 28, 2020, from https://bit.ly/3hT25vl

Jerusalem Post. (2014). *Infections from hospitals continue to kill thousands.* Accessed November 26, 2020, from https://bit.ly/3fE6Qb5

Kaase, M. (2011). Nachweis von Carbapenemasen im Jahr 2010. Bericht des NRZ für gramnegative Krankenhauserreger. *Epidemiologisches Bulletin, 32.* Accessed November 25, 2020, from https://bit.ly/3pZiB0k

Kaase, M. (2013). Zur aktuellen Situation bei Carbapenemase-bildenden gramnegativen Bakterien. Ein Bericht des NRZ für gramnegative Krankenhauserreger. In German. *Epidemiologisches Bulletin, 19.* Accessed November 25, 2020, from https://bit.ly/3l62kTI

Kentikelenis, A., Karanikolos, M., Reeves, A., et al. (2014). Greece's health crisis: From austerity to denialism. *The Lancet, 383*(9918), 748–753. https://doi.org/10.1016/S0140-6736(13)62291-6.

KI-Media. (2008). *Vietnam second in Southeast Asia in counterfeit drugs.* Accessed November 16, 2020, from https://bit.ly/3np5B1G

Klein, E. Y., Van Boeckel, T. P., & Martinez, E. M. (2018). Global increase and geographic convergence in antibiotic consumption between 2000 and 2015. *PNAS, 115*(15), E3463–E3470. https://doi.org/10.1073/pnas.1717295115.

Köck, R., Daniels-Haardt, I., Becker, K., et al. (2018). Carbapenem-resistant *Enterobacteriaceae* in wildlife, food-producing, and companion animals: A systematic review. *Clinical Microbiology and Infection, 24*(12), 1241–1250. https://doi.org/10.1016/j.cmi.2018.04.004.

Kumarasamy, K. K., Toleman, M. A., Walsh, T. R., et al. (2010). Emergence of a new antibiotic resistance mechanism in India, Pakistan, and the UK: A molecular, biological, and epidemiological study. *The Lancet Infectious Diseases, 10*(9), 597–602. https://doi.org/10.1016/S1473-3099(10)70143-2.

Leenstra, T., Bosch, T., Vlek, A. L. et al. (2017). Carbapenemase producing Enterobacteriaceae in the Netherlands: Unnoticed spread to several regions. *Nederlands Tijdschrift voor Geneeskunde, 161,* D1585 English abstract. Accessed from https://bit.ly/2LhOhyp

Li, R., Van Doorn, H. R., Wertheim, H. F. L., et al. (2016). Combating antimicrobial resistance: Quality standards for prescribing for respiratory infections in Vietnam. *The Lancet Global Health, 4*(11), E789. https://doi.org/10.1016/S2214-109X(16)30267-4.

Lübbert, C. (2014). *Was lernen wir aus dem Leipziger KPC-Ausbruch? Krankenhaushygiene Up2Date 09*(01), 13–20. https://doi.org/10.1055/s-0034-1365033. In German. Accessed from https://bit.ly/2XpilKU

Lübbert, C., & Rodloff, A. C. (2014). *Der Leipziger KPC-Ausbruch – was man aus den Fehlern lernen kann.* Oral presentation in German at the Bad Honnef Symposium, 14–15 April 2014 Königswinter. Accessed November 25, 2020, from https://doi.org/10.3205/14bhs14

Lübbert, C., Lippmann, N., Busch, T., et al. (2014). Long-term carriage of *Klebsiella pneumoniae* carbapenemase–2-producing *K pneumoniae* after a large single-center outbreak in Germany. *American Journal of Infection Control, 42*(4), 376–380.

Munoz-Price, S., Poirel, L., Bonomo, R. A., et al. (2013). Clinical epidemiology of the global expansion of *Klebsiella pneumoniae* carbapenemases. *The Lancet Infectious Diseases, 13*(9), 785–796. Accessed from https://bit.ly/3q1l2yO

Nethmap/Maran. (2016). *Consumption of antimicrobial agents and antimicrobial resistance among medically important bacteria in the Netherlands/Monitoring of antimicrobial resistance and antibiotic usage in animals in the Netherlands in 2015.* Accessed November 26, 2020, see page 98 https://bit.ly/3mbicFT

Nethmap/Maran. (2017). *Consumption of antimicrobial agents and antimicrobial resistance among medically important bacteria in the Netherlands/Monitoring of antimicrobial resistance and antibiotic usage in animals in the Netherlands in 2016.* Accessed November 26, 2020, see page 112 https://bit.ly/2K0G5SK

Nethmap/Maran. (2018). *Consumption of antimicrobial agents and antimicrobial resistance among medically important bacteria in the Netherlands/Monitoring of antimicrobial resistance and antibiotic usage in animals in the Netherlands in 2017.* Accessed November 26, 2020, see page 108 https://bit.ly/3nsWMDO

Nethmap/Maran. (2019). *Consumption of antimicrobial agents and antimicrobial resistance among medically important bacteria in the Netherlands/Monitoring of antimicrobial resistance and antibiotic usage in animals in the Netherlands in 2018.* Accessed November 26, 2020, see page 109 https://bit.ly/39hB7LB

Nethmap/Maran. (2020). *Consumption of antimicrobial agents and antimicrobial resistance among medically important bacteria in the Netherlands/Monitoring of antimicrobial resistance and antibiotic usage in animals in the Netherlands in 2019.* Accessed November 26, 2020, see page 104 https://bit.ly/2XlP5F9

Nguyen, K. V., Thi Do, N. T., Chandna, A., et al. (2013). Antibiotic use and resistance in emerging economies: A situation analysis for Viet Nam. *BMC Public Health, 13*, 1158. https://doi.org/10.1186/1471-2458-13-1158.

Ni, W., Cai, X., Wei, C., et al. (2015). Efficacy of polymyxins in the treatment of carbapenem-resistant enterobacteriaceae infections: A systematic review and meta-analysis. *The Brazilian Journal of Infectious Diseases, 19*(2), 170–180. https://doi.org/10.1016/j.bjid.2014.12.004.

NRDC (Natural Resources Defence Council). (2013). *Press release. FDA's New Antibiotics Policy Fails to Protect Health.* NRDC: FDA Gives Industry a Free Pass on Antibiotic Misuse. Accessed from https://www.nrdc.org/media/2013/131211

Ostholm-Balkhed, A., Tärnberg, M., Nilsson, M., et al. (2013). Travel-associated faecal colonization with ESBL-producing enterobacteriaceae: Incidence and risk factors. *The Journal of Antimicrobial Chemotherapy, 68*(9), 2144–2153. https://doi.org/10.1093/jac/dkt167.

Otters, H. B. M., Van der Wouden, J. C., Schellevis, F. G., et al. (2004). Trends in prescribing antibiotics for children in Dutch general practice. *The Journal of Antimicrobial Chemotherapy, 53*(2), 361–366. https://doi.org/10.1093/jac/dkh062.

PEW. (2013). *PEW charitable trusts. Press release FDA Acts to Fight Superbugs.* Accessed from https://bit.ly/2J1M3lV

Pfennigwerth, N. (2017). Bericht des NRZ für gram negative Krankenhauserreger. *Epidemiologisches Bulletin, 26,* 229–233. https://doi.org/10.17886/EpiBull-2017-034.2. Accessed from https://bit.ly/393gt1p

Pfennigwerth, N. (2018). Bericht des Nationalen Referenzzentrums (NRZ) für gramnegative Krankenhauserreger. *Epidemiologisches Bulletin, 28,* 263–267. https://doi.org/10.17886/EpiBull-2018-034. Accessed from https://bit.ly/335EmBX

Pfennigwerth, N. (2019). Bericht des Nationalen Referenzzentrums für gramnegative Krankenhauserreger, 2018. *Epidemiologisches Bulletin, 31*, 289–294. https://doi.org/10. 25646/6210. Accessed from https://bit.ly/3pKv9bL

Pfennigwerth, N. (2020). Bericht des Nationalen Referenzzentrums für gramnegative Krankenhauserreger, 2019. *Epidemiologisches Bulletin, 29*, 3–10. https://doi.org/10.25646/ 6920. Accessed from https://bit.ly/2IU1vjO

Qureshi, Z. A., Hittle, L. A., O'Hara, J. A., et al. (2015). Colistin-resistant *Acinetobacter baumannii*: Beyond carbapenem resistance. *Clinical Infectious Diseases, 60*(9), 1295–1303. https://doi.org/10.1093/cid/civ048.

Reuland, E. A., Al Naiemi, N., Kaiser, A. M., et al. (2016). Prevalence and risk factors for carriage of ESBL-producing enterobacteriaceae in Amsterdam. *Journal of Antimicrobial Chemotherapy, 71*(4), 1076–1082. https://doi.org/10.1093/jac/dkv441.

Reuters. (2012). *Basic hygiene at risk in debt-stricken Greek hospitals.* Accessed November 29, 2020, from https://reut.rs/3lmWnlf

Rico, A., Phu, T. M., Satapornvanit, K. et al. (2013). Use of veterinary medicines, feed additives and probiotics in four major internationally traded aquaculture species farmed in Asia. *Aquaculture, 412*(413), 231–243. Accessed from https://bit.ly/3s9kxUY

RIVM (Rijksinstituut voor Volksgezondheid en Milieuhygiëne). (2012). *Nationale surveillance van MRSA en CPE t/m wk 52 2011.* In Dutch. Accessed November 26, 2020, from https://bit.ly/ 3q7MoDv

RIVM (Rijksinstituut voor Volksgezondheid en Milieuhygiëne). (2013). *Nationale surveillance van MRSA en CPE t/m wk 52 2012.* In Dutch. Accessed November 26, 2020, from https://bit.ly/ 3q5XVTN

RIVM (Rijksinstituut voor Volksgezondheid en Milieuhygiëne). (2014). *Nationale surveillance van MRSA en CPE t/m wk 52 2013.* In Dutch. Accessed November 26, 2020, from https://bit.ly/ 2Xpue3M

RIVM (Rijksinstituut voor Volksgezondheid en Milieuhygiëne). (2015). *Nationale surveillance van MRSA en CPE t/m wk 52 2014.* In Dutch. Accessed November 26, 2020, from https://bit.ly/ 2XkZ659

Ruppé, E., Armand-Lefèvre, L., Estellat, C. et al. (2014). Acquisition of carbapenemase-producing Enterobacteriaceae by healthy travellers to India, France, February 2012 to March 2013. *Eurosurveillance, 19*(14). Accessed from https://bit.ly/2JWN9j7

Santé Publique France. (2018). *Enquête nationale de prevalence des infections nosocomiales et des traitements anti-infectieux en établissements de santé France mai-juin 2017.* In French. Accessed November 29, 2020, from https://bit.ly/37gH4Wy

Schar, D., Klein, E. Y., Laxminarayan, R., et al. (2020). Global trends in antimicrobial use in aquaculture. *Scientific Reports, 10*, 21878. https://doi.org/10.1038/s41598-020-78849-3.

Schwaber, M. J., & Carmeli, Y. (2008). Carbapenem-resistant enterobacteriaceae. A potential threat. *Journal of the American Medical Association, 300*(24), 2911–2913. https://doi.org/10. 1001/jama.2008.896. Accessed from https://bit.ly/2JZGCEs

Schwaber, M. J., Lev, B., Israeli, A., et al. (2011). Containment of a country-wide outbreak of Carbapenem-resistant *Klebsiella pneumoniae* in Israeli hospitals via a nationally implemented intervention. *Clinical Infectious Diseases, 52*(7), 848–855. https://doi.org/10.1093/cid/cir025.

SFK – Stichting Farmaceutische Kerngetallen. (2020). *Data en feiten 2020.* In Dutch Accessed November 16, 2020, from https://bit.ly/3bhrEF3

Singh, B. R. (2009). Prevalence of vancomycin resistance and multiple drug resistance in enterococci in equids in North India. *The Journal of Infection in Developing Countries, 3*(7). https://doi.org/10.3855/jidc.467.

Statista. (2020a). *Number of hospital beds in Greece from 2000 to 2018.* Accessed November 23, 2020, from https://bit.ly/3nvB5Dc

Statista. (2020b). *Greece: Unemployment rate from 1999 to 2020.* Accessed November 29, 2020, from https://bit.ly/2Jm5rd9

Steinmann, J., Kaase, M., Gatermann, S. et al. (2011). Outbreak due to a *Klebsiella pneumoniae* strain harbouring KPC-2 and VIM-1 in a German university hospital, July 2010 to January 2011. *Eurosurveillance 16*(33). Accessed from https://bit.ly/3pZ95cQ

Stoesser, N., Sheppard, A. E., Peirano, G. et al. (2017). Genomic epidemiology of global *Klebsiella pneumoniae* carbapenemase (KPC)-producing *Escherichia coli*. *Scientific Reports, 7*, 5917. Accessed from https://bit.ly/39bGLgt

Tängdén, T., Cars, O., Melhus, Å. et al. (2010). Foreign travel is a major risk factor for colonization with *Escherichia coli* producing CTX-M-type extended-Spectrum β-lactamases: A prospective study with Swedish volunteers. *Antimicrobial Agents and Chemotherapy, 54*(9), 3564–3568. https://doi.org/10.1128/AAC.00220-10. Accessed from https://aac.asm.org/content/54/9/3564

The Economic Times. (2015). *Indian medical tourism industry to touch $8 billion by 2020: Grant Thornton.* Accessed November 16, 2020, from https://bit.ly/35yOiW0

The New York Times. (2013). *How austerity kills. Opinion.* Accessed November 29, 2020, from https://nyti.ms/38sO44u

UKL- Universitätsklinikum Leipzig. (2012). Pressemitteilung vom 24.05.2012. In *Eindämmung eines seltenen multiresistenten Keims am Universitätsklinikum Leipzig (UKL).* Accessed November 25, 2020, from https://www.uniklinikum-leipzig.de/presse/Seiten/Pressemitteilung_399.aspx

UKL- Universitätsklinikum Leipzig. (2013). Pressemitteilung vom 24.06.2013. In *KPC-Ausbruchsgeschehen erfolgreich beendet.* Accessed November 25, 2020, from https://www.uniklinikumleipzig.de/presse/Seiten/Pressemitteilung_5215.aspx

Van der Bij, A. K., & Pitout, J. D. D. (2012). The role of international travel in the worldwide spread of multiresistant Enterobacteriaceae. *Journal of Antimicrobial Chemotherapy, 67*(9), 2090–2100. https://doi.org/10.1093/jac/dks214.

Van der Bij, A. K., Van Mansfeld, R., Peirano, G., et al. (2011). First outbreak of VIM-2 metallo-β-lactamase-producing *Pseudomonas aeruginosa* in the Netherlands: Microbiology, epidemiology and clinical outcomes. *International Journal of Antimicrobial Agents, 37*(6), 513–518. https://doi.org/10.1016/j.ijantimicag.2011.02.010.

Van der Bij, A. K., Van der Zwan, D., Peirano, G., et al. (2012). Metallo-β-lactamase-producing *Pseudomonas aeruginosa* in the Netherlands: The nationwide emergence of a single sequence type. *Clinical Microbiology and Infection, 18*(9), E369–E372. https://doi.org/10.1111/j.1469-0691.2012.03969.x.

Việt Nam News. (2010). *Counterfeit drugs challenge pharma industry.* Accessed November 16, 2020, from https://bit.ly/38O6YDt

VietnamNet Bridge. (2017). *Experts sound the alarm over counterfeit drugs in Vietnam.* Accessed November 16, 2020, from https://bit.ly/3kDcVoM

Voor in 't Holt, A. F., Severin, J. A., & EMEH, L. (2014). A systematic review and meta-analyses show that Carbapenem use and medical devices are the leading risk factors for Carbapenem-resistant *Pseudomonas aeruginosa*. *Antimicrobial Agents and Cehemotherapy, 58*(5), 2626–2637. https://doi.org/10.1128/AAC.01758-13.

WAAAR (World Alliance Against Antiotic Resistance). (2014). *The WAAAR declaration against antibiotic resistance.* Accessed November 20, 2020, from https://bit.ly/35nMnDd

Wakker Dier. (2014). *Resistente bacteriën op garnalen en vis.* In Dutch with many references in English. Accessed November 17, 2020, from https://bit.ly/3pD1VeQ

Walsh, T. R., Weeks, J., Livermore, D. M., et al. (2011). Dissemination of NDM-1 positive bacteria in the New Delhi environment and its implications for human health: An environmental point prevalence study. *The Lancet Infectious Diseases, 11*(5), 355–362. https://doi.org/10.1016/S1473-3099(11)70059-7.

Webb, H. E., Bugarel, M., Den Bakker, H. C., et al. (2017). Carbapenem-resistant bacteria recovered from faeces of dairy cattle in the High Plains region of the USA. *PLoS One, 11*(1), e0147363. https://doi.org/10.1371/journal.pone.0147363.

Wendt, C., Schütt, S., Dalpke, A. H., et al. (2010). First outbreak of *Klebsiella pneumoniae* carbapenemase (KPC)-producing *K. pneumoniae* in Germany. *European Journal of Clinical Microbiology & Infectious Diseases, 29*(5), 563–570. https://doi.org/10.1007/s10096-010-0896-0.

Wertheim, H. F. L. (2011). *Inappropriate antibiotic use and resistance in Asia and its global impact; a delicate balance of antibiotic accessibility.* Oral presentation at the spring meeting of the NVMM (Dutch Society for Medical Microbiology), Arnhem 18–20 Apr 2011. Accessed November 9, 2020, See pages S39 and S40, abstract Oo60 https://bit.ly/3k9Z3SJ

Wertheim, H. F. L., Chandna, A., Vu, P. D., et al. (2013). Providing impetus, tools, and guidance to strengthen National Capacity for antimicrobial stewardship in Vietnam. *PLoS Medicine, 10*(5), e1001429. https://doi.org/10.1371/journal.pmed.1001429.

Weterings, V., Zhou, K., Rossen, J. W., et al. (2015). An outbreak of colistin-resistant *Klebsiella pneumoniae* carbapenemase-producing *Klebsiella pneumoniae* in the Netherlands (July to December 2013) with inter-institutional spread. *European Journal of Clinical Microbiology and Infectious Diseases, 34*, 1647–1655. https://doi.org/10.1007/s10096-015-2401-2.

WHO. (2010). *Growing threat from counterfeit medicines.* Accessed April 4, 2021, from https://www.who.int/bulletin/volumes/88/4/10-020410/en/

WHO. (2014). Sixty-seventh world health assembly. *Antimicrobial Resistance.* Accessed November 25, 2020, from https://bit.ly/3nqGHi9

WHO – World Health Organization. (2018). *Substandard and falsified medical products.* Accessed November 16, 2020, from https://bit.ly/3hTcgQz

WHONET Greece. (2021, updated every 6 months). *Choose: Cumulative results [select desired period], Klebsiella pneumoniae, blood isolates.* Data available from 1996 until last biannual update. Accessed April 4, 2021, from http://www.mednet.gr/whonet/

Widmann-Mauz, A. (2013). *Answer to written parliamentary question of German MP Bärbel Höhn.* In German. Accessed November 20, 2020, from https://bit.ly/2JVtOPi

Won, S. Y., Munoz-Price, L. S., Lolans, K., et al. (2011). Emergence and rapid regional spread of *Klebsiella pneumoniae* carbapenemase–producing enterobacteriaceae. *Clinical Infectious Diseases, 53*(6), 532–540. https://doi.org/10.1093/cid/cir482.

World Bank. (2020a). *Current health expenditure (% of GDP).* Latest data. Accessed November 24, 2020, from https://bit.ly/3i2Lfu4

World Bank. (2020b). *Out-of-pocket expenditure (% of current health expenditure).* Latest data. Accessed November 24, 2020, from https://bit.ly/2JZIUU4

Yigit, H., Queenan, A. M., Anderson, G. J., et al. (2001). Novel carbapenem-hydrolyzing β-lactamase, KPC-1, from a carbapenem-resistant strain of *Klebsiella pneumoniae. Antimicrobial Agents and Chemotherapy, 45*(4), 1151–1161. https://doi.org/10.1128/AAC.45.4.1151-1161.2001.

# Looking Behind the Figures

## 8

For years the Netherlands has topped the list of countries with the lowest use of antibiotics in human medicine.[1] In the veterinary sector, the situation was precisely the opposite. For years the Netherlands ranked high on the list of intensive users. Cattle in the Netherlands were given large doses of antibiotics as a preventative measure, in order to stop the animals from becoming sick. At the same time the antibiotics stimulated the animals' growth. Until 2006, antibiotics important for treating human beings were also used as animal growth promoters throughout Europe. Then a European law forbidding this came into force. The use of antibiotics as growth promoters immediately declined sharply. But their therapeutic use increased to the same extent. From this moment on, animals were given massive doses of antibiotics as a preventative measure.[2] And if animals became ill, then all the animals in the building were treated at the same time, not just those who were sick. This was referred to as herd treatment.[3] In all honesty, it should also be mentioned that meat prices are so low that farmers can scarcely afford sick animals. This naturally encourages improper use and abuse of antibiotics. Only recently have data on antibiotics use in livestock farming been centrally collated in the EU. In April 2010, the European Medicines Agency (EMA) launched the ESVAC Project, the European Surveillance of Veterinary Antimicrobial Consumption. A year later, the EMA published an initial report containing antibiotics sales data for veterinary medicine from 2005 and 2009 in nine EU countries that were able to provide data for several successive years. The report contains absolute figures for the quantities of antibiotics bought from pharma companies in the veterinary sector, as well as figures corrected to reflect the estimated stock of cattle. 'Actually they should also be corrected with respect to animal types', says veterinary microbiologist Professor

---

[1] Of course, the lowest use of antibiotics is not necessarily the best use. Underdosing is also possible.

[2] See also Chap. 5, *A thin layer of faeces on everything you touch.*

[3] A herd is a group of animals that is admitted to a livestock farm at a certain time and looked after as a group.

R. van den Brink, *The End of an Antibiotic Era*,
https://doi.org/10.1007/978-3-030-70723-1_8

Dik Mevius. 'Then the figures would be truly comparable'. Mevius works at the Central Veterinary Institute of Wageningen University and is on the faculty for veterinary medicine at Utrecht University. From early 2011 to 1 January 2014 he was Chairman[4] of the SDa veterinary medicines authority, whose remit includes publishing standards for the use of antibiotics in veterinary medicine. In the first ESVAC report, the Netherlands really stick out. From 2006, the Dutch farmers were right out in front. After correction to reflect livestock numbers, they give their livestock more than three times as many antibiotics as their Danish colleagues. Even the British farmers use two and a half times fewer antibiotics. Well-known intensive users, such as the Czechs or Swiss, use fewer than half as many antibiotics as the Dutch. Only the French and the Belgians[5] come anywhere near the Dutch (EMA 2011). From 2010, a more positive picture of the Netherlands began to emerge (EMA 2012). In this year antibiotics use fell, a trend that continued until 2016. At the end of October 2017 the seventh ESVAC report was published, containing data that included 2015. The veterinary usage of antibiotics in the Netherlands had decreased sharply since 2010, from 165 milligrammes of antibiotics per PCU (kilogramme) to 64 milligrammes.[6] The Netherlands was the fifteenth largest user of veterinary antibiotics out of 30 EU/EEA countries. Cyprus was the no. 1 user, with 434 milligrammes per PCU, followed by Spain (402), Italy (322) and Hungary with 211 milligrammes per PCU (EMA 2017). A year later the eight ESVAC-report in the year 2016 still put the Dutch on the fifteenth rank using 53 milligrammes per PCU (EMA 2018). The top users in 2017 of veterinary antibiotics were once more Cyprus (453), Spain (363), Italy (295), Portugal (208) and Hungary with 187 milligrammes per PCU (EMA 2019). The latest data published in 2020 show that Cyprus remained top user with 466 milligrammes per PCU, followed by Italy (244), Spain (219), Portugal (187) and Hungary (181). The Netherlands rank again fifteenth on this list. Overall, the use of antibiotics in the European livestock industry decreased between 2011 and 2018 by more than a third (EMA 2020).

---

[4]On 1 January 2014 Mevius was succeeded by Jaap Wagenaar, Professor of Clinical Infectious Diseases at Utrecht University and veterinary surgeon.

[5]In 2010, the use of antibiotics in the veterinary sector in Belgium decreased to 299.3 tonnes, compared with 304 tonnes in 2009: The use of certain antibiotics important for humans has vastly increased: cephalosporin by 8.8%, quinolone by 2.8% and macrolide by 16.3%. The doses of these antibiotics are also considerably lower (BelVet-SAC 2010).

[6]The amounts of veterinary antimicrobial medicines sold in different countries are linked to the animal demographics of each country, among other factors. In this report, the annual sales figures in each country were divided by the total estimated weight of livestock at the time of treatment and of slaughtered animals for the corresponding year, taking into account the import and export of animals to other member states for fattening or slaughter. The population correction unit (PCU) is the term used for the estimated weight. The PCU is purely a surrogate for the animal population at risk, in order to normalise sales by animal population in individual countries: 1 PCU equals 1 kg.

## The Swann Report

Sweden was the first country to take measures against the unnecessary use of antibiotics. 'We started with animals', says Christina Greko, Professor at the Statens Veterinärmedicinska Anstalt (SVA), Sweden's national veterinary institute. 'Only thereafter we began working on the problem systematically in human medicine as well. In the veterinary sector, everything started in 1986 with the ban on the use of antibiotics as growth promoters. 20 years later this ban was extended to cover the European Union. When we joined the European Union in 1995 there were two options: either we adapted our laws to the European ones, or the EU adapted its laws to ours. The latter took place. The Swann report of 1969 played an important role in the Swedish ban.[7] The key recommendation of the Swann report was that antibiotics used for therapeutic purposes in humans must not be used as growth promoters (Swann et al. 1969). The result of this was that certain antibiotics were actually no longer used as growth promoters in Europe. The Swann report instigated a discussion in Sweden, and journalists played a key role in this. It was then that we started to compile statistics on the use of antibiotics. Very soon one of the biggest Swedish newspapers came out with the headline: '30 tonnes of antibiotics for healthy animals'. The debate flared up again, and in 1986 a ban on the use of antibiotics as growth promoters was implemented'. At the end of 2014, Swedish farmers used 9.3 tonnes of antibiotics for their animals annually. That corresponds to 11.5 milligrammes per kilo of meat. Only Iceland and Norway perform better, using 5.2 and 3.1 milligrammes per kilo respectively (EMA 2016). But by the end of 2018 the Swedes were using 9.8 tonnes of antibiotics for all animals—a clear increase on the 9.3 tonnes used in 2014, but at 12.5 milligrammes per PCU still a very low figure. Only Norway (2.9 milligrammes per PCU) and Iceland (4.9) continued to perform better (EMA 2020).

## The Danish Model

In contrast to Sweden, the livestock industry in Denmark mainly consists of intensive livestock farming. The Danes have three times fewer inhabitants than Holland in a somewhat larger land area, and fewer livestock. In Denmark, the big business is pig farming. For a long time antibiotics were used liberally in Danish intensive livestock farming as well, but not on the same scale as in the Netherlands. Since the sharp reduction of antibiotics used for livestock in the Netherlands the figures for the two countries have come closer together. In 2010, the Danes used 47.5 milligrammes of antibiotics per PCU. The Dutch used 146.1 milligrammes per PCU (EMA 2020). By the end of 2018, the Danish usage of antibiotics had decreased to 38.2 milligrammes per PCU and the Dutch usage tot 57.5 milligrammes per PCU (EMA 2020). More

---

[7] A commission set up in 1968 by the British Ministers for agriculture and health, presided over by Professor Swann, was given the task of investigating the use of antibiotics in livestock farming.

than at any other time, the use of antibiotics in Danish pig farming rose steeply at the beginning of the 1990s. This was accompanied by ever more frequent infections by bacteria that were resistant to several antibiotics. The use of the antibiotic avoparcin as a growth promoter resulted in VRE being detected more and more frequently. VREs are Enterococci that are resistant to the antibiotic vancomycin. They can be dangerous for severely enfeebled patients.[8] This caused the Danish government to take action. In 1994, the Danes decided to take radical measures. New legislation made it so financially unattractive for veterinarians to run their own pharmacies that the practice that had existed for years, whereby veterinarians not only prescribe medicines but also supply them to farmers, disappeared. The measures—which included a ban on default preventative use of antibiotics—had an astonishing effect. The documented use of antibiotics in intensive livestock farming declined by 40 per cent. In subsequent years, the Danes began to ban the use of antibiotics as growth promoters, and reduce the use of the most important antibiotics for humans in livestock farming.[9]

'If veterinarians earn a large part of their income from prescribing antibiotics and other medicines', says Annette Cleveland Nielsen, 'then they are much more willing to prescribe them. It seems to me that it's a human characteristic to try and increase your income'. Cleveland Nielsen was for more than 11 years Head of the veterinary advice department at the Danish Ministry for Food, Agriculture and Fisheries. Since May 2019 she is Pharmacovigilance Officer and Special adviser at Lægemiddelstyrelsen (Danish Medicines Agency). 'In order to compensate for the veterinarians' loss of income, we have introduced a system in which they sign agreements with the farmers. Under this system, the veterinarians have become more like health consultants, and they are paid for it. If they prescribe medicines, the farmers must obtain these from a pharmacy. Precise records are kept of what veterinarians prescribe, and why'. All veterinarians are checked every 2 years. 'We have 400 veterinarians involved in food production. Every year we visit 200 and check everything'.

Cleveland Nielsen's authority not only monitors the veterinarians' activity, but also that of the livestock farmers. 'If we establish that farmers are regularly asking new veterinarians to visit them, we carry out an additional check and ask both parties why this is so. This might be connected with the fact that the farmers want the veterinarians to prescribe more antibiotics. But up to now the agreements have been functioning well, and we rarely see cases where people change their veterinarian for no good reason'. Cleveland Nielsen says that larger agribusinesses are usually safer. 'They have better methods for preventing illnesses, partly because they are stronger economically. They work with fixed suppliers and customers, which reduces risks. There are more diseases in farms that get their piglets from several suppliers, and

---

[8]Many Dutch hospitals had to combat VRE outbreaks in 2012. See Chap. 5 *A thin layer of faeces on everything you touch.*

[9]This section on the change in Danish policy is based on a study carried out by Berenschot (Beemer et al. 2010).

more antibiotics are used. Very large livestock farms have so many animals that they drive them to the abattoir themselves in big livestock trucks. In this way, the animals can't be contaminated in transit by contact with animals from other farms'.

Frank Møller Aarestrup is a Professor at the Technical University of Denmark in Copenhagen and head of the Division for Global Surveillance and the Research Group for Genomic Epidemiology. He is one of the architects of this Danish policy. In addition to his post as government adviser in Copenhagen, he also advises the European Commission and the World Health Organisation (WHO). Møller Aarestrup finds it hard to understand why veterinarians in the Netherlands—and also in Germany—continue to be pharmacists at the same time.[10] 'That shouldn't be allowed. It is a perverse incentive that leads to unnecessary use of antibiotics and other medicines'.

The so-called Danish model is universally approved. Nikolaj Nørgaard, Director of the *Videncenter for Svineproduktion*, a research institute for pig farming, also supports this position. 'And I say this on the basis of my experience'. The figures speak for themselves. The radical reduction in the use of antibiotics has not damaged Danish pig farms. After a short period in which piglet mortality rose, when the farmers did not yet know how to keep them healthy without preventative use of antibiotics, the sector has performed better than before the Danish model was introduced. Yields have increased. The total production of pigs in Denmark increased by almost a half between 1992 and 2008. In the same period, the use of antibiotics in pigs fell by more than a half. The percentage of resistant bacteria in pigs and broiler chickens has fallen by values ranging from 60 to 100 per cent, and current values are now less than 20 per cent. Animal health has not been affected by the major reduction in antibiotics use. The number of piglets per sow has even increased, and fewer chicks died than they did before the use of antibiotics was restricted (Aarestrup et al. 2010; Kovács 2011).

In 2012, the use of antibiotics in the Danish livestock industry rose by 4 per cent to 112 tonnes (DANMAP 2013). Three quarters of this was given to pigs. They received 5 per cent more antibiotics in 2012 than in 2011. But despite the increase in 2012, 11 per cent fewer antibiotics were used in this year than in 2009. By this means the Danish farmers achieved their aim of reducing the use of antibiotics by 10 percent between 2009 and 2012 (Levy 2014). In 2013, there was a further 4 per cent rise of antibiotics use in intensive livestock farming, to 116.3 tonnes. In pig farming, the increase was 6 per cent. 78 per cent of all antibiotics used in intensive livestock farming were administered to pigs. Antibiotics use in Danish intensive livestock farming equals a third of the average use in the EU (DANMAP 2014). Over the course of 2014, Danish farmers used 106.8 tonnes of antibiotics (DANMAP 2015). The renewed decrease in the veterinary use of antibiotics that began in 2014

---

[10]According to information supplied by veterinary microbiology expert Jaap Wagenaar at Utrecht University and his Danish colleague Henrik Wegener of the Danish Institute for Food and Veterinary Research in Søborg, the situation in the Nordic countries is exceptional. In other countries veterinary surgeons sell the medicines they prescribe themselves.

continued at a relatively slow pace in the years 2015 to 2018 in which, according to the tenth ESVAC report, the Danes used 93.6 tonnes of antibiotics (EMA 2020).

## Berenschot Does Not Believe in It

For years one question has persistently been asked: what is keeping the Dutch from adopting the Danish model?[11] In 2009, the Berenschot consultancy firm was commissioned by the Dutch agriculture minister to investigate whether the Danish model ought to be introduced in the Netherlands as well. The reason for this was the sharp increase of MRSA bacteria in livestock that concerns both animals and humans. The frequent occurrence of MRSA amongst livestock farmers and their families meant that all sorts of extra measures were required if they had to be admitted to hospital. There was a panic fear of MRSA or other (multi)resistant bacteria in hospitals.[12]

The deterioration of the MRSA situation over the years has been caused by the excessive use of antibiotics in livestock farming. And this was partly encouraged by the fact that medicines sales made a substantial contribution to the revenues of veterinary practices. The differences between practices are considerable, but sales of medicines account for between 30 and 75 per cent of veterinarians' turnover. Although they described the success of the Danish model, despite this Berenschot has little faith in a separation of the roles of veterinarian and pharmacist in the Netherlands. They list all the possible objections to this separation, which in Denmark have largely been resolved already. It might indeed be possible that veterinarians would not prescribe antibiotics so often if they did not earn extra as a result. But the pressure on veterinarians to prescribe antibiotics remains the same. And if one veterinarian is not prepared to do what the livestock farmer wants, then the latter can go to another one. The loss of medicine sales would cause veterinarians' income to fall sharply. This would have to be compensated for by increasing the prices for consultations, and might result in farmers calling on the services of veterinarians less frequently. For farmers, antibiotics remain an attractive option for keeping their business profitable. Berenschot fears that livestock farmers would therefore look for opportunities to give their animals preventative antibiotics all the same. They could obtain antibiotics illegally and give them to their animals without any veterinarian being involved. Berenschot recommends meticulous surveillance of the use of antibiotics and veterinarians' prescription habits, as well as the use of antibiotics by farmers. He thus supports a plan by the Royal Dutch Society for Veterinary Medicine (KNMvD) to establish a veterinary medicines authority. In

---

[11]With or without the Danish model, the sales of antibiotics fell from 495 tonnes in 2009 to 176 tonnes in 2016, which is also a considerable decrease compared to the 150 tonnes sold in 2019 (SDa 2020a).

[12]Specific isolation rules apply to pig farmers and their families until it is confirmed that they are not infected with MRSA.

concrete terms, Berenschot proposes concentrating mainly on the veterinarians who prescribe the most medicines. 'It is estimated that fewer than five per cent of Dutch veterinary practices prescribe more than 80 per cent of the total quantity of antibiotics. These are veterinarians who have specialised in intensive livestock farming, and who therefore cater for the large majority of animals' (Beemer et al. 2010).

## Task Force

The agriculture minister of the time accepted Berenschot's conclusions. She had made a prior agreement with veterinarians that by the end of 2011 the use of antibiotics had to be reduced by 20 per cent compared with 2009, in which year 495 tonnes of antibiotics had been used in intensive livestock farming. One month later, on 9 April 2010, the minister once again sent parliament a letter about antibiotic resistance and antibiotics use, this time in conjunction with her colleagues from the health ministry at that time. In this second letter, the ministers demanded that by the end of 2013 the use of antibiotics must be reduced by at least a half in comparison with 2009 (Verburg and Klink 2010). The 'Antibiotic Resistance in Livestock Farming' task force had to work out appropriate proposals for this.[13] Six months later the task force made a series of suggestions. These included founding a veterinary medicines authority, which should determine standards for a good antibiotics policy, and setting up a system to make veterinarians' prescription habits and the use of antibiotics in livestock farming transparent. This veterinary medicines authority (SDa) was founded in spring 2011 (SDa 2020b). The SDa's first success was to publish a series of guidelines in summer 2011. 'Antibiotics use in agribusinesses is very varied', Dik Mevius said at the time (NOS 2011). 'There are some that use very little. Here little needs to be done. We have established a signal value and a reaction value. Famers whose antibiotics use exceeds the reaction value must do something to counteract this at once. And we also monitor this. The signal value does not require them to reduce their use. But if farmers' antibiotics use exceeds the signal value, this can be a hint that they need to do something about it. Initially we're concentrating on the big users and the veterinarians who prescribe large amounts. If we compel these to reduce their antibiotics use, the average use falls as well. Where lots is being used it's easy to cut down a bit. Additionally, by this means the risk for public health can be reduced as quickly as possible'. The SDa cannot impose any sanctions. Mevius thought this was a shame. 'In my view it would be good if we had more say where veterinarians are concerned – if we at the SDa could hold those who prescribe a lot responsible for it'.

---

[13]The 'Antibiotic Resistance in Livestock Farming' task force, presided over by agriculture specialist and former Managing Director of Radboud University Medical Centre Jos Werner, was created in 2008 by Minister of Agriculture Gerda Verburg. Werner was at the time also sitting on the supervisory board of the pharma company Merck, which has a large veterinary medicine department.

The target of halving the use of antibiotics was achieved in 2014, 1 year sooner than agreed. In the economics ministry's 2014 budget, which now included agriculture as well, the government demanded that antibiotics used in livestock farming must be reduced further. In 2015, use would have to decrease by 70 per cent compared with 2009. This goal has not been achieved. After the years of rapid decrease, antibiotics use in the veterinary sector declined only slightly in 2014 and 2015. In 2015, use fell to almost 206 tonnes, a reduction of around 58% by comparison with 2009. In 2016, the decrease in use of veterinary antibiotics was once again more marked. It fell from 206 to 176 tonnes, bringing the total decrease compared to 2009 to 64.4%. In 2017 there was a 3% increase in the sales of veterinary antibiotics, which rose to 182 tonnes. The total tonnage of livestock in the Netherlands decreased from 2.63 million tonnes in 2016 to 2.44 million in 2017. By the end of 2017, the total decrease in the use of veterinary antibiotics compared to 2009 was 63.4%. In 2018, the usage of veterinary antibiotics dropped slightly again to 179 tonnes. This reduction was realized in all sectors except broilers. Finally, in 2019, the sales of antibiotics for livestock farming decreased further to 150 tonnes, a reduction compared to 2009 of 69.6% (SDa 2020a; EMA 2020).

To obviate the problem of figures that revealed little, in 2012 the SDa produced its own data on the use of antibiotics in the various livestock farming sectors for the first time. Since 2011 farmers have had to document the use of antibiotics in their operations. At the end of June 2012, the SDa published its first report with detailed figures on the use of antibiotics in intensive livestock farming (SDa 2012; Bos et al. 2013). Not in tonnes per sector, but in kilogrammes per business unit. 'Basically this enabled us to see what was going on behind the figures for total use', explains Mevius. 'The use of antibiotics per business unit varies considerably across all sectors. And in all sectors there is a group of operators that deviate considerably from the middle value and use large quantities of antibiotics'. Depending on the sector, the big users give their animals between four and 15 times more antibiotics than the average user. This high level of use cannot be explained by the health status of the animals. There are also agribusinesses that use hardly any antibiotics. 'In the beginning we wanted to investigate the ten per cent of agribusinesses with the highest levels of use first', said Mevius. 'But these figures were terrifying, and so we immediately decided to extend our investigations to the top 25 per cent of users'. Livestock farmers who use too many antibiotics are reported to the relevant sector. Many large-scale users are asked by their sector to draw up a plan for reducing the use of antibiotics, and to implement it. The SDa can forward the data to the NVWA (the Netherlands Food and Consumer Product Safety Authority), which can then launch an investigation and impose monetary fines. It is the same for veterinarians. First, they are given the chance to change their prescription practices in consultation with their own industry association. If they do not do this, the SDa can annul the agreements between these veterinarians and the farmers.

One year later, when the SDa published its report on the use of antibiotics in livestock farming in 2012, it became clear that many farmers' use of antibiotics per animal was still considerably above the average. Moreover, the SDa reports a slight shift in the use of antibiotics towards medicines that can be administered in smaller doses and whose therapeutic effects last longer. One antibiotic does not always equal another. The number of agribusinesses that use many more antibiotics than the average of the relevant sector, and the number of veterinarians who prescribe above-average amounts of antibiotics have clearly decreased. In the pig farming sector, slightly more than 3 per cent of business units use too many antibiotics structurally, and in the veal farming sector the figure is almost 3 per cent. The use of antibiotics important for humans declined sharply in 2012: third- and fourth-generation cephalosporins by 76 per cent, fluoroquinolones by 50 per cent, aminoglycoside 40 per cent and colistin 35 per cent—a trend that continued in subsequent years (SDa 2013). In 2013, 2014 and 2015 a small number of farming enterprises still continued to use antibiotics on a large scale (SDa 2014, 2015, 2016). At the end of 2016, it became known that the SDa had reported the data relating to the intensive users of antibiotics to the NVWA. It is not known whether data concerning veterinarians who are major suppliers were also shared with the NVWA. In 2016, the total sale of veterinary antibiotics decreased considerably by roughly 18% (SDa 2017), followed by an 8% increase in 2017 (SDa 2018) and a 1% decrease in 2018 (SDa 2019). The last available data in 2019 show a sharp decrease again of 16% bringing the total sales volume at 150 tonnes (SDa 2020a).

## Illegal Antibiotics

Both the FIDIN data on sales of antibiotics in the veterinary sector and the figures in the SDa reports only reflect sales and prescriptions of antibiotics that were registered. There is no doubt that there is an illegal market for antibiotics in the veterinary sector, whose extent is unknown. However, the quantities of antibiotics occasionally confiscated suggest that the illegal market is a significant one. In spring 2011, the food safety authority (NVWA) confiscated 4000 kilogrammes of illegal antibiotics for the poultry sector in the north of the Netherlands (Bleker and Schippers 2012). In the Dutch poultry sector as a whole, 35 tonnes of antibiotics were used legally in 2011. The illegal antibiotics were supplied to poultry breeders. The investigators think that '45 per cent of broiler chicken farmers were guilty of uncontrolled use of antibiotics. The medicines were imported from China and India and presumably brought into the Netherlands via Poland'. The subsequent trial of the suspects for endangering public health ended in disaster. According to the court in Groningen, the public prosecutor had committed a grave error of procedure. The statements by senior officers from the criminal investigation department—the most important witnesses—had been agreed with him in advance. The court was only prepared to pursue the case if the presiding judge could question the police informants about the start of the investigation. The public prosecutor refused to allow this, since in this case the safety of the informants could not be guaranteed. The court, therefore, decided not to continue proceedings against the six suspects.

At the end of July 2012 the NVWA confiscated another large quantity of illegal antibiotics (De Telegraaf 2012). This time, after a tip-off from Belgium, the NVWA agents were able to withdraw 1000 kilogrammes of the antibiotic virginiamycin from circulation.[14] The illegal antibiotics were found at a loading facility in the south of the Netherlands, near the Belgian border. The NVWA presumes that the antibiotics were meant to be mixed in with cattle feed as growth promoters. One thousand kilogrammes of antibiotics would have been sufficient to 'enrich' a million kilogrammes of feed. At the same time as the antibiotics were confiscated in the Netherlands, 1000 kilogrammes of illegal virginiamycin were also found on the other side of the border in Belgium. The use of this medicine as an additive for livestock feed has been banned in the European Union since 1998. After the stir caused by ESBL in chickens in the Netherlands at the beginning of spring 2010, a similar commotion occurred in Belgium—above all in Flanders. Moreover at the end of March 2010, after a tip-off from the Netherlands about the use of ceftiofur in a Dutch chicken hatchery with a sister company in Belgium, raids were carried out in 20 hatcheries.[15] Ceftiofur is an antibiotic of the cephalosporin group that is very important to human beings, and its use for the treatment of poultry has been forbidden. The antibiotic was found in three of the 20 Belgian chicken hatcheries. One-day-old chicks were sprayed with ceftiofur. Other illegal antibiotics were found in four of the hatcheries. At the end of December 2013, the Dutch food safety authority again took action against the illegal use of antibiotics. This time a veal fattening farm was involved. During regular checks, a banned antibiotic was found in 54 of the animals on the farm. The meat was destroyed and the farm, together with its 2400 calves, was placed under supervision (Feednavigator.com 2014). In summer 2014, the NVWA shut down a livestock feed production facility where the antibiotic furazolidone was mixed in with the feed. It appears that the feed had been sent to at least 100 pig and veal fattening farms. The meat was delivered to food outlets in the Netherlands, Germany, France and Italy (Boerderij 2014). In a number of farms where livestock feed containing the banned substance was still found, the animals were culled. Antibiotics are also regularly found in consignments of illegal medicines during random checks by customs officials at airports. The Internet makes it possible not only for individuals, but also for dealers or farmers to order practically any medicine desired by illegal means.

Even if illegal use of ceftiofur is not a hot topic in Holland or Germany, this antibiotic can nevertheless be traced in chicken meat, explains Dik Mevius, until 2014 Head of the SDa (Dutch Veterinary Medicines Authority). 'There's something like a "poultry production pyramid". The great-grandparent birds come from pure breeding lines. There are in fact only two major breeds worldwide—Cobb and Ross—and besides these there's also Hubbard. The great-grandparent birds are bred in relatively small numbers by small outfits in the US and UK. They are delivered as eggs or chicks to farms, including Dutch farms, where grandparent birds are produced. These in turn are used to produce the parent birds, which are used

---

[14]A bacteriostatic antibiotic from the group of streptogramins, which is isolated from cultures of *Streptomyces virginiae*.

[15]In a hatchery, eggs are artificially hatched using incubators. The female chicks are delivered to breeding farms by the hatcheries.

for the production of broiler chickens and laying hens. All over the world, very large quantities of cephalosporins are used in this production chain. However, since March 2010 this has no longer been the case in the Netherlands. At that time I became very involved with this issue, until the practice of spraying with ceftiofur was curtailed. The spraying was carried out on broiler chickens. But with the exception of the European Union, the use of cephalosporins is internationally approved, in order to prevent early deaths of chicks'. In January 2012 the FDA also banned this form of cephalosporin use (FDA 2012). The main reason for this was the fear that resistances to this important class of antibiotics could spread to humans via the food chain.

## Simple and Inevitable

Mevius thinks that in certain ways the size of poultry farms, and their working practices, contribute towards the dismantling of barriers against the illegal use of antibiotics. 'Poultry farms are very big undertakings', he says. 'These companies often have subsidiaries abroad. It might be the case that some poultry farmers bring antibiotics into the country themselves. It might be equally possible that certain veterinarians do it. In my opinion, illegal use is not the biggest problem in this sector. But of course, you can quite easily get all kinds of antibiotics delivered from China via the internet. Now that there have been demands for more transparency about the use of antibiotics, there are of course people who therefore look for opportunities to acquire them illegally. This danger arises when you start to register everything. Then at the same time you create a demand for illegal practices'. Mevius has no information about the extent of this. 'There are only anecdotal reports. Earlier you used to hear stories about hauliers who took chicks to the Czech Republic and came back with a load of antibiotics. Such practices exist. Earlier, the hatcheries used to deliver the antibiotics along with the chicks. That occurred in order to prevent compensation claims. They gave a guarantee of quality, and losses above a certain percentage in the first ten days were charged to the supplier of the chicks. Nowadays they deliver a chick passport with the chick, giving details of its parents, other batches of chicks from these parents, information about confirmed pathogens etc., so that they can receive targeted treatment. But the hatchery, propagator, fattener and slaughterer all act independently. In Denmark they document the supply chain. All the details of the production process are transparent there. The chick passport is an attempt to make this process more transparent, but in reality it's just a makeshift measure that doesn't really work. We have to set up a system here similar to the one they have in Denmark.'

Mevius' Swedish colleague Christina Greko cannot say much about the extent of illegal antibiotics use in her country either. 'Some years ago, in a scientific journal, there was an attempt to put the black market for antibiotics in Europe under the microscope. There are vast differences in the data for individual countries. Nevertheless it is possible to identify a general tendency for illegal use in the northern countries to be lower than in those of the south. Buying antibiotics over the internet is totally forbidden in Sweden'. In Denmark, too, little is known about the extent of illegal antibiotics use. 'Our impression is that it's only a small problem in Denmark', explains Frank Møller Aarestrup. 'We at the university cannot get access to agricultural businesses. The food safety authority does have an investigative service of this kind, but they normally announce their visits to these businesses in advance. There is no doubt that there's an illegal market for antibiotics, but I don't believe that this illegal market is a large one. And here I'm supported by the fact that Denmark is a very small country with a small number of large-scale farmers. If a farmer were to use illegal antibiotics, it wouldn't remain hidden for long. It would become known. One of the rumours going round is that the present illegal use of antibiotics originates from Dutch farmers. We have some of these in Denmark. Perhaps they've brought their bad habits with them. I can't say whether this rumour is true'.

## Globalised (Lack of) Food Safety

'There's a global movement of people, animals and meat', says Aarestrup. 'Denmark exports 90 per cent of all the pigs it produces. As far as I know, 60 per cent of the pork that we consume ourselves is imported. That sounds illogical, but it's a consequence of globalisation. If you're eating salmon in Denmark today, then this salmon has probably been bred in Norway, then sent to Vietnam to be processed as salmon fillet and packaged. The salmon has therefore been transported all over the world before it ends up here on our plates. This is because of the cheap labour force in Vietnam. That's why I always try to stress that this is a worldwide problem. If farmers in the Netherlands use lots of antibiotics for their animals it's not just a problem for the Dutch, but also for the rest of the world. And so we in Denmark must also have a say in what happens in the Netherlands. Norway and Sweden use only very few antibiotics, and to a certain extent Denmark is also doing quite well in this respect. We export food safety, but we also import problems with foodstuffs from other countries'. Aarestrup's statement is nicely illustrated by an event that took place in February 2013. It involved hamburgers and kebabs that had to be withdrawn from the market in Sweden because they were contaminated with EHEC (The Local 2013). The meat came from a Dutch meat processor in Enschede, which had delivered a consignment of 12,000 kilogrammes of meat strips to a Swedish hamburger manufacturer in October 2012. The meat from which the strips had been produced originated from six different abattoirs in Latvia, the United Kingdom, Poland and Hungary (The Irish Times 2013). In turn, these abattoirs sourced their animals from different farmers. It is therefore impossible to say where the meat batch became infected. Most of the hamburgers and kebabs were sold on the Swedish market, but some of them were also exported from Sweden to Finland and Spain. Helena Storbjörk Windahl of the *Livsmedelsverket* (Swedish food authority) told me that the Dutch meat supplier's documents proved that they had complied with all the regulations. 'Everything indicates that the meat was tested for the presence of bacteria', she said. 'But actually only a few samples are ever tested, and with such a large quantity of meat originating from so many different sources any contamination can easily be overlooked. Only one piece of meat has to be contaminated with EHEC. The more sites are involved in meat production, the greater the risks for food safety'.

The contamination of salmon produced by the Dutch fish processing firm of Foppen with *Salmonella* is another good example of what Aarestrup means. Smoked salmon was contaminated with *Salmonella Thompson* at a Foppen production site in Greece. It was mainly sold in the Netherlands, but some of it ended up on the American market. An estimated 23,000 people were colonised and infected by the bacterium. In the case of 1149 patients, a *Salmonella* infection was confirmed in the laboratory (Friesema et al. 2012). Four people died of this infection. The bacterium was able to nestle in packaging trays that a design fault had made too porous. The trays were stored in a non-refrigerated room at Foppen's Greek subsidiary. The Greek heat did the rest (OvV 2013). The fish processor has frequent hygiene problems. The company had to pay fines in 2010, 2011 and 2012, and in 2014 Foppen was again placed under heightened supervision owing to deficient hygiene (Schippers 2014).

## Chicken Meat as a Risk for MRSA-Colonisation

A study carried out in 16 Dutch hospitals between 2009 and 2011 showed that consumption of chicken meat by people with no known classic risk factors represents a risk factor for colonisation with MRSA. Traditionally, risk factors have included recent admission to a hospital abroad or contact with pigs or calves. This was the first time it was established that consumption of chicken is also a risk for colonisation by MRSA (Van Rijen et al. 2013). Before this, several Dutch research teams had established that a large proportion of the chicken in Dutch shops is contaminated with ESBL. ESBL was found in many other kinds of meat as well, but in much smaller quantities than in chicken. It was therefore not possible to ascertain whether the animals came into contact with ESBL-producing bacteria at the abattoir, or whether they had already been carriers prior to this (Overdevest et al. 2011; Leverstein-van Hall et al. 2011). 'People can in fact become infected with ESBL while preparing or consuming chicken meat', Dik Mevius confirms, 'but that's not the only means of transfer. It only partly explains the ESBL problem. Not all ESBLs that we find in people actually correspond genetically to the strains that we can identify in chickens'. This is confirmed by various studies, for example those by scientists at the VU University Medical Centre in Amsterdam or the team headed by Maurine Leverstein-van Hall.

## Governments Must Take Responsibility

Behind one country's problems with food safety there very often lurks a problem that concerns all countries. These problems, therefore, need to be tackled on a global level, says Frank Møller Aarestrup. 'If we could guarantee that the salmon I spoke about earlier were filleted and packaged under the same conditions and regulations in Vietnam that apply here, then there wouldn't be a problem any more. But we haven't yet got that far. Traditionally, food safety is the responsibility of individual countries. This must change, because it does not correspond to reality. The primary production of foodstuffs takes place in one country, the processing of a product suitable for consumption in another, and the problems with food safety then occur in a third country. We need institutions that draw up rules with universal validity. In fact some already exist, for example the European Food Safety Authority (EFSA)[16] and the Codex Alimentarius Commission,[17] which draw up global standards for food safety. The biggest problem is national governments' lack of willingness to take responsibility for the problem and to recognise that they are part of a globalised world. More than anywhere else, this is a problem in emerging and developing countries—where primary and secondary production often takes place, and where the risks for food safety are much greater. We must provide these people with more information about possible solutions, and agree on standards that are good for everybody. And if this takes too long or doesn't work, we can argue that, if you don't fulfil these safety requirements, we won't import your food products any more. This threat is a good spur to motivation. In India you often hear people say: "Why should we talk about food safety? Perhaps we should first talk about how we can guarantee that everyone has something to eat." And naturally I understand that. But one shouldn't stop talking about food safety just because there's a shortage of food', thinks Aarestrup. 'It is fully justified if we say to other countries: "If you want to export your products to us, you must fulfil our safety standards. It is also a way of ensuring that developing countries don't make the same mistakes that we did in the past. They may also decide to produce for the local market only, and thus fulfil their own safety standards. In the EU, restaurants can put raw meat on the menu. In the US that's not allowed. There's a much greater fear of EHEC over there. But it's also connected with the legislative culture there. In the US, if someone falls ill after going to a restaurant, the restaurant owner is swiftly taken to court. That's very easy over there. The standards for food safety in the US and Europe aren't really that different. But the way in which they're used certainly is'.

## Unfortunate Circumstances

One day in 2003, as Eric and Ine van den Heuvel were leaving the Radboud University Medical Centre in Nimwegen with their critically ill 2-year-old daughter Eveline, and reflecting on what had happened to them, it became clear that quite a lot

---

[16]Most of the work of the European Food Safety Authority is done in response to requests from the European Commission, the European Parliament or EU member states, as the EFSA website states (EFSA 2020).

[17]The Codex Alimentarius Commission (Codex) is an international forum of 188 member states and one memberorganisation (the European Union) coordinated by the FAO (the UN Food and Agriculture Organisation) and the WHO (World Health Organisation) (Codex Alimentarius 2020).

of things had already been going wrong for some time without their being aware of it. Their daughter was supposed to undergo open heart surgery for a second time, but then it emerged she was carrying an MRSA. Hospitals have a real fear of MRSA. If the bacterium appears in a hospital, a lot of money and effort is needed to get rid of it again. But above all, MRSA is especially dangerous for vulnerable patients. It was therefore not possible to carry out the necessary operation. As with every other carrier of *Staphylococcus aureus,* the doctors recommended that Eveline and her parents should first try to get rid of the bacteria by decolonisation,[18] in order to prevent postoperative wound infections. Finally, Eveline underwent the operation all the same. By February 2004, 18 months after her first heart operation, the situation had worsened and was now life threatening. After the operation, she was treated for several weeks under isolation conditions. Visitors were only allowed near her in special protective clothing. At first, the Van den Heuvels had no idea where their daughter could have come into contact with MRSA. The link to their own pig-fattening farm only became apparent to them when, in a group of pig farmers that had stayed at the Van den Heuvels' house for a training session, MRSA was found 730 times more frequently than amongst the general population. The fact that four out of five members of the family were also carrying MRSA is not particularly significant. This is the case with more than a half of MRSA-positive patients. This case of livestock-associated MRSA, the first known case in a human being in the Netherlands, was discovered by clinical microbiologist Andreas Voss from Nijmegen (Voss et al. 2005). 'At the same time similar events occurred in three other places in the Netherlands, which triggered immediate investigations', Professor Jan Kluijtmans reported during a meeting on the occasion of European Antibiotic Awareness Day 2011. More and more cases of livestock-associated MRSA are occurring in people who have never had contact with animals. MRSA carriers in the general public represent a threat to successful MRSA policy in the Netherlands. The basis of this policy is that the risk groups—patients who have recently been in a hospital abroad, or farmers and their families—are carefully screened before they are admitted to hospital (Kluijtmans 2011; Sikkens and van Agtmael 2012). According to Jan Kluijtmans, the MRSA policy costs the Amphia Hospital in Breda 5.54 euros per admission. But as a result the hospital also saves 10.11 euros that would otherwise have to be spent on colonised or infected patients. And, moreover, more than 15 deaths are avoided every year (Van Rijen and Kluytmans 2009). The more MRSA spreads among the general population, the fewer benefits the screening provides. Members of the general public do not fulfil the criteria for the risk groups, and so are not identified by the screening policy.

In a 2-year study of the incidence of MRSA in 17 Dutch hospitals, 1023 cases of MRSA were identified (RIVM 2012). In almost 60 per cent of these cases, the germ

---

[18]'Decolonisation' is a way of eradicating or reducing considerably the asymptomatic carriage of MRSA. The procedures are carried out for at least 5 days. The nares, the nasopharynx, the skin (especially folds of the skin), the gastrointestinal tract and the perineum are the main sites of colonization by MRSA and, thus, for decolonization. After this, new cultures are taken to see if the treatment has been effective.

could be traced back to contact with animals. In almost 15 per cent of cases, a recent admission to a hospital abroad may have been the cause. In over a quarter of cases the source of the infection or colonisation could not be identified. Livestock-associated MRSA is found not only in pigs and calves, but also in poultry. 15 per cent of the meat consumed in the Netherlands is contaminated with MRSA. This may possibly play a role in the infection of people who have no other risk factors.[19] For some years now, the number of actual infections by MRSA in the Netherlands has been slightly increasing. In 2011 the figure was 1060 (RIVM 2012), in 2012 slightly more, with 1067 cases (RIVM 2013), and in 2013 there were 1110 cases (RIVM 2014). In 2014, this trend was interrupted: the national reference centre identified 859 invasive MRSA isolates, a clear decline by comparison with the previous year (RIVM 2015). In 2015, the national reference centre only recorded 709 invasive MRSA isolates, more than 80 per cent of which were not livestock associated (Nethmap/Maran 2016). It is assumed that more than 85 per cent of all the MRSA isolates are sent to the reference centre from laboratories in the Netherlands. In 2016, the number of invasive MRSA-isolates identified by the national reference laboratory at the RIVM decreased again to 518, more than two-thirds of these invasive ones originating from pus or wounds (NethMap/MARAN 2017). In 2017 there was a slight increase in the number of MRSA-isolates to 560 (NethMap/MARAN 2018). In 2018 the number of invasive MRSA-isolates increased again to 634 out of 31.266 diagnostic isolates (2%). Since the use of selective culture media strongly favours the isolation of MRSA over methicillin-susceptible *S. aureus* the MRSA-prevalence in the population may be lower than expected based on these data. In blood isolates the MRSA prevalence was 1.2% (NethMap/MARAN 2019). In 2019 621 out of 30,661 diagnostic isolates were MRSA, again 2% (NethMap/MARAN 2020).

In Denmark, the Statens Serum Institutet confirmed a total of 1.981 *S. aureus* infections in 2016. The number of cases has stabilized at this level after a steep increase from approximately 1500 annual cases before 2014. Forty (2.1%) of the cases were caused by MRSA. Thus, the MRSA frequency among *S. aureus* blood isolates continues to be very low compared to most other countries. Seven of the 40 MRSA cases were caused by LA-MRSA (compared to three in 2015) (DANMAP 2017). The number of bacteraemias with *Staphylococcus aureus* increased to 2104 cases in 2017. The share of methicillin-resistant *Staphylococcus aureus* (MRSA) bacteraemias was 2.2% in 2017, and thus remained low. The total number of new MRSA cases recorded in 2017 (3.579) was in line with the 2016 level (3555 cases), which is more than four times the 2008 level (853 cases). The strong increase seen in the past 10 years is, in part, due to the introduction of new screening practices, including the introduction of livestock MRSA into the screening programme. However, it is also due to an increase in the number of community-acquired cases and the development of livestock MRSA. Livestock MRSA comprised the largest single group (34%) of the total number of MRSA cases in 2017 (DANMAP 2018). In 2019

---

[19]Data from an oral communication in 2012 of Professor Jan Kluijtmans to the author.

3.657 cases of Methicillin-Resistant *Staphylococcus aureus* were registered, of which around 30% were due to LA-MRSA. Out of 2.233 bacteraemia caused by *S. aureus*—susceptible and resistant to methicillin combined—2.1% were due tot MRSA (DANMAP 2019).

In Germany, the number of MRSA infections is at a much higher level than in the Netherlands, with approximately 14,000 cases per year (Gastmeier 2013). It did not change very much between 2007 and 2012, although the number of methicillin-resistant *Staphylococcus aureus* isolates decreased (Meyer et al. 2014). According to Matthias Pulz, Head of the regional health authority in Lower Saxony: 'In a lot of respects we in Lower Saxony are of course an integral part of the tendency seen in Germany. And we can see that MRSA has passed its peak'. In 2007, 33% of all invasive *S. aureus* isolates were MRSA; by 2012 that number had decreased to 27% (Meyer et al. 2014). According to ECDC data published in 2018 the MRSA-rate in Germany decreased from 12.9% in 2014 to 9.1% in 2017. (ECDC 2018). And, according to the latest ECDC-data published in November 2020, it decreased further to 6.7% in 2019 (ECDC 2020).

'At the beginning of the 1990s the incidence of MRSA in the Netherlands and Germany was about the same', says Jörg Hermann, Director of the Institute for Hospital Hygiene in Oldenburg. 'It was around one per cent'. When MRSA appeared in those days, the Dutch tackled the problem directly with their 'search and destroy' strategy. They said: 'This is scary for us. We don't want these pathogens in our hospitals. We're going to isolate all the patients carrying them, and try to eradicate these pathogens so that they don't spread further'. The Germans believed that whenever a new form of resistance appeared, all you had to do was develop a new antibiotic and the problem would be under control. To understand this you have to look at their tradition of antibiotics discovery and production—because Germany, with its big companies like Bayer, was the heartland of antibiotics development. This was an enormous mistake. Because of it, patients were not isolated early on and the germs were not destroyed. They always believed that you only had to give infected patients the right antibiotic and everything would work out all right. But it did not. In the 1960s, there were editorials in major international newspapers claiming that 'we have now concluded the chapter on infectious diseases'. Antibiotics would control all of that. And then the bacteria taught us that they were considerably quicker and more capable of adaptation than we are'.

---

## Good Bacteria

Like so many pig breeders Van den Heuvel used large quantities of antibiotics, but was not aware of the risks they might pose for his own health and that of his family. What happened to Eveline, and what the Van den Heuvels found out about the dangers of excessive antibiotics use afterwards, occasioned a radical shift in their thinking. As a first step, the Van den Heuvels ensured that the hygiene in the livestock buildings was optimised. For example, the feeding dishes and other objects they used to tend their animals were moved around less. They used separate clothing for each herd. The piglets from different sows were no longer kept together, and when they were given iron, new needles were used for each litter. Since they had learnt that antibiotics are of no use against viruses, they stopped giving the animals antibiotics as a treatment against swine flu. They were only treated with aspirin powder. Animal feed enriched with antibiotics was also out of the question now. This package of measures led to a reduction of antibiotics uses by more than a half. That was in 2009. Afterwards the Van den Heuvels began to use probiotics on a large scale.[20] They cleaned with probiotics, added them to the drinking water in order to purify the water system probiotically and keep it clean, and they sprayed the animals' stalls with it.

In this way, they created a completely different climate in the sty, with mainly good bacteria instead of pathogenic ones. The result, says Van den Heuvel, was that by 2011 antibiotics use on their farm was 95 per cent lower than in 2008. And the financial results gave them no cause for complaints either, he says. There are several other pig breeders like the Van den Heuvels. And now there are also intensive poultry breeders who get by (almost) without antibiotics.

Jan Kluijtmans thinks that this is the path we have to pursue further. 'Reducing antibiotics use in intensive livestock farming by a half is of course a good start, and the sector seems to be on the right track', he says 'But we must aim at a much greater reduction of antibiotics use. I envisage a value of around 90 per cent'. In an interview published in the fourth quarter of 2011 by *Wageningen World*—a quarterly periodical produced by the Wageningen University agricultural department—Jan Kluijtmans goes one step further. 'Ideally we must aim at intensive livestock farming without antibiotics. Wageningen has the expertise needed to implement sustainable livestock farming, with vaccines against veterinary contagions, better animal feed and better livestock barns'. But consumers will then have to pay more for meat, because the present system of intensive livestock farming with its low margins cannot work sustainably (Sikkema 2011).

The ideal scenario described by Professor Kluijtmans is still a long way off. On 19 March 2015, an unsettling study appeared in PNAS, the *Proceedings of the National Academy of Sciences* (Van Boeckel et al. 2015). In 2010, 228 countries across the entire world used a total of 63,151 tonnes of antibiotics for livestock breeding. The big users were China, with 23 per cent of total use, the United States (13%), Brazil (9%), India (3%) and Germany (3%). Between 2010 and 2030 the total use of antibiotics in intensive livestock farming will increase by 67 per cent, to 105,596 tonnes. Two-thirds of this increase are attributable to growing animal stocks, the rest to the expansion of intensive livestock farming. In China, Brazil, Russia, India and South Africa, the use of antibiotics in intensive livestock farming will actually double up until 2030. In these countries, their use in human medicine will rise by around 13 per cent in the same period. By 2030, the list of the top five users of antibiotics in intensive livestock farming will look somewhat different from

---

[20]According to the Food and Agriculture Organization of the United Nations and the World Health Organization, probiotics are living microorganisms that benefit the host organism's health if administered in sufficient quantities (FAO/WHO 2002).

the way it did in 2010. China will still head the list, with 30 per cent of total use. It will be followed by the United States with 10 per cent, Brazil with eight, India with four and Mexico with 2 per cent.

In his office in Hanover, Matthias Pulz, President of the Lower Saxony Regional Health Authority, comments on the important developments that are taking place in Germany and the Netherlands. 'Medical doctors and veterinarians have come a bit closer together. Earlier there was only opposition between them, but now I believe a certain mutual understanding is developing. They know that they can only solve this together. It is not going to work if each excludes the other. As the regional health authority we're in very close contact with the State Office for Consumer Protection and Food Safety in Oldenburg, our counterpart in the veterinary sector. Many people believe that the antibiotic resistance problem is only connected with agriculture. However, I don't believe this. There are reciprocal effects between the two areas. The problem of antibiotic resistance in intensive livestock farming naturally has an impact on the human domain. The key problem, however, is without doubt selection. The way I use my antibiotics also affects whether any germs I introduce find particularly good conditions for multiplying. We're still in the initial stages, but we now have a chance to give the matter of "antibiotics use" the attention it deserves. We've been talking about it for 20 or 30 years, but now we could perhaps succeed, because we also have the legal requirements'.

Guido Werner of the RKI also sees opportunities to take action and reduce antibiotic resistances. 'A very small staff/patient ratio, for example in an intensive care unit, can certainly be an important factor for preventing the spread of multiresistant pathogens. Moreover this has already been proven by the relevant studies'. In fact the staff/patient ratio could be a decisive factor. On 19 March 2015 issue of *PLOS Computational Biology,* a study appeared that seems to confirm this explicitly. At a hospital in the French spa resort of Berck-sur-Mer, the movements of patients and nursing staff were registered by radio sensors. The interactions of 590 participants in the study were recorded every 30 seconds over a period of 4 months. Analysis of the data collected showed that the many contacts between nursing staff and patients were the channel through which *Staphylococcus aureus* was transferred. The more patients a nurse has to look after, the greater the probability that they will spread the bacteria in their patient group (Obadia et al. 2015).

---

## Reserved for Humans

Professor Jan Kluijtmans was a member of the Health Council of the Netherlands commission that published the report 'Antibiotics in intensive livestock farming and resistant bacteria in humans' on 31 August 2011 (Gezondheidsraad 2011). It named the top three resistant bacteria that were suspected to have a possible causal connection with antibiotics use in intensive livestock farming. The report mentioned bacteria producing vancomycin-resistant Enterococci (VRE), methicillin-resistant *Staphylococcus aureus* (MRSA) and extended spectrum beta-lactamases (ESBL).

'The problems with VRE and MRSA', the Health Council wrote, 'play a role in hospitals in particular, and are kept under control through an intensive programme of infectious disease management. In the case of MRSA this is called a "search and destroy" policy (identification of carriers, isolation of patients and eradication of their carrier status) [...] Livestock-associated MRSA is still well controlled in hospitals, but now it also seems to be occurring amongst the general population. ESBL-producing bacteria are the biggest problem. These bacteria quickly gain ground and are not confined to hospitals, but are also found in other places, above all as causal agents for urinary tract infections that are difficult to treat'. Although the extent to which livestock farming is involved in the spread of ESBL is not precisely known, according to the commission ESBL-producing bacteria pose the greatest microbial threat to public health arising from livestock farming, both now and in the near future.

The Council declares that antibiotics that are used as a last resort against human infections by ESBL-producing bacteria must be reserved exclusively for this purpose. The Health Council commission recommends that the relatively new antibiotic tigecycline[21] should not be approved for the veterinary medicines market, and advises against the use of carbapenem antibiotics in veterinary medicine.[22] The problems with carbapenems in intensive livestock farming predicted by the Health Council in 2011 were not long coming. In January 2014 the German Federal Institute for Risk Assessment reported on the first carbapenemase-producing *Enterobacteriaceae* in livestock, with an update 2 years later (BfR 2016). And this was not the last report on the topic.[23] In the long term, an alternative for the use of colistin in veterinary medicine will have to be found. In the short term a ban is not possible, since colistin is the first choice for treatment of certain animal diseases. In summer 2013 the European Medicines Agency (EMA) published a recommendation that the European Commission should restrict the use of colistin in veterinary medicine as far as possible. Only sick animals and animals which come in contact with sick animals should still be treated with colistin. Preventative use must be prohibited (EMA 2013). The Dutch Health Council also demands a ban on the use of third- and fourth-generation cephalosporins for group treatment of animals. 'In order to make actual reductions in resistance development over the long term, the use of all beta-lactam antibiotics for preventative and systematic interventions in livestock farming should be forbidden'. The Health Council commission also proposes that all new antibiotics and all presently available antibiotics that are no longer used in intensive livestock farming, or not used there at all, should be reserved for human

---

[21]If a bacterium is resistant to antibiotics of the carbapenem class, there are still two other medicines left that can be used: tigecycline and colistin.

[22]If no approved medicine is available for a specific disease the veterinary surgeon must act according to a decision tree, which can lead to their using a medicine approved for humans on animals.

[23]For more on this topic see Chap. 7 *The end in sight.*

use.[24] 'When limiting the use of antibiotics in intensive livestock farming, in the commission's view it is of decisive importance that the agreements are carried out: it must be clear which authority is monitoring compliance and is entitled to punish abuses. Good, transparent recording of antibiotics use in intensive livestock farming is an indispensable part of this' (Gezondheidsraad 2011).

A few days after the Health Council's statement, a similar report appeared from the Van Doorn Commission. This had been commissioned to carry out an investigation into the future of intensive livestock farming by the province of North Brabant. The President, Daan van Doorn, had formerly been a senior manager at VION, the biggest meat processing firm in the Netherlands. Like the Health Council, van Doorn and his team support the idea of banning the preventative use of antibiotics in intensive livestock farming. The Van Doorn Commission also proposes drawing up a blacklist of the antibiotics that are important for human beings, and may no longer be used in livestock farming. Nutreco, the largest supplier of animal feeds in the Netherlands, supports the approach suggested by Van Doorn. Market leader Albert Heijn and 16 other supermarket chains support this strict antibiotics policy. Animal protection, environmental and consumer groups should also be invited to support it. Albert Heijn and LTO are following the example of the Van Doorn Commission. On 1 September 2011, 27 parties[25] signed the so-called 'Den Bosch Agreement'. In it they promised that all meat in supermarkets would be antibiotic free by 2020 (Commissie Van Doorn 2011). Major interest groups such as *Natuur en Milieu* (Nature and Environment), the Dutch Society for the Protection of Animals and the Brabant Environmental Federation did not sign the Den Bosch Agreement because it does not abolish factory farming and says nothing about the number of factory farms which will be allowed to continue operating.

## References

Aarestrup, F. M., Jensen, V. F., Emborg, H. D., et al. (2010). Changes in the use of antimicrobials and the effects on productivity of swine farms in Denmark. *American Journal of Veterinary Research, 71*(7), 726–733. https://doi.org/10.2460/ajvr.71.7.726.

Beemer, F., Van Velzen, G., Van den Berg, C., et al. (2010). *Wat zijn de effecten van het ontkoppelen van voorschrijven en verhandelen van diergeneesmiddelen door de dierenarts?* In Dutch. Accessed November 30, 2020, from https://edepot.wur.nl/133692

BelVet-SAC. (2010). *Belgian Veterinary Surveillance of Antimicrobial Consumption National consumption report 2010.* Accessed November 29, 2020, from https://bit.ly/3gwRdCw

BfR. (2016). *Bundesinstitut für Risikobewertung. Antibiotikaresistenz: Carbapenemase-bildende Keime in Nutztierbeständen. Aktualisierte Mitteilung Nr. 036/2016 des BfR vom 23.12.2016.* In German. Accessed December 9, 2020, from https://bit.ly/2LqG6zP

---

[24]Besides tigecycline (already mentioned in connection with ESBL-producing bacteria), the commission also includes in this category glycopeptides (e.g. vancomycin), daptomycin, oxazolidinone (linezolid) and mupirocin.

[25]These included supermarket chains, abattoirs, farmers' associations and animal feed suppliers.

Bleker, H., & Schippers, E. I. (2012). *Antibioticagebruik in de veehouderij. Letter to parliament.* In Dutch. Accessed December 3, 2020, from https://bit.ly/3otkMbr

Boerderij. (2014). *Bedrijf en woning diervoerfabrikant doorzocht.* In Dutch. Accessed December 6, 2020, from https://bit.ly/2VMieZf

Bos, M. E. H., Taverne, F. J., Van Geijlswijk, I. M., et al. (2013). Consumption of antimicrobials in pigs, veal calves, and broilers in The Netherlands: quantitative results of nationwide collection of data in 2011. *PLoS One, 8*(10), e77525. https://doi.org/10.1371/journal.pone.0077525.

Codex Alimentarius Commission. (2020). *International food standards.* Accessed December 6, 2020, from https://bit.ly/33Ou5dE

Commissie Van Doorn. (2011). *Al het vlees duurzaam De doorbraak naar een gezonde, veilige en gewaardeerde veehouderij in 2020.* In Dutch. Accessed December 9, 2020, from https://edepot.wur.nl/176874

DANMAP. (2013). *DANMAP 2012 - Use of antimicrobial agents and occurrence of antimicrobial resistance in bacteria from food animals, food and humans in Denmark.* Accessed November 30, 2020, from https://bit.ly/3qcgMgB

DANMAP. (2014). *DANMAP 2013 - Use of antimicrobial agents and occurrence of antimicrobial resistance in bacteria from food animals, food and humans in Denmark.* Accessed November 30, 2020, from https://bit.ly/3oeLowl

DANMAP. (2015). *DANMAP 2014 - use of antimicrobial agents and occurrence of antimicrobial resistance in bacteria from food animals, food and humans in Denmark.* Accessed November 30, 2020, from https://bit.ly/36n7k28

DANMAP. (2017). *DANMAP 2016 - use of antimicrobial agents and occurrence of antimicrobial resistance in bacteria from food animals, food and humans in Denmark.* Accessed December 7, 2020, from https://bit.ly/39Ozp4D

DANMAP. (2018). *DANMAP 2017 – Use of antimicrobial agents and occurrence of antimicrobial resistance in bacteria from food animals, food and humans in Denmark.* Accessed December 7, 2020, from https://bit.ly/33PgLWg

DANMAP. (2019). *DANMAP 2019 - Use of antimicrobial agents and occurrence of antimicrobial resistance in bacteria from food animals, food and humans in Denmark.* Accessed April 5, 2021, from https://www.danmap.org/reports/2019

De Telegraaf. (2012). *1000 kilo illegale antibiotica in Brabant.* In Dutch. Accessed December 3, 2020, from https://bit.ly/3npeOqB

ECDC (European Centre for Disease Prevention and Control). (2018). *Surveillance of antimicrobial resistance in Europe – Annual report of the European Antimicrobial Resistance Surveillance Network (EARS-Net).* Accessed December 8, 2020, from https://bit.ly/2L69ICM

ECDC (European Centre for Disease Prevention and Control). (2020). *Data from the ECDC Surveillance Atlas – Antimicrobial Resistance.* Accessed December 8, 2020, from https://bit.ly/35lcsTm

EFSA (European Food Security Authority). (2020). Accessed December 6, 2020, from https://www.efsa.europa.eu/

EMA (European Medicines Agency). (2011). *Trends in the sales of veterinary antimicrobial agents in nine European countries (2005-2009).* Accessed November 29, 2020, from https://bit.ly/2VgYBrS

EMA (European Medicines Agency). (2012). *Sales of veterinary antimicrobial agents in 19 EU/EEA countries in 2010.* Accessed November 29, 2020, from https://bit.ly/3mfdOFP

EMA (European Medicines Agency). (2013). *Use of colistin products in animals within the European Union: development of resistance and possible impact on human and animal health.* Accessed December 9, 2020, from https://bit.ly/3n3Pl6S

EMA (European Medicines Agency). (2016). *Sales of veterinary antimicrobial agents in 29 European countries in 2014.* Accessed November 30, 2020, from https://bit.ly/2Jue05G

EMA (European Medicines Agency). (2017). *European Surveillance of Veterinary Antimicrobial Consumption. Sales of veterinary antimicrobial agents in 30 European countries in 2015.* Accessed November 29, 2020, from https://bit.ly/36jnqKg

EMA (European Medicines Agency). (2018). *European Surveillance of Veterinary Antimicrobial Consumption. Sales of veterinary antimicrobial agents in 30 European countries in 2016.* Accessed from https://bit.ly/3oaaJXY

EMA (European Medicines Agency). (2019). *European Surveillance of Veterinary Antimicrobial Consumption. Sales of veterinary antimicrobial agents in 31 European countries in 2017.* Accessed November 29, 2020, from https://bit.ly/2HT1fkG

EMA (European Medicines Agency). (2020). *European Surveillance of Veterinary Antimicrobial Consumption. Sales of veterinary antimicrobial agents in 31 European countries in 2018.* Accessed November 29, 2020, from https://bit.ly/2JnO6An

FAO/WHO. (2002). *Guidelines for the evaluation of probiotics in food.* Accessed December 8, 2020, from https://bit.ly/3s3L32a

FDA - US Food and Drug Administration. (2012). *Cephalosporin order of prohibition questions and answers.* Accessed from https://bit.ly/2JDQqDK

Feednavigator.com. (2014). *Dutch feed maker could face sanction over banned antibiotic in veal supply chain.* Accessed December 6, 2020, from https://bit.ly/3lQhHQx

Friesema, I. H., De Jong, A. E., Fitz James, I. A., et al. (2012). . Outbreak of Salmonella Thompson in the Netherlands since July 2012. *Eurosurveillance, 17*(43). Accessed from https://bit.ly/3hTOYtI

Gastmeier, P. (2013). *Nosokomiale Infektionen in Deutschland und Häufigkeit von Infektionen durch multiresistente Erreger. Oral presentation (in German) at the Bad Honnef symposium 2013 on 25 and 26 March 2013 in Königswinter Germany.* Accessed December 7, 2020, from https://bit.ly/2VRll1U

Gezondheidsraad. (2011). *Health Council of the Netherlands. Antibiotica in de veeteelt en resistente bacteriën bij mensen. Summary in Dutch.* Accessed December 8, 2020, from https://bit.ly/39TBkF6

Kluijtmans, J. (2011). *Oral presentation on livestock associated MRSA.* Bilthoven 18 Nov 2011. No link available.

Kovács, E. (2011). *Lessons from the Danish Ban on Antimicrobial Growth Promoters. Interfaith Centre on Corporate Responsibility.* Accessed November 30, 2020, from https://bit.ly/3hUcDtW

Leverstein-van Hall, M. A., Dierikx, C. M., Cohen Stuart, J., et al. (2011). Dutch patients, retail chicken meat and poultry share the same ESBL genes, plasmids and strains. *Clinical Microbiology and Infection, 17*(6), 873–880. https://doi.org/10.1111/j.1469-0691.2011.03497.x.

Levy, S. (2014). Reduced Antibiotic Use in Livestock: How Denmark Tackled Resistance. *Environmental Health Perspectives, 122*(6), A160–A165. https://doi.org/10.1289/ehp.122-A160.

Meyer, E., Schröder, C., Gastmeier, P., et al. (2014). The reduction of nosocomial MRSA infection in Germany. An analysis of data from the hospital infection surveillance system (KISS) between 2007 and 2012. *Deutsches Ärzteblatt International, 111*(19), 331–336. https://doi.org/10.3238/arztebl.2014.0331. Accessed from https://bit.ly/39dDltM.

NethMap/MARAN. (2016). *Consumption of antimicrobial agents and antimicrobial resistance among medically important bacteria in the Netherlands/Monitoring of Antimicrobial Resistance and Antibiotic Usage in Animals in the Netherlands in 2015.* Accessed December 7, 2020, from https://bit.ly/2VPpTWA

NethMap/MARAN. (2017). *Consumption of antimicrobial agents and antimicrobial resistance among medically important bacteria in the Netherlands/Monitoring of Antimicrobial Resistance and Antibiotic Usage in Animals in the Netherlands in 2016.* Accessed December 7, 2020, from https://bit.ly/3ous8v5

NethMap/MARAN. (2018). *Consumption of antimicrobial agents and antimicrobial resistance among medically important bacteria in the Netherlands/ Monitoring of Antimicrobial Resistance and Antibiotic Usage in Animals in the Netherlands in 2017.* Accessed December 7, 2020, from https://bit.ly/2JVXoEk

NethMap/MARAN. (2019). *Consumption of antimicrobial agents and antimicrobial resistance among medically important bacteria in the Netherlands/Monitoring of Antimicrobial Resistance and Antibiotic Usage in Animals in the Netherlands in 2018.* Accessed December 7, 2020, from https://bit.ly/37B3GRu

NethMap/MARAN. (2020). *Consumption of antimicrobial agents and antimicrobial resistance among medically important bacteria in the Netherlands/Monitoring of Antimicrobial Resistance and Antibiotic Usage in Animals in the Netherlands in 2019.* Accessed December 7, 2020, from https://bit.ly/3s4q7bf

NOS. (2011). *Normen voor antibiotica voor dieren.* In Dutch. Accessed December 1, 2020, from https://bit.ly/35lUSin

Obadia, T., Silhol, L., Opatowski, L., et al. (2015). Detailed contact data and the dissemination of *Staphylococcus aureus* in hospitals. *PLoS Computational Biology, 11*(3), e1004170. https://doi.org/10.1371/journal.pcbi.1004170.

Overdevest, I., Willemsen, I., Rijnsburger, M., et al. (2011). Extended-spectrum β-Lactamase Genes of *Escherichia coli* in Chicken Meat and Humans, the Netherlands. *Emerging Infectious Diseases, 17*(7), 1216–1222. https://doi.org/10.3201/eid1707.110209.

OvV - Onderzoeksraad voor Veiligheid -Dutch Safety Board. (2013). *Salmonella in smoked salmon. English summary.* Accessed December 6, 2020, from https://bit.ly/3gpBoh6 For the complete report, in Dutch, see https://bit.ly/3hTPQP0

RIVM. (2012). *Nationale surveillance van MRSA en CPE t/m week 52 2011.* In Dutch. Data on both 2010 and 2011. Accessed December 6, 2020, from https://bit.ly/2MIbVo9

RIVM. (2013). *Nationale surveillance van MRSA en CPE t/m week 52 2012.* In Dutch. Accessed December 6, 2020, from https://bit.ly/35nnMhS

RIVM. (2014). *Nationale surveillance van MRSA en CPE t/m week 52 2013.* In Dutch. Accessed December 7, 2020, from https://bit.ly/399I2om

RIVM. (2015). *Nationale surveillance van MRSA en CPE t/m week 52 2014.* In Dutch. Accessed December 7, 2020, from https://bit.ly/2JXGRzT

Schippers, E. I. (2014). *Beantwoording Kamervragen over salmonella en gezondheidsrisico's bij de firma Foppen.* In Dutch. Accessed December 6, 2020, from https://bit.ly/2LfPGp9

SDa. (2012). *Autoriteit Diergeneesmiddelen. Beschrijving van het antibioticumgebruik bij vleeskuikens, zeugen en biggen, vleesvarkens en vleeskalveren in 2011 en benchmarkindicatoren voor 2012. Rapportage van het expertpanel van de SDa, Autoriteit Diergeneesmiddelen.* In Dutch. Accessed December 1, 2020, from https://bit.ly/3ocU5r0 See also: Bos et al. 2013.

SDa. (2013). The Netherlands Veterinary Medicines Institute. *Usage of antibiotics in livestock in the Netherlands in 2012.* Accessed December 3, 2020, from https://bit.ly/2I6ZjFa

SDa. (2014). The Netherlands Veterinary Medicines Institute. *Usage of antibiotics in agricultural livestock in the Netherlands in 2013. Trends and benchmarking of livestock farms and veterinarians.* Accessed December 3, 2020, from https://bit.ly/3lEhbVy

SDa. (2015). The Netherlands Veterinary Medicines Institute. *Usage of antibiotics in agricultural livestock in the Netherlands in 2014. Trends and benchmarking of livestock farms and veterinarians.* Accessed December 3, 2020, from https://bit.ly/3qsik6v

SDa. (2016). The Netherlands Veterinary Medicines Institute. *Usage of antibiotics in agricultural livestock in the Netherlands in 2015. Trends and benchmarking of livestock farms and veterinarians, and a revision of the benchmarking method.* Accessed December 3, 2020, from https://bit.ly/39DsDyz

SDa. (2017). The Netherlands Veterinary Medicines Institute. *Usage of antibiotics in agricultural livestock in the Netherlands in 2016. Trends and benchmarking of livestock farms and veterinarians.* Accessed December 3, 2020, from https://bit.ly/3qqjkrG

SDa. (2018). The Netherlands Veterinary Medicines Institute. *Usage of antibiotics in agricultural livestock in the Netherlands in 2017. Trends and benchmarking of livestock farms and veterinarians.* Accessed December 3, 2020, from https://bit.ly/2JJJzZn

SDa. (2019). The Netherlands Veterinary Medicines Institute. *Usage of antibiotics in agricultural livestock in the Netherlands in 2018. Trends and benchmarking of livestock farms and veterinarians.* Accessed December 3, 2020, from https://bit.ly/2L55dYF

SDa. (2020a). The Netherlands Veterinary Medicines Institute. *About SDa*. Accessed December 1, 2020, from https://bit.ly/3bkkxLU

SDa. (2020b). The Netherlands Veterinary Medicines Institute. *Usage of antibiotics in agricultural livestock in the Netherlands in 2019. Trends and benchmarking of livestock farms and veterinarians*. Accessed December 1, 2020, from https://bit.ly/39wKWoU

Sikkema, A. (2011). Boeren zonder antibiotica. *Wageningen World, 2*(4), 10–15. In Dutch Accessed December 8, 2020, from https://edepot.wur.nl/218419

Sikkens, J. J., & van Agtmael, M. A. (2012). *Verslag Europese antibioticadag 2011: Antibiotica op het humaanveterinaire grensvlak*. In Dutch. Accessed December 6, 2020, from https://bit.ly/3bkT6Sd

Swann, M. M., Baxter, K. L., Field, H. I., et al. (1969). Report of the Joint Committee on the use of Antibiotics in Animal Husbandry and *Veterinary Medicine*. Accessed November 30, 2020, from https://bit.ly/3bkpdBs

The Irish Times. (2013). *Swedish government withdraws hamburgers*. Accessed December 6, 2020, from https://bit.ly/3hVnHHt

The Local. (2013). *Meat recalled over E. coli faeces fears*. Accessed December 6, 2020, from https://bit.ly/3hYXpUH

Van Boeckel, T. P., Brower, C., & Gilbert, M. (2015). Global trends in antimicrobial use in food animals. *PNAS, 112*(18), 5649–5654. https://doi.org/10.1073/pnas.1503141112.

Van Rijen, M. M., & Kluytmans, J. A. (2009). Costs and benefits of the MRSA search and destroy policy in a Dutch hospital. *European Journal of Clinical Microbiology and Infectious Diseases, 28*(10), 1245–1252. https://doi.org/10.1007/s10096-009-0775-8.

Van Rijen, M. M. L., Kluytmans-van den Bergh, M. F. Q., Verkade, E. J. M., et al. (2013). Lifestyle-associated risk factors for community-acquired methicillin-resistant *Staphylococcus aureus* carriage in the Netherlands: An exploratory hospital-based case-control study. *PLoS One*, (8), 6, e65594. https://doi.org/10.1371/journal.pone.0065594.

Verburg, G., & Klink, A. (2010). *Deskundigenberaad RIVM en reductie antibioticumgebruik. Letter to the Parliament with as supplement an expert advice on the reduction of the antibiotic use in livestock farming*. In Dutch. Accessed December 1, 2020, from https://bit.ly/2KO8NpO

Voss, A., Loeffen, F., Bakker, J., et al. (2005). *Methicillin-resistant Staphylococcus aureus* in pig farming. *Emerging Infectious Diseases, 11*(12), 1965–1966. https://doi.org/10.3201/eid1112.050428.

# The Role of Microbiology

9

To be able to react to an outbreak rapidly and adequately, you need microbiologists. And in Germany, surprisingly, that is a problem. In German hospitals, microbiological laboratories have been outsourced on a vast scale. And microbiologists have been made redundant. In some federal states, there is no longer a public health laboratory. When they make decisions concerning public health, health authorities have to rely utterly and entirely on the diagnoses and information of private laboratories and other providers. 'Because of the cuts in microbiology departments, the entire structure that previously existed to prevent infectious diseases has practically disappeared', says Professor Alex Friedrich, Head of the Department for Medical Microbiology and Hospital Hygiene at the University Medical Centre Groningen. Friedrich is German and worked in his homeland until the end of 2010. 'At the very most, ten per cent of the approximately 2000 hospitals in Germany still employ microbiologists. And even fewer hospitals have their own microbiological laboratory. Half of university hospitals no longer have a professor of hygiene, and big university hospitals such as Aachen have outsourced their medical microbiological diagnoses to a private laboratory'.[1] In all, there are less than 300 microbiologists left in German hospitals, and a number of these hold a management position. Some 200 microbiologists more work in other healthcare institutions and in private practices. In addition to this some 500 microbiologists, Germany counted 72 medical specialists for hygiene, so-called *Fachärzte für Hygiene*. That was the situation in 2012.

By 2020 the number of active microbiologists has increased. Hospitals in Germany employ 337 microbiologists, 317 more work in a private practice outside a hospital-setting and another 157 in different medical institutions. That brings the total of active microbiologists in Germany in 2020 to 811 (Ärztestellen 2020a). The number of active *Fachärzte für Hygiene* has also increased considerably to 227 (Ärztestellen 2020b). 'We see a clear increase in the number of microbiologists

---

[1]This conversation with professor Friedrich took place late 2012.

R. van den Brink, *The End of an Antibiotic Era*,
https://doi.org/10.1007/978-3-030-70723-1_9

and medical specialists for hygiene in Germany. That is good news', says professor Alex Friedrich in December 2020. The number of microbiologists per population is still higher in the Netherlands but the gap is narrowing. In 2018, the Netherlands counted 321 active microbiologists of whom 45% were female (Prismant 2019). That means that the Netherlands count 18 microbiologists per million inhabitants, whereas Germany counts 13 microbiologists per million inhabitants. Germany has 83.2 million inhabitants per 1 October 2020 (Destatis 2020a), almost five times as many as the Netherlands. There are 498,000 hospital beds in Germany, 6 for every 1000 inhabitants (Destatis 2020b). That is more than twice as many as the 2,3 beds per 1000 inhabitants in the Netherlands, with a total of 39,900 hospital beds end 2018 (De Staat van Volksgezonheid en Zorg 2020) for a population of roughly 17.5 million (CBS 2020). Of the 69 independent Dutch hospital-organisations, with 116 hospitals and 129 outpatient clinic facilities, 50 have their own laboratory (Volksgezondheidenzorg.info 2020; NVMM 2012).

The remaining hospitals rely on laboratories that work for several hospitals in the region for their medical microbiology needs. With the exception of laboratories in university medical centres (UMCs), generally speaking, the laboratories also work for resident doctors. A number of microbiological laboratories have specialised in specific problems. This applies particularly to the RIVM, the university medical centre laboratories and some larger peripheral laboratories. In the public healthcare sector, the RIVM has the leading role in the field of infectious diseases. There is a network that includes the RIVM, the health authorities and the microbiological laboratories contracted by the health authorities to perform this work.

## Lack of Cooperation

Friedrich was not alone in criticising the infrastructure for the prevention and control of infectious diseases in Germany. Professor Jürgen Heesemann, former President of the German Society for Hygiene and Microbiology, works at the Max von Pettenkofer Institute of the Ludwig Maximilian University in Munich. 'Microbiology is no longer part of hospital routine', he told me in 2012. 'Hospitals often have no microbiological departments at all, or only very limited ones. This has been caused by cuts'. Jörg Hermann is Director of the Institute for Hospital Hygiene in Oldenburg. The institute is responsible for hospital hygiene in all three medical centres in the north German university town. 'That's something quite special', says Hermann. 'There are public, private, catholic and protestant hospitals. For a long time this has meant that they don't cooperate with one another, and that's still the case today. On paper, the way we do things in Oldenburg looks very simple. One hygiene institute with a microbiological laboratory takes care of the three hospitals in Oldenburg. Then you go to the next town, and there the hospitals do not cooperate with one another at all. They don't work with competitors, neither in hygiene nor in microbiology. And of course that doesn't work'. This lack of cooperation between the hospitals has certainly not been beneficial for the position of medical microbiology in hospitals. As Hermann says, 'Even in the 1990s, attempts were already being made to outsource specific services from the hospitals owing to cost pressures. This is now the biggest problem. Microbiology has become more and more remote from the hospital. And we can no longer just reverse this situation at the drop of a hat. What's working so well in the Netherlands nowadays—the fact that there's an in-house microbiologist in the hospital, that they carry out diagnoses, that they can take the results to the ward and say, "I give antibiotics advice and I also have a hygiene specialist on hand, and you need to isolate the patient (or you don't)"—you hardly find this in Germany outside university medical centres. We only have equivalent microbiologists and specialist hygiene doctors who deal with this problem in five per cent of German hospitals, whereas such experts are to be found in over 90 per cent of hospitals in the Netherlands'.

Karsten Becker is a professor at the Friedrich Loeffler-Institute of Medical Microbiology at the medical faculty of the University of Medicine in Greifswald, in northeast Germany, since November 2019. For over 20 years, he served as a Professor at the Institute of Medical Microbiology at the University Hospital Münster. 'There was a shift of awareness that said that hygiene and microbiology were drivers and causes of costs. That is of course very dangerous, because the reality is the precise opposite. Those who take prophylactic measures, i.e. the hospital hygienists, and those who diagnose diseases—especially infections in our case—are those who save money in the long term if provided with appropriate staff and resources. This structurally determined awareness shift decisively contributed to the way the problem of multiresistant pathogens was ignored for a long time. Policymakers finally woke up again and took countermeasures only as a result of the pressure of practical effects. In other words, as a result of the fact that we have increasing numbers of multiresistant pathogens, at the moment gram-negative ones in particular, although we should by no means forget the gram-positive ones either. However, the idea that well-equipped diagnostic and prophylactic systems, i.e. hospital hygiene, saves money has still not penetrated the economic side of hospital management. Awareness of this is largely still lacking. And all this is still further intensified by the fact that, as a result of technological developments and market development trends, we are seeing a concentration of, for example, diagnostic systems. Hospitals that previously had microbiological laboratories and other laboratories, even university medical centres, now outsource these services. In this way they lose the close and, above all, necessary contacts between doctors working in diagnosis and those working in treatment, at the cost of patient safety. Added to this there are of course other factors, such as longer transport times or information loss. In my view this is a very, very dangerous development. And it isn't counteracted by the opposing trend of developing a so-called "point of care" diagnostic system, where you say "we're going to perform the diagnosis right by the sick bed". Because if that isn't carried out by trained staff it leads to incorrect assessment of the results. And—what's far worse still—in that case you lose the interconnections with the other diagnoses that are normally brought together in a microbiological laboratory. There is a fragmentation of facts, which then makes it more difficult to assemble a complete picture of the patient's situation. Of course, it's difficult to rebuild all this. Once the damage has been done it's obviously expensive to put it right again. It's very important to proceed in a coordinated, integrated manner. Prophylaxis, diagnostics, therapy and follow-up care—all these belong closely together. When you remove a building block because you think it will save costs, then you fall flat on your face'.

In some ways, a large outbreak can be a blessing in disguise. The major outbreak of enterohaemorrhagic *E. Coli* (EHEC) in Germany in 2011 claimed many victims, but in the end, it led to some important reforms of health laws.

On Thursday, 19 May 2011 the Robert Koch Institute (RKI) in Berlin received a message from Hamburg. In the first two weeks of May, there had been a strikingly large increase of EHEC infections with the dangerous complication HUS (haemolytic uremic syndrome) there. An EHEC infection is accompanied by severe, bloody diarrhoea. The bleeding is caused by haemorrhagic colitis—a colonic inflammation—which is accompanied by haemorrhages. In a small percentage of colonic infection cases, a so-called HUS can develop—an acute kidney failure that can become life-threatening. Three children had become infected with HUS at the same time. EHEC infections are normally caused by consumption or processing of contaminated food, or through contact with infected animals. On 20 May, a team from the RKI travelled to the university medical centre in Hamburg and spoke to 60 EHEC-positive patients there. More or less under the RKI specialists' very eyes, the number of HUS cases rose dramatically. In 3 months, 3842 patients fell ill with a gastrointestinal infection that had been caused by the particularly virulent EHEC strain O104:H4. Of the nearly 4000 people with an EHEC infection, 855 developed an HUS, and 2987 an EHEC gastroenteritis. This was the biggest HUS epidemic that had been known anywhere in the world so far. More than two-thirds of the HUS patients were female. In contrast to the EHEC variants that had been going around in previous years, EHEC O104:H4 was detected mainly in adults. Fifty-three patients died, of which 35 had suffered from HUS and 18 had a gastrointestinal infection. The size of this outbreak was unusually large. In the 5 years preceding this, an average of 218 cases of gastrointestinal infection by EHEC and 13 cases of HUS were reported in the same period (RKI 2011). In the years following the outbreak, the number of cases of EHEC gastroenteritis and HUS infections stabilised again at a much lower level, although it was still considerably higher than in the years preceding the outbreak. There were also patients outside Germany who were infected by the same strain as that of the German outbreak. As early as 25 May, Sweden reported nine HUS patients, all of whom had been in Germany shortly before. The Netherlands reported 11 patients suffering from an infection by the German EHEC strain. Four of them developed an HUS. In other parts of the European Union, a further 65 people contracted an infection by the same EHEC strain. Forty-nine of them developed an HUS. On 22 July 2011, 76 patients who were carrying an infection by the German EHEC strain were known to the ECDC in Stockholm, and as well as in Sweden, Denmark, France, the Netherlands and Norway, there were also similar patients in Austria, Poland, Spain, the Czech Republic and the UK. One of these patients died (European Commission 2011).

The message to the Robert Koch Institute concerning the cluster of HUS- and EHEC-positive patients was late arriving. The first patient was diagnosed on 2 May.

The first report did not come until 16 days later. Doctors and laboratories must report EHEC or HUS cases to their local health authorities within 24 hours. There the reports are checked and entered into an electronic database. All cases that fulfil the criteria listed by the RKI must then be reported to the health authority of the relevant federal state within three working days of the report to the local authority. Every case is then checked again, and reported to the RKI within a week. This process is meant to prevent duplicate or false reports from occurring. At the same time, it means that it can take up to two and a half weeks before the RKI are informed about HUS cases and possible outbreaks.

On 11 May 2012, a press conference was held at the University Hospital Münster on the occasion of the first anniversary of the big outbreak. The bacteria strain that had been responsible for so many deaths and enormous financial damage in 2011 was typed in Münster. But, once again, after a long delay. The first isolate of the outbreak strain did not arrive in Münster until Monday, 23 May 2011. Two days later, the strain was identified as O104:H4. 'There is no regulation in Germany requiring strains to be sent to the national reference laboratory', says Professor Helge Karch, Germany's leading EHEC specialist. Shortly after the press conference, I spoke with Professor Karch. 'Unfortunately I received this O104:H4 strain far too late. It took one to two weeks longer than necessary. The earlier it's possible to confirm which type of EHEC we're looking at, and whether the same strain is involved in several cases, the sooner we know whether we have to deal with an outbreak or with several simultaneously occurring individual cases. In this case particular urgency was demanded, because the strain was so pathogenic. And because, as intestinal bacteria, *E. coli* are very easily transferred. It's best to obtain a bacteria strain immediately from the first patient. But for that you need a functioning microbiology system where research and diagnosis are linked to one another'.

## Already Divided

Professor Martin Mielke is Head of the Department for Infectious Diseases at the Robert Koch Institute. At the beginning of 2014, he explained his views on the management of the 2011 EHEC outbreak to me at his office in Berlin. He expressed himself in less critical terms than some of his colleagues but acknowledged things could have been handled better. 'The first sample we received in connection with this went to the laboratory on Friday and on Monday the diagnosis was ready. By Tuesday it was clear which strain was present. It was a new strain that had not yet been described. In other words, after the material was received the pathogen was identified extraordinarily quickly. Herr Karch received the pathogen at the same time as us. We forwarded it immediately. There was no delay there'. But the outbreak strain took its time before arriving at the RKI. 'That's the main point', Mielke says. 'In Germany—but I think it's the same in the Netherlands—the diagnosis of EHEC is based on toxin identification. You don't include the culture automatically; first, you need to perceive an accumulation. When the accumulation had been detected, the material also came. We now know that the receipt of material for microbiological fine analysis occurred at a time when the food which triggered everything was already in circulation. Exactly the same would happen in an analogous case in another country. With EHEC you have an incubation time of up to ten days, and the food had been circulating for a long time before the patients developed symptoms'. After the RKI received the outbreak strain the diagnosis went very swiftly, but the outbreak had already been raging for some time before this strain was sent. There were no reports that anything unusual was going on. 'This is a hot topic', says Professor Mielke. 'A number of things were changed afterwards, for example the speed with which reports are passed on. With cases of diarrhoea, the moment a laboratory receives a stool sample a toxin test is also carried out, and that already triggers the report. There is an obligation to report such an action. The time interval until this report is forwarded is speeded up. That's actually one feature that was worse before the EHEC crisis than it is now. Fast-tracking the reporting channels was a direct reaction to the EHEC problem. When accumulations are observed, or in cases of EHEC, it's now the case that confirmation of a toxin-forming E. coli results in the stool being forwarded to the federal state laboratory. These are reactions to the crisis. And there, isolation and further type identification are carried out. The crucial feature of EHEC diagnosis is that isolating the pathogens that form the toxin is very time-consuming. And this isn't routinely carried out by the laboratories on-site. Therefore the process has now been organised so that the primary laboratories forward such a case to the federal state laboratory, and then they take responsibility for it. In this way, everything comes together there. The state laboratory gets an overview of everything, and can then carry out the relevant further diagnosis. This takes place with the support of the reference laboratory, which in our case is located at the RKI. And this speeds up the process'.

Professor Martin Mielke explains that, since 2011, still further changes have been carried out in the field of infection prevention in Germany, in addition to those he mentioned in connection with the EHEC outbreak. 'What's often lacking is the possibility of giving advice on-site. We amended the infection prevention law again in 2011, and microbiological and pharmaceutical advice are explicitly enshrined in legislation there. In large, well-managed hospitals, microbiologists definitely carry out antibiotics visits. But that doesn't happen in all hospitals. That's why, when amending the infection protection law, it was explicitly emphasised that this should be increasingly carried out and implemented. Infectiologists from the German Society for Infectiology, in other words actual clinicians who deal with infections, regard antibiotics advice as an important component of this. And as far as microbiology is concerned, there too it's accepted that we cannot achieve things just by carrying out laboratory investigations, but that it's a matter of on-site advice as well. This point can actually be found now in the hygiene regulations of the federal states. All 16 federal states have now responded to this aspect of the infection protection law, and during their inspections now consider whether such advice is available on-site. A lot of things have been set in motion here'.

Even before the EHEC outbreak, problems with MRSA in particular, but also with ESBL and other antibiotic-resistant bacteria made it clear that the prevention of infectious diseases in Germany was not functioning correctly. The German Bundestag recognised this problem. On 20 March 2011, the governing parties (CDU/CSU) and the FDP proposed a change to the infection protection law which would make the 400 largest hospitals in Germany, those with more than 400 beds each, legally obliged to reappoint hospital hygienists, with a particular view to preventing infection (BMG 2011). In July 2011, the change to the law was passed (Bundesamt für Justiz 2011). The new law says that the guidelines must be observed.[2] One of these guidelines stipulates that hospitals with more than 400 beds must employ a hospital hygienist (KRINKO 2009). Among other things, the justification for the new law states that between 400,000 and 600,000 of the more than 17 million patients in German hospitals contract a healthcare-related infection every year. These are usually caused by bacteria that are resistant to various types of antibiotics. According to estimates, 7500–15,000 patients die of these infections. Various interest groups of infectiologists and doctors working in public healthcare who were affected by the new law welcomed it, but in a joint declaration pointed out that at least 700,000 healthcare-associated infections occur annually, and that at last 30,000 deaths per year are connected with this (DGKH 2011). They emphatically demanded that sufficient financial resources should be provided to enable the new responsibilities to be implemented as well.

## Abstract Problems Versus Collective Problems

'The privatised laboratories are definitely a problem', says Heesemann. 'Their prices are low and they work very quickly, but they don't give any advice to doctors treating patients in hospitals. They send their results, that's all. Moreover when the EHEC outbreak occurred, this led to delays'. In her office in Münster Annette Jurke, who is responsible for infection prevention in North Rhine-Westphalia, expresses similar views. 'I wasn't in North Germany at the time. But I heard that fighting the outbreak wasn't helped very much by the fact that there were no microbiologists in the hospitals. There's no argument against outsourcing microbiological laboratories per se. But when that means you also outsource surveillance of (resistant) bacteria and hygiene expertise, then the quality of the whole thing changes. If I ask a hospital how many MRSA cases they have and they tell me that I must address this question to a laboratory in far-off Augsburg, then I know that they've taken outsourcing too far here. This information must be available in every hospital, in order to be able to interpret the results of the laboratories' cultures and tests. We have a vast number of hospitals in Germany. Far too many to have laboratories everywhere. And so it's all the more important to have specialists everywhere who can function as bridges between laboratories and clinics'. Professor Alexander Mellmann from Münster puts

---

[2]The RKI's Commission for Hospital Hygiene and Infection Prevention (KRINKO) draws up the guidelines.

it like this. 'For a big laboratory situated a few hundred kilometres from the hospital sending it a bacteria strain, a pathogenic bacterium of this sort is an abstract problem. They themselves are, of course, unaffected by it. This is a completely different situation from that in a hospital that has its own laboratory. There it's a collective problem'.

Besides the microbiological laboratories in hospitals, many laboratories in German regional health authorities have also been closed. The work they used to perform is now done by big laboratories as well. Since there are hardly any more regional or hospital laboratories, the bar for GPs who, for example, send in samples from patients with diarrhoea has been raised. Not because of the prices the big laboratories demand—they actually work more cheaply—but because there is no longer any laboratory in the local or regional healthcare network. In the Netherlands, the doctors send the isolates to their local GPs' or hospital laboratory. The short distances also guarantee quick results. The doctors can simply contact the microbiologists. The microbiologists from the hospital laboratories are available to answer their colleagues' queries and, if needed, go to visit the patients themselves. On top of this, they have the structures of the Centre for Infectious Disease Control at the RIVM at their disposal.

'Around 1000 staff work at the Robert Koch Institute in Berlin', says Alex Friedrich. 'That's far fewer than at the RIVM, where 1500 staff share a similar workload. But the RKI is responsible for five times as many people. The RKI's recommendations must also be implemented in the federal states. The authority to make decisions rests with the health authorities of the federal state. The local health authorities then put them in practice. Scaled up to a size equivalent to the RIVM's, the RKI would have to employ approximately 7000 staff distributed across the entire country. And here the few staff in the federal states do not make a great difference. Even though North Rhine-Westphalia has increased its staffing provision in recent years, the number of staff still falls far short of that in the Netherlands. And the few that there are in North Rhine-Westphalia don't have their own laboratory any more either. Which means that in practice they can only talk, add up figures, give advice and write e-mails. And then there are also 55 regional health authorities. The large ones, such as those in Cologne and Dusseldorf, still have their own laboratory. But the others don't. And in North Rhine-Westphalia there's no central laboratory like the RIVM in the Netherlands. Even though more people live there than in the Netherlands'. Alexander Mellmann mentions another sore point. 'The benefits of preventative measures aren't so easily expressed in terms of sums of money. What is the profit if you stop someone becoming ill? That's very difficult to calculate. No-one questions the benefits of car seat belts, even though the probability that something will happen to people driving without one is very small. The benefits of seat belts are difficult to calculate. We see the same problem in the case of infection prevention. What benefits do investments in this area bring? It's our task to explain this. Here in Münster, the management of the university hospital is convinced that investments in prevention pay off'.

# Help

According to Alex Friedrich of the University Medical Centre Groningen, purely in terms of hard figures, 800 new hospital hygienists had to be trained in Germany as a result of the new law from 2011. But to do this, the training opportunities first needed to be created. To cope with this need in Münster, the Westphalian Academy for Hospital Hygiene was founded in spring 2012. 'There we offer course places in the fields of infection prevention, medical microbiology and hospital hygiene for young doctors', says Mellmann. Many hospitals now train other specialist doctors, for example surgeons and specialists in internal medicine, who take a condensed form of the training course in hygiene. These trained specialist doctors can then take on the functions of a hospital hygienist as well. 'We offer help to some of our colleagues in Germany', says Friedrich. 'We go back to German hospitals and carry out work there. At the same time we try to find interested candidates whom we can train, so that they can then take over this work themselves. We're trying to set up a cross-border academy for postdoctoral training in microbiology and hospital hygiene in our Euregio'.[3] Ron Hendrix, who has been working as a clinical microbiologist since 2013 at Certe, the microbiology laboratory in Groningen, provides 'development aid' in Germany. He also works at the UMC Groningen, where he is involved in cross-border studies on antibiotics use. 'At the moment microbiology is an export winner for us. From our base at the UMC Groningen, we're training some of the staff at a large German hospital that's one and a half hours away.[4] And we give them distance advice. The management board of this hospital has understood that you can make money out of good infection prevention. In several hospitals we are now setting up a system that gives doctors time for this work. We train them, and we're standing in the wings ready to advise them if they get stuck. And we're getting more and more similar requests from Germany. This problem won't be solved in the next 10 years—no chance', says Hendrix. Alex Friedrich hopes that, for the first time, fully trained microbiologists and hospital hygienists will be newly appointed in the hospitals of the border region. 'In the border region we care for the patients collectively across the border. Therefore the quality of infection prevention on the German side of the border must achieve the same level as quickly as possible'. The latest data on the number of medical microbiologists and hygiene specialists show a positive trend regarding the number of specialised staff in German hospitals (Ärztestellen 2020a).

---

[3]This 'Euregio' (the Ems-Dollart region) comprises the Dutch provinces of Groningen, Friesland, Drenthe and Overijssel, and the north-western part of the German states of Lower Saxony and North Rhine-Westphalia.

[4]This refers to the Herford Clinics group, with a total of 800 beds. In addition a number of hospitals in the Münsterland—the area around the city of Münster—are given advice.

## IGZ Against Outsourcing of Laboratories and Microbiologists

The Netherlands' sound infection prevention and treatment structures, including their comprehensive network of medical microbiology laboratories, are envied around the world. And yet this successful model is the topic of debate. In December 2010, the Plexus management consultancy published a report on outpatient diagnosis for the Dutch Health Ministry (Plexus 2010). 'Compared with neighbouring countries', the authors wrote, 'the laboratory landscape in the Netherlands is highly fragmented, with the result that it is hardly possible to achieve savings. Observers from abroad speak of an "archaic structure" in which operational management lags far behind international developments'. In Plexus' view, outpatient diagnostic centres (ADZ) would be able to fulfil this role not just much more cheaply, but also to a quality standard that would be at least the same, or even higher. Depending on the assumptions made, Plexus arrives at savings of between 690 million and 1.14 billion euros per year. The Plexus report was naturally received very sympathetically by the leading officials at the health ministry.

'The way to continue in the future is for Dutch microbiology to continue functioning as it does now', was the reaction of Edwin Boel, former President of the Dutch Society for Medical Microbiology since November 2013, who works at the UMC Utrecht and who was appointed to lead the National Coordination Team Diagnostic Chain at the Health Ministry during the outbreak of SARS-CoV-2. 'The ministry is looking primarily at the costs of medical microbiology. How high is the price for a laboratory result? We have to make it much clearer what happens to the test results if we want to keep microbiology alive'.

## Buy Cheaply, Pay Dearly

Boel and the NVMM fear developments like those in Germany, where commercial laboratories take over the work of hospital laboratories. 'I can predict that it will be much more expensive if there is a development in the Netherlands comparable to that we've seen in Germany. In order to avoid this, we need to do a lot more to emphasise the added value of our work', says Boel. 'I have heard that the ministry has had talks with a series of large commercial laboratories abroad, including several in Germany and one in Antwerp. We also know that the Australian firm of Sonic is very interested in the European market. They have taken over a big commercial laboratory in Antwerp and are starting to build one in Nimwegen'. There are also several large commercial laboratories in the Netherlands already, for example a big laboratory for GPs in Etten-Leur. At the end of 2011, Maurine Leverstein-van Hall moved from the UMC Utrecht to the Haaglanden Medical Center (HMC) in the Hague. 'By centralising microbiological diagnosis in large commercial laboratories you can work more efficiently, because better use is made of the equipment. But medical microbiology has three functions, not just diagnosis. Above all else, a microbiologist is a kind of watchdog. They must make sure that no pointless diagnostic tests are demanded. But also that too little diagnosis isn't carried out either. Then, of course, they must perform their work in the laboratory, the actual diagnosis, and manage the lab. But they're also involved in direct care of the patients. And on top of this the microbiologist is also responsible for infection prevention. All these tasks are included in the price for a culture that is carried out in a hospital laboratory. In a commercial laboratory, all of these functions except pure diagnosis are omitted. Naturally that makes it cheaper. But also worse. Just look at the percentage of MRSA in the Netherlands and Germany, with their commercial laboratories.[5] And of course, you also lose the overview of what's going on in your own immediate surroundings. The GPs send their cultures to the GPs' laboratory in Etten-Leur, or even to Germany. If we admit a patient to hospital under such circumstances, we have no idea what they might already have had. And of course there's also a delay, because the material for the culture also has to be despatched. In cases of emergency diagnosis, short distances from the doctor submitting the sample are very important. This simply doesn't work at larger distances', says Leverstein-Van Hall.

This debate flared up in the spring and summer of 2020 as the Dutch laboratories for medical microbiology lacked the capacity to perform the required number of SARS-CoV-2 tests. It took several months before the Health Ministry decided to contract a number of large laboratories, specifically those in Germany, to perform part of the testing. The desire to protect the close-knit Dutch infrastructure of many smaller laboratories for medical microbiology against powerful market intruders—as the huge laboratories from abroad are perceived—certainly played a role in the slow decision-making in this respect in the Netherlands. The fear for a lesser quality of the diagnostic work proved to be not unrealistic. Some of the commercial labs did not automatically report positive tests to the public health authorities as required, making it impossible to track and trace the contacts of persons that contracted SARS-CoV-2 and undermining the containment of the outbreak (NOS 2020).

## What Do You Get for Your Money?

Within the NVMM, Gijs Ruijs—also a former president of the society—is intensively engaged in the discussion about the concentration of microbiological laboratories. Ruijs works as a clinical microbiologist at the Isala Clinics in Zwolle. 'I find that there's a dimension missing in the discussion about microbiology', says Ruijs. 'What do you get for the money you put into clinical microbiology? Even the

---

[5]For a long time, MRSA occured roughly 20 times more frequently in hospitals in Germany than in the neighbouring countries of Denmark and the Netherlands (Van Gemert-Pijnen 2011). See Foreword by Professor Alex Friedrich. A comparison between the Netherlands and North Rhine-Westphalia reveals even more favourable figures for the Netherlands. In the Netherlands, the percentage of MRSA in blood cultures is 0.9%. In North Rhine-Westphalia, the value is 32 times higher (Van Cleef et al. 2012): Since then number of MRSA blood isolates had considerably decreased in Germany to 11.3% in 2015 and further to 6.7% in 2019. But the MRSA-rate remained three times higher than in Denmark and even four times higher than in the Netherlands (ECDC 2020).

authorities aren't concerned about this. That's striking, to put it mildly. This content is lacking in the whole discussion about centralisation of laboratories. High volumes enable lower prices, but naturally you can't take part in patient visits in the intensive care unit when you work several 100 kilometres away from it. You need a good relationship with your colleagues, so that occasionally you can tell them you have an MRSA problem and must implement an admissions ban. You can't do that by e-mail'. Ruijs visited several laboratories abroad with his colleague Thijs Tersmette of the St. Antonius Hospital in Nieuwegein: Sonic Healthcare's AML in Antwerp—the largest commercial laboratory in Belgium—LABCO in Madrid[6] and *Labor Mönchengladbach MVZ Dr Stein + Kollegen*. 'In the laboratory in Mönchengladbach we were told they catered for 60 hospitals with five microbiologists. There are three of us in our hospital in Zwolle. On our tour of the laboratory we also visited the room containing the equipment used for processing blood cultures. They had one and a half times the number of devices that we had in the Isala Clinics. There can be no question that the diagnosis being carried out there is seriously inadequate. How can you carry out consultations in intensive care units with five microbiologists for 60 hospitals? Of course that's just not on. What you see in Germany isn't comparable with this specialism as we know it here. No way. And the decisions that are made in Germany have considerable effects. This is what happens when the whole discussion revolves around money, and not what you get for your money. I see vast potential in regional partnerships that include several hospitals. And as part of this, of course, you have to talk about the quality requirements a laboratory needs to fulfil'. By autumn 2013, the discussion on the centralisation of laboratories had moved a step closer towards becoming actual everyday practice. The VGZ health insurance firm—with 4.3 million policyholders a very important stakeholder—announced that it was aiming towards centralisation of microbiological laboratories. The VGZ wanted to make financing of laboratory diagnosis dependent on this. After talks in which Professor Alex Friedrich, on behalf of the Netherlands Society for Medical Microbiology, once again made it clear that the model proposed by the VGZ had foundered in Germany, and that they were now trying to reverse these developments, the representatives of the health insurer promised to think again about their new policy. The insurance firm is aware of the quality of microbiology in the Netherlands. 'The Netherlands possess a good microbiological network, with microbiologists in practically every hospital. This creates a tightly meshed network, which can be helpful in possible crisis situations'. The VGZ's conclusion is unambiguous: 'Microbiology is therefore less suited for concentration of service providers. An important point here is the difference between the presence of a microbiologist in a hospital and microbiological testing. A microbiologist fulfils other tasks besides just carrying out tests. They are involved in infection prevention, crisis situations etc. We do not desire a situation such as they have in Germany, where in many laboratories only a few microbiologists cater for

---

[6]The laboratories LABCO and Synlab has merged. The new name of the group is SYNLAB and it is market leader in Europe.

more than 50 or 100 hospitals. The question therefore remains, whether there should be several microbiologists in each hospital. [...] With regard to microbiology, we are now trying to find out what level of organisation is desirable. The results found will be decisive in determining what form future financing will take'. At the end of February 2015, Gijs Ruijs spoke out again. 'What is unpalatable about this discussion is that the insurance companies simply postulate something without saying what these statements are based on. Moreover they're describing a situation that applied around 30 years ago. They're completely forgetting that many peripheral activities form part of diagnosis nowadays, such as MRSA policy, local working agreements, extra sample diagnosis for GPs, training programmes for GPs and medical assistants, and much more still. None of that can be carried out by a German laboratory 200 km away. Because over there they have no idea what the working structures between the local GPs, medical specialists and health authorities are like. But the health insurers are all-powerful. They can operate as a cartel with impunity, and don't have to answer to anybody. There is no balance of power, and that is decidedly unhealthy'.

Health insurance company VGZ pushed again for concentration of clinical microbiological and other diagnostics in the fall of 2019 during the negotiations for the 2020 contracts. According to VGZ, the concentration of diagnostics is necessary because the tightly meshed network of laboratories for medical microbiology, clinical chemistry, pathology and for thrombosis care, add up to an overall overcapacity and a loss of efficiency. VGZ decided, very much against the will of the Dutch Society for Medical Microbiology (NVMM) and other scientific organisations, to contract one organisation responsible for all diagnostics, in each region. In the main regions where VGZ has an important position in the health insurance market, VGZ did as it announced and contracted one partner for all diagnostics (VGZ 2019).

## Complicity in the Charges

Roel Coutinho was the Director of the Centre for Infectious Disease Control in the Netherlands for many years. He knows his specialist area like few others. 'The efforts to outsource laboratories and have the work carried out in large central laboratories are all founded on the desire to make the whole thing cheaper. Microbiologists are not innocent here, because for a long time they have been one of the big earners.[7] This applies to self-employed microbiologists, not contractually

---

[7]When a new financing system, the so-called DBC system, was introduced in 2005, the incomes of many tenured microbiologists and other medical specialists, for example radiologists, anaesthetists and clinical chemists, rose dramatically. This was the result of a failure in the DBC system. In every DBC it is defined that for a combination of one diagnosis and the corresponding treatment, all the cost components connected with this diagnosis are included. In the case of many diagnoses, for example, this also includes a blood or urine culture. Therefore, the DBC contains a default amount for such a culture—regardless of whether this is carried out or not. In 2010, the system was partly corrected.

employed ones.[8] This created a specific landscape, and it wasn't a healthy one. I find this a great shame. Because the specialism itself is in fact very valuable if it's integrated with the therapeutic disciplines and collaborates closely with them. When you see what's coming towards us in the matter of antibiotic resistance, then there's all the more reason to retain the status quo. Those who think that it might also be possible to do things more cheaply are in error. This is a typical example of trying to make savings in the wrong place. The responsibilities of clinical microbiologists will continue to increase, and a smoothly running microbiology system will become ever more important'. The former CIB director is inspired by the new generation of clinical microbiologists. 'The younger generation is more interested in public healthcare and scientific research. This is a trend that can be observed right across the medical sciences'.

## Clinical Microbiology: A Sine Qua Non of Good Treatment

Until the end of 2016, Jan van Wijngaarden was Chief Inspector for Public Health in the Netherlands. 'A system like the one we have in the Netherlands, with doctors who have specialised in clinical microbiology and therefore also know the subject from the laboratory side, who know about infection prevention and also contribute to patient treatment, is an important asset. The supervisory authority believes that the presence of clinical microbiologists in a hospital is a sine qua non of responsible medical care. In other words, if a hospital wants to abolish these posts, then we will take measures against it. We have already done this several times in the past few years. There were hospitals that wanted to outsource the clinical microbiology service. Up to now we've been able to resist this. But with the increasing pressure to make everything cheaper, it's questionable how long we can continue to succeed in this. If everybody's against us, and there's a lot of money involved, we could lose the battle. That would mean losing a unique system that is actually becoming more and more important in our present situation, with resistance problems increasing.' The supervisory authority has the support of the biggest health insurer in the country. When negotiating contracts with hospitals for 2013, Achmea/Zilveren Kruis included necessary requirements for infection prevention in hospitals for the first time. This was a direct consequence of the OXA-48 *Klebsiella* outbreak at the Maasstad Hospital. The fact that the biggest insurance provider stipulated its demands for the quality of infection prevention in hospitals is a clear sign of support for clinical microbiology. Or maybe was, because from 2022 Achmea/Zilveren

---

[8]Self-employed microbiologists came under fire during the SARS-CoV-2 pandemic. The high volume of PCR tests performed to establish whether people were SARS-CoV-2 positive or not meant a considerable rise of their income. This increase was all the more criticised because several of these self-employed medical microbiologists were also advising the government on (testing) policies, because they are considered to be (among) the best in their profession. Some of them agreed to a claw-back of their extra income to the public health funds.

Kruis follows the example set by VGZ and will only contract one partner for all diagnostics as well (Kruis 2021).

## Recommendations

Until 2014, Paul Huijts was General Director for Public Health at the Dutch health ministry (VWS). Today he is secretary-general at the Ministry of Foreign Affairs. 'The conversation about outsourcing and centralising microbiology provision wasn't started by us', he says. 'That came from the hospitals. The IGZ must stipulate limits if primary healthcare provision is in danger. In our opinion, outsourcing a laboratory for clinical microbiology presupposes that the hospital will retain its in-house microbiological expertise. And by that we mean staff who understand what's written in a laboratory report. And who occupy a position in the hospital that allows them to initiate the necessary measures. Strictly speaking, we do not have any particular opinion regarding the outsourcing of laboratories, or where the tests are carried out. But in the hospitals, a functioning system of hospital hygiene must be guaranteed. And the IGZ is keeping an eye on this'.

In an IGZ report from 2013, Van Wijngaarden draws up further requests for Edith Schippers, the Dutch health minister at that time. 'If we wish to keep hospitals free of dangerous microorganisms for as long as possible, we need to mobilise all our resources. And we'll have urgent need of our available expertise, which is unique in the world. At the moment it's irresponsible to take risks in these matters. We need experts who can assess what's coming into hospitals, how it spreads and what it means for the patients. These experts must also be able to type bacteria strains and have the necessary authority to carry out good infection prevention. They must also be in a position to communicate the events in the hospital to the outside world and keep the public health aspects of the situation in sight. We need experts who have sufficient authority to enable them to be heard. For all these tasks we'll continue to need clinical microbiologists in hospitals in future'. The supervisory body formulated some clear requirements for the hospitals. 'Monitor whether germs are coming into the hospital. Establish whether they're spreading. And comply with the guidelines of the Working Group for Infection Prevention (WIP) meticulously, in order to prevent the spread of microorganisms as far as possible. And we request that the use of antibiotics be handled with greater care'.

## 'Antimicrobial Stewardship'

The supervisory body has asked the *Stichting Werkgroep Antibioticabeleid* (Working Group for Antibiotics Guidelines) for advice. At the SWAB symposium on 20 June 2011, the organisation's chairman Jan Prins gave an outline of his reply to Van Wijngaarden. A key feature of this reply was a new guideline that prescribed rules for the restricted use of antibiotics and included an obligation to introduce a so-called 'antimicrobial stewardship' programme that is still at the heart of Dutch antibiotic policies (SWAB 2020). In addition to this, increased attention must be paid to (hand) hygiene. The guideline on restricted use of antibiotics stipulates when specific antibiotics must be used, and includes both outpatient and inpatient treatment. Depending on the antibiotic chosen, the reasons for using it must be given, including the indication and required diagnosis procedures. This is important if the hospital is aiming to make more frequent targeted use of antibiotics, rather than just prescribe them on an empirical basis. In addition to this, the guideline stipulates that only a limited number of experts may prescribe the most important antibiotics. 'In the last analysis, not every internal medicine specialist can prescribe every type of chemotherapy either', says Prins. A so-called 'A-team' must be formed in every hospital, which includes at least one internist-infectiologist, one clinical microbiologist, one hospital pharmacist and one or more hygiene experts. This team must be given control of hospital hygiene and antibiotics prescription. The 'antimicrobial stewardship' programme must lead to standardisation of the measures and activities which, in many hospitals, are already being carried out by antibiotics commissions, or the department of clinical microbiology or hospital hygiene. Each hospital must then meet the standards that have been prescribed in this way. When drawing up its proposals, the SWAB used important features of model initiatives in other countries whose effectiveness had already been proven (Dellitt et al. 2007). The team's task is to monitor the use of antibiotics and the emergence of resistance, and report these to the national surveillance systems. The decisive factor in all this is that the hospital management equips its A-team with the requisite competencies and financial resources. Van Wijngaarden incorporated the SWAB's recommendations in his report, which was sent to the minister at the end of February 2013. Van Wijngaarden was forceful in his advocacy of the microbiologists. 'Medical microbiologists are indispensable. The best evidence for this is seen in Germany. Here infection prevention has been neglected. We were able to see this clearly during the EHEC outbreak'.

The first antibiotics teams were formed as early as the end of 2012. The MC Zuiderzee in Lelystad and the Canisius Wilhelmina Hospital in Nijmegen were among the first institutions to assemble such teams. At Lelystad, a successful pilot project was carried out in autumn 2012. According to statements by internist-infectiologists Sebastiaan Weijer and Rachida El Moussaoui, the project delivered impressive results. Patients were less often treated with antibiotics for no good reason, or with the wrong antibiotic. And if this happened all the same, then they were given the medicine for a shorter period than before. Because of the reduced use of antibiotics, there were also less antibiotic resistance. The new approach also had financial effects, because unnecessary use of antibiotics was reduced and patients were treated with effective medicines sooner. After the success of this pilot project at the MC Zuiderzee, a start was made on introducing the new guideline in all hospitals (NOS 2012). The Canisius Wilhelmina Hospital in Nijmegen estimated the cost-saving of its A-team to be € 40.000 a year (Oberjé et al. 2017).

Stichting Werkgroep Antibiotica Beleid (SWAB) and the Werkgroep Infectiepreventie (WIP) play a decisive role in the Dutch infection prevention system. They draw up the guidelines, and the SWAB monitors the use of antibiotics and the emergence of resistance. Both organisations are mainly based on collaborations of clinical microbiologists, hygiene specialists and infectiologists. Up to now, the WIP has drawn up 130 guidelines, says former Chair of the Supervisory Board of the WIP Gijs Ruijs. These guidelines are all monitored and, if needed, updated. 'We must organise the WIP on a more professional basis, in order to constantly optimise the process of creating new guidelines and updating the existing library of guidelines. The financial support we receive from the Dutch health ministry (VWS) at the moment is insufficient for this. If we turn to the Dutch Hospital Association, which is actually the target group for our universally praised guidelines, then we discover to our disappointment that they decline to make any financial contribution. This poses a threat to the long-term survival of the WIP'. The working group for infection prevention has therefore sounded the alarm bell. In a letter to health minister Schippers, they announced that the group would suspend its activities if no additional financial resources were made available. In the summer of 2014, there was an initial meeting with senior ministry staff, and others followed in 2015 and 2016. A minister who makes antibiotic resistance such an important topic, who praises Dutch antibiotics policy all over the world, and who made it a key topic during the Netherlands' EU presidency in 2016, cannot afford to demolish such an important pillar of their policy. Schippers' spokesperson, therefore, announced that the minister would prevent this work from being suspended. At the end of 2016, these sanctimonious words were proven to be false. On 16 December 2016, the WIP announced that their successful group would be shutting down. Neither hospitals nor ministers wanted to make up for the lack of funds. In 2017, the WIP stopped all its activities (RIVM 2017). A new structure has to be built to replace the WIP. In this new organisation the RIVM—the Netherlands National Institute for Public Health and the Environment—will work together with the Federation of Medical Specialists (FMS) and the future Institute for the Quality of Long-term Care (LZ) to develop and update guidelines for the proper use of antibiotics (Schippers 2017). The RIVM is temporarily functioning as a helpdesk for professionals in the field of infection prevention. However, the guidelines are for the time being no longer being updated. The Samenwerkingsverband Richtlijnen Infectiepreventie (SRI, Partnership Guidelines Infectionprevention) is due to take over the role played until 2017 by the WIP (RIVM 2020). At the beginning of April 2021, this SRI was still not active.

## Additional Funding

On 2 July 2013, minister Schippers sent a letter to the Dutch parliament, in which she explained how she aimed to combat the growing problem of antibiotic resistance (Schippers 2013). For this purpose, the minister adopted some of the proposals of the SWAB—such as forming antibiotics teams—and the IGZ. Minister Schippers' letter also contained parts of a document by the Dutch Society for Medical Microbiology (NVNM) that made a number of statements about the current status and role of clinical microbiologists. In the document, the NVMM acknowledges that measures to increase cost-efficiency are important, but also warned against the dangers of outsourcing laboratories. 'When outsourcing diagnosis facilities, the following conditions must be observed. First, the clinical microbiologists must advise the laboratory and be closely involved in their in-house activities. Only this can guarantee that all laboratory activities are closely coordinated with events at the clinic or in the region (e.g. outbreaks). Second, it is of the greatest importance that the clinical microbiologist is present in the hospital. Only in this way can they directly coordinate their activities in the clinic with the latest information from the laboratory. This ensures transparent and therefore successful collaboration, and quick agreement procedures. The same applies for microbiologists who do not work in a hospital. They can only work efficiently and effectively when they are closely networked with the laboratory and the institutions for which they are working, e.g. nursing homes and organisations for outpatient treatment. If this cannot be guaranteed when outsourcing services to independent laboratories, then the collaboration that is so important for the quality of microbiological provision in the Netherlands is put at risk. The patients would suffer the most from this' (NVMM 2012).

The minister announced that additional funds would be provided to improve surveillance. Besides the reporting centre for outbreaks, in addition a national system would be set up that would enable the development of bacterial resistance to be monitored at the molecular level. The new system was intended to give better insights into where the resistances were coming from and how they spread. The ministry would also provide additional financial resources for the network for monitoring infectious diseases in nursing homes (SNIV). 'To sum up', the minister writes in her letter to parliament, 'it can be said that a common approach to infection prevention, surveillance, antibiotics use and the control of outbreaks must be implemented in care facilities, regardless of whether the bacteria in question are resistant or non-resistant'.

And, according to Schippers' statement, the IGZ would be responsible for monitoring compliance with the guidelines on infection prevention. On 19 December 2013, the IGZ published two reports on infection prevention in hospitals and nursing homes. The verdict of the supervisory body was harsh. 'The hospitals are not well prepared for the increase in HRMOs.[9] The guidelines are inadequately observed' (IGZ 2013). As for the nursing homes, the supervisory body's comments included: 'During an initial inspection tour of 21 elderly care facilities, it emerged that compliance with hygiene and infection prevention measures was inadequate. In the senior care homes there were considerable risks of infection and spread of resistant microorganisms' (Tweede Kamer 2013). Doctors and nurses frequently violated the most basic rules, for example wearing watches or jewellery during their work. The supervisory body was also dissatisfied with the personal hygiene of staff and patients. Doctors, nursing staff and auxiliary staff washed their hands much less often than is required. Good hand hygiene is one of the most important factors for preventing the spread of (resistant) bacteria. According to the supervisory board's

---

[9]HRMO stands for 'highly resistant microorganism'.

statements, the measures taken with regard to cleaning and disinfection, in both the hospitals and the nursing homes or senior care facilities, left much to be desired.

At the end of June 2019, the RIVM published a short report on a point prevalence study of antibiotic resistance in nursing homes. More than 4400 inhabitants of 159 elderly homes participated in the study. None of them carried a carbapenemase-producing *Enterobacteriaceae*. ESBL-producing *Enterobacteriaceae* were more of a problem. In a third of the participating homes, the ESBL rate was over 10%, which is considered to be the maximum 'normal' rate. They were advised on intensifying infection prevention measures (Van Kleef et al. 2019).

## 'Results Say More Than Process Indicators'

On 3 March 2014, a commentary on the IGZ reports of December 2013 by six leading microbiologists appeared in the Dutch journal *Nederlands Tijdschrift voor Geneeskunde* (NTvG). The commentary bore the pregnant title 'Results say more than process indicators'. The microbiologists first discuss some statements by the authorities. 'At the University Medical Centre Utrecht, for example', they write, 'it was discovered that the cleaning staff who cleaned the patients' rooms decided for themselves whether they moistened their cleaning cloths, and how often. There were no measuring cups for adding water, as a result of which the hospital was evaluated "inadequate" in the "cleaning" category. Moreover, several forms containing the results for hand hygiene checks were missing; nor was every emergency patient asked about risk factors for HRMO when admitted. In themselves these are interesting facts, but their significance for the patients' safety is unclear. Issues such as "How high is the risk of infection by an HRMO in a Dutch hospital?" or "Has the risk increased in recent years" were not investigated. The supervisory authority limited itself to recording process indicators, while the relevant and available results indicators were not investigated'. And it is precisely these results indicators that give a favourable picture of infection prevention in Dutch hospitals. Nowhere in the world are there so few serious healthcare-associated infections as in Dutch and Scandinavian hospitals, the microbiologists write in their commentary. The authors fear that the supervisory authority's actions could have counterproductive effects and that hospitals could spend large sums of money to fulfil formal requirements whose benefits have not always been proven. They fear this could happen at the cost of the pragmatic initiatives currently being carried out by experts in infection prevention. They end with a clear appeal to the minister and the supervisory body. 'We are thoroughly aware that the rise in antibiotic resistance constitutes a genuine threat, and that hospitals must prepare themselves for it. And also that the IGZ needs instruments to enable them to check the hospitals. And we know that even in Dutch hospitals there is still more room for improvement. We therefore emphatically call on the supervisory body, in consultation with the professional groups affected, to stipulate objective indicators that are relevant to patient safety, so that safety in

Dutch hospitals in the field of infection prevention and spread of HRMOs can be secured' (Bonten et al. 2014).

# References

Ärztestellen. (2020a). *Der Stellenmarkt des Deutschen Ärtzeblattes. Facharzt -Weiterbildung Hygiene und Umweltmedizin: Dauer, Inhalte Perspektiven.* In German. Accessed December 10, 2020, from https://bit.ly/3gBP3kY

Ärztestellen. (2020b). *Der Stellenmarkt des Deutschen Ärtzeblattes. Facharzt-Weiterbildung Mikrobiologie, Virologie und Infektionsepidemiologie.* In German. Accessed December 10, 2020, from https://bit.ly/3gxaHqC

BMG – Bundesministerium für Gesundhuit. (2011). *Kabinett beschließt Entwurf eines "Gesetzes zur Änderung des Infektionsschutzgesetzes und weiterer Gesetze".* In German. Accessed December 12, 2020, from https://bit.ly/383kfpM

Bonten, M. J. M., Friedrich, A. W., Kluytmans, J. A. J. W., et al. (2014). *Infection prevention in Dutch hospitals; results say more than process indicators* (English abstract). Accessed December 13, 2020, from https://bit.ly/2MRrwlD full text in Dutch https://bit.ly/3ow9K50

Bundesamt für Justiz. (2011). *Gesetz zur Verhütung und Bekämpfung von Infektionskrankheiten beim Menschen.* In German. Accessed December 12, 2020, from https://bit.ly/35n6Vvy

CBS. (2020). Bevolkingsteller. Accessed December 10, 2020, from https://bit.ly/39vsHij

De Staat van Volksgezonheid en Zorg. (2020). *Ziekenhuisbedden.* Accessed December 10, 2020, from https://bit.ly/35kskWr

Dellitt, T. H., Owens, R. C., McGowen, J. E., Infectious Diseases Society of America and the Society for Healthcare Epidemiology of America, et al. (2007). Guidelines for developing an institutional program to enhance antimicrobial stewardship. *Clinical Infectious Diseases, 44*(2), 159–177. https://doi.org/10.1086/510393.

Destatis. (2020a). *Current population.* Accessed April 6, 2021, from https://bit.ly/3qEtVPX

Destatis. (2020b). *Six hospital beds per 1,000 inhabitants in 2017.* Accessed December 10, 2020, from https://bit.ly/3bkGF96

DGKH. (2011). *Gemeinsame Stellungnahme der Deutschen Gesellschaft für Krankenhaushygiene (DGKH), der Gesellschaft für Hygiene, Umweltmedizin und Präventivmedizin (GHUP) und des Bundesverbandes der Ärztinnen und Ärzte des Öffentlichen Gesundheitsdienstes e. V. (BVÖGD) zum Entwurf eines Gesetzes zur Verbesserung der Krankenhaushygiene und zur Änderung weiterer Gesetze.* In German. Accessed December 12, 2020, from https://bit.ly/3saq0uH

ECDC. (2020). *Country summaries - antimicrobial resistance in the EU/EEA 2019.* Accessed December 12, 2020, from https://bit.ly/3owalDM

European Commission. (2011). *SANCO. Lessons learned from the 2011 outbreak of Shiga toxin-producing Escherichia coli (STEC) O104:H4 in sprouted seeds.* Accessed December 12, 2020, from https://bit.ly/3479txh

IGZ. (2013). *Health Care Inspectorate. Keten van infectiepreventie in ziekenhuizen breekbaar: meerdere zwakke schakels leiden tot onveilige zorg.* In Dutch, English summary. Accessed December 13, 2020, from https://bit.ly/2W7uS5j

KRINKO. (2009). *Personelle und organisatorische Voraussetzungen zur Prävention nosokomialer Infektionen Empfehlung der Kommission für Krankenhaushygiene und Infektionsprävention. Bundesgesundheitsblatt, 9*(52), 951–962. https://doi.org/10.1007/s00103-009-0929-y. In German. Accessed December 12, 2020, from https://bit.ly/3oLTNaU

Kruis, Z. (2021). *Beleid en contract eerstelijnsdiagnostiek & trombosezorg.* Accessed April 6, 2021, from https://www.zilverenkruis.nl/zorgaanbieders/zorgsoort/eld/beleid-en-contract

NOS. (2012). *Antibiotica-team in elk ziekenhuis.* In Dutch. Accessed December 13, 2020, from https://bit.ly/2Xr959m

NOS. (2020). *Van commerciële tests op het coronavirus is alleen topje van ijsberg bekend.* In Dutch. Accessed January 9, 2021, from https://bit.ly/3nuTdx9

NVMM. (2012). *Tussen Laboratorium en Kliniek. De geïntegreerde taakset van de arts-microbioloog.* In Dutch. Accessed December 13, 2020, from https://bit.ly/2L742IF

Oberjé, E. J. M., Tanke, M. A. C., & Jeurissen, P. P. T. (2017). Antimicrobial stewardship initiatives throughout Europe: proven value for money. *Infectious Disease Report, 9*(1), 42–47. https://www.pagepress.org/journals/index.php/idr/article/view/6800/6776

Plexus. (2010). *Rapportage Business Case Eerstelijns Diagnostiek.* In Dutch. Accessed December 12, 2020, from https://bit.ly/3nvz2Po

Prismant. (2019). *Aantal werkzame specialisten per specialisme en uitstroom van Specialisten in de komende 20 jaar. Onderzoeksverslag voor het Capaciteitsorgaan.* In Dutch. Accessed December 10, 2020, from https://bit.ly/3ouE5kC. See page 9.

RIVM. (2017). *Beëindigen operationele activiteiten Stichting WIP.* In Dutch. Accessed December 13, 2020, from https://bit.ly/3oGDBru

RIVM. (2020). *Informatie over het SRI.* In Dutch. Accessed December 13, 2020, from https://bit.ly/38tieVb

RKI - Robert Koch Institute. (2011). *Report: Final presentation and evaluation of epidemiological findings in the EHEC O104:H4 outbreak, Germany 2011.* Accessed December 12, 2020, from https://bit.ly/37c8kGL

Schippers, E. I. (2013). *Letter to Parliament of 2 July.* In Dutch. Accessed December 13, 2020, from https://bit.ly/3npoaTb

Schippers, E. I. (2017). *Letter to Parliament. Verzamelbrief Samenwerkingsmodel Richtlijnontwikkeling infectiepreventie.* In Dutch. Accessed December 13, 2020, from https://bit.ly/3mgGkG8

SWAB – Working Group for Antibiotics Guidelines. (2020). *Antimicrobial stewardship.* Accessed December 13, 2020, from https://bit.ly/39i8vA6

Tweede Kamer der Staten Generaal. (2013). *Verbetering van hygiëne en infectiepreventie in ouderenzorg snel realiseerbaar.* In Dutch. Accessed December 13, 2020, from https://bit.ly/3hZ5dpt

Van Cleef, B. A. G. L., Kluytmans, J. A. J. W., Van Benthem, B. H. B., et al. (2012). Cross border comparison of MRSA bacteraemia between the Netherlands and North Rhine-Westphalia (Germany): A cross-sectional study. *PLoS One, 7*(8), e42787. https://doi.org/10.1371/journal.pone.0042787.

Van Gemert-Pijnen, J. E. W. C. (ed.) (2011). *Eursafety it is your safety: EurSafety Health-net – Euregionaal netwerk voor patiëntveiligheid en bescherming tegen infecties Rapportage over de periode 2009-2011.* In Dutch. Accessed December 13, 2020, from https://bit.ly/3gGxQqG

Van Kleef, E., Wielders, L., Bijkerk, P., et al. (2019). *Puntprevalentieonderzoek naar antibioticaresistentie in verpleeghuizen.* In Dutch. See page 7 for English synopsis. Accessed December 13, 2020, from https://bit.ly/3ouFcki

VGZ. (2019). *Overeenkomsten.* In Dutch. Accessed December 13, 2020, from https://bit.ly/3blrVGT

Volksgezondheidenzorg.info. (2020). *Aantal instellingen voor medisch specialistische zorg.* In Dutch. Accessed Decemebr 10, 2020, from https://bit.ly/3gxxjay

# INTERREG-Projects: 'Pathogens Don't Recognise Any Borders'

10

'I'll have to take this call', says Ron Hendrix as his mobile rings. He switches from Dutch to German. He is listening attentively. 'I wouldn't do that', says Hendrix to the caller. 'I'd do a culture first'. Afterwards, he explains to me what the conversation was all about. 'It was about a patient in the intensive care unit of a big German hospital that I often visit as a supervisor. The patient has already been given meropenem and linezolid, and now they want to give him tigecycline as well. Those are all reserve medicines, and they wanted to prescribe the drug simply on the basis of the clinical picture, without carrying out any kind of culture. That didn't seem like a very good idea to me, because afterwards they won't have anything in reserve any more. It's a 1000-bed hospital, but it doesn't have its own laboratory or medical microbiology department. For four years now, they've had four doctors who function as hygiene officials. We train these hygiene staff'. It is a perfect example of what EurSafety Health-net actually involves in practice (EurSafety Health-net 2020a). Cross-border collaboration, professional advice, education and training of colleagues. Here is another example. On 31 March 2015, the University Medical Centre Groningen (UMCG) and the Leer Clinic signed a cooperation agreement (Klinikum Leer 2015). With this deal their collaboration in the field of infection prevention, which had already been in place for a year, was formally established and extended at the same time. Microbiologist Berry Overbeek has been based in Leer so that he can support his German colleagues in their work (Klinikum Leer 2019). 'Pathogens don't recognise any borders—and therefore it has to be the same with infection prevention', writes Professor Alex W. Friedrich in his Foreword to 'EurSafety– It's your safety', a report on the period 2009–2011 by EurSafety Health-Net—a Euregional network for patient safety and infection prevention (Van Gemert-Pijnen 2011). The EurSafety Health-Net project forms part of INTERREG, which is roughly half-financed by the European Regional Development Fund of the European Union. The other half of funding comes from the states and provinces taking part and the project participants themselves. EurSafety Health-net is one of the so-called 'A projects'. These involve cross-border collaboration between neighbouring regions that are separated from one another by a national border. In this case, the regions in question are the Dutch provinces of Friesland, Drenthe, Overijssel, Gelderland and Limburg and the German federal states of Lower Saxony and North Rhine-Westphalia. Together they form the Euregions of Ems-Dollart, Gronau-Enschede, Rhine-Waal, Rhine-Maas North and Maas-Rhine.[1] The last of these, which also includes the Belgian provinces of Limburg and Liege, does not formally belong to the EurSafety Health-net, but is running a similar project with euPrevent EMR. EurSafety Health-Net started in 2009 under auspicious circumstances, because the project had a solid foundation from day one onwards. It was able to build on the pioneering work of the MRSA-Net, which had already been successful (EurSafety Health-net 2020b).

The MRSA-net—or, to give it its full name, the Euregion MRSA-net Twente/ Münsterland—was founded in 2005 as a cross-border partnership between the University of Twente, the regional microbiological laboratory for Twente and Achterhoek (LabMicta), the University Hospital Münster and the state institute for the public health service in North Rhine-Westphalia at that time.[2] Ron Hendrix still remembers the beginnings very well. 'Back then, when I was still Director of LabMicta, I was already working on studies of protocols and how people handle them. Along with the University of Twente, I started research there for a new doctoral thesis on this topic'. Lisette van Gemert-Pijnen has already been working with Euregional projects for around fifteen years. She is a psycholinguist and Professor in the Department of Communications Sciences of the Faculty of Behavioural Management and Social Sciences at the University of Twente. She is an expert on communications processes in network structures. 'One of the things with which MRSA-net is involved is creating a system that makes it easier to deal with protocols at the workplace', she says. 'This involves setting up a digital environment for protocols, because the existing protocols haven't been working for healthcare staff so far. Finally, an antibiotics advice service was introduced alongside this. We discovered that an MRSA protocol of this kind is all very well and good, but that the main problem is concealed behind it. And that's the improper use of antibiotics. Since the staff in my research group mainly come from the fields of behavioural science and health technology, my principal role is to find out why people aren't carrying out in practice the things you'd expect them to do on the basis of the protocols. Why do doctors and nurses behave differently from the way prescribed in all these wonderful protocols on infection prevention? We're discovering more and more indications that the expert-oriented approach of hygiene specialists and microbiologists simply doesn't work in practice. One of the reasons for this is the discrepancy between expert knowledge and workplace behaviour. The protocols contain a whole range of things that you're forbidden to do, and a wealth of expertise. But they don't contain very much about the roles, tasks and

---

[1]The first Euregion was formed in 1958 in Gronau-Enschede.
[2]The new name of the institute is the *Landeszentrum Gesundheit Nordrhein-Westfalen* (LZG. NRW).

responsibilities of people in the workplace. Nobody knows what they're supposed to do.'

Let us go back to the year 2001. A new microbiologist was starting work at the University Hospital Münster—Alex Friedrich. He had come from the University Hospital of Würzburg. 'In Münster he immediately noticed that there was a big difference between the prevalence of MRSA there and that found in south Germany, and an even bigger difference in comparison with the values on the Dutch side of the border,' says Hendrix. 'Back then, Alex tried to find an opportunity to establish contact with a large laboratory on our side. On the one hand that was mere curiosity, but on the other hand it was also very practical, because he wanted to submit a project proposal, and needed a Dutch partner for it. A mutual friend of ours organised a meeting. Within five minutes we were deeply engaged in our conversation, and we hit if off right away.' This initial conversation was followed by further talks about a common project on MRSA. 'Alex was enthusiastic and full of drive,' recalls Hendrix. 'And, true to form, he wrote an exceptionally ambitious project proposal, at least by the standards of its time. This was MRSA-net. This was submitted to the European Union via EUREGIO, and to our astonishment we received 900,000 euros for four years'.

## Back to the Past

Today, Alex Friedrich is Head of the Department of Medical Microbiology and Hospital Hygiene at the University Medical Centre Groningen (UMCG). 'In 2001 I came to Münster from Bavaria. I noticed that the percentage of MRSA in the Münsterland was lower than I had been used to in southern Germany. But then the figures started to rise there as well. It was as though I'd gone back five years in time. In south Germany I had just been through an epidemic we couldn't deal with. It simply went on and on. Everything we did or said didn't really help, because often it wasn't even implemented. In Münster I actually got a second chance. There we didn't have 12 per cent MRSA, as in the south, but only two per cent. But the prevalence was increasing. And so I said: Let's try something else'. By this time Friedrich already had several international contacts. Including some in the Netherlands—and that played an important role. At that time, the European Antimicrobial Resistance Surveillance System (EARSS) for antibiotic resistance was still attached to the RIVM.[3] Before Friedrich went to Würzburg, he worked at the Istituto Superiore di Sanità in Rome, the Italian counterpart of the RIVM, the RKI or the CDC. 'I worked alongside the bacteriologists. Among the epidemiologists working there was Stef Bronzwaer, who had been sent to Rome from the RIVM. When I went to Germany, he went back to the Netherlands and became Coordinator of EARSS. In

---

[3]European Antimicrobial Resistance Surveillance System, founded in 1999. At that time it was administered by the RIVM. In the meantime it has been renamed the EARS-Net and incorporated into the ECDC in Stockholm.

Rome we had become friends—in part because we were both married to an Italian. I learned a great deal from him, and therefore knew sooner than most that there was such a great difference between the Netherlands and Germany'. Friedrich and Bronzwaer visited each other regularly. 'And then', Friedrich recalls, 'I said to myself: That can't be right. You go from Münster to Enschede to do your shopping, and suddenly there's 20 times less MRSA there. There were always lots of Germans there, and so MRSA must simply come over the border. Therefore, it seemed, either it couldn't be transferred from person to person, or the transfer took place in a quite different way from what we'd thought up to then. And we were situated on the border of a country where obviously they were already doing things much better. Years before I came to Münster, Georg Peters had introduced a kind of 'search and destroy' policy for MRSA there (MRSA-net 2020a). By means of these screening tests, he brought all the affected patients to light. I remember that once when we were sitting together I said: 'That's not acceptable—another 150 MRSA-positive patients in 3 months. Where are they all coming from?' After that I made a list of all these patients, and we saw that 90 per cent of them had been transferred from other hospitals to the University Hospital Münster. I then gave a presentation in front of all the hygiene staff from the nine hospitals in Münster, where I told them that we had got almost all the MRSA cases in our hospital from them. To which they replied: 'And we get the MRSA patients from you'. I then suggested that we should collaborate, in order to discuss how we could achieve an MRSA-free Münster. I had already written my project proposal. We then contacted the microbiologists responsible for the neighbouring Dutch border region via the ESG—the Euregional Service Centre for Health (ESG), an EUREGIO project whose aim was to initiate cross-border healthcare projects.[4] I had a project proposal, but no connections with Dutch experts in the border territory, and no experience with INTERREG projects. The ESG had both. The Dutch microbiologist I met subsequently in Enschede was big and blond, and greeted me with the words: 'My name is Ron Hendrix, we can do great things together'. And then we began to collaborate. That worked well right from the start. I then asked Inka Daniels-Haardt to take part in the project, because we needed a German state health authority or a Dutch health authority (GGD) for the project. And Ron invited the University of Twente, since we also need a university to work with'.

## Bringing Others on Board

Inka Daniels-Haardt is a medical specialist for hygiene and environmental medicine, and Head of the specialist division for health protection at the North Rhine-Westphalia regional health centre (LZG.NRW, at that time still in Münster, since 2018 in Bochum). 'The fact that the University Hospital Münster was close was a great help. We're practically neighbours, and knew each other very well. That's

---

[4]The ESG has now become the Euro Health Connect (EHC) Foundation.

always an important starting point, this personal relationship. And when we started thinking about the MRSA-net, it was clear from the outset that the project would have to involve all three pillars: science, healthcare institutions and the public health service. We constructed the project in such a way that it rests on all three pillars, and that also the health authorities in the region—at the time this was only Twente-Münsterland—were brought on board immediately. I am responsible for the entire North Rhine-Westphalia region. That meant I had good access to the regional health authorities. The EUREGIO MRSA-net officially started in 2005 in the Twente and Münsterland regions. The aim was to protect the inhabitants of the Dutch-German border regions from MRSA infections as far as possible. The big differences in MRSA prevalence between the Netherlands and Germany are not predetermined by nature. In the Netherlands a 'search and destroy' policy has been practised for years, and you can see the fruits of it in the very low MRSA prevalence compared to other countries. One of the main aims of the MRSA-net was to share knowledge about this procedure. As Ron Hendrix says, 'We've set up a system where we ask hospitals to show that they're complying with the guidelines. So we haven't invented anything new. It's only been about complying with the existing rules and regulations. Hospitals that do this, and can prove it, can get the MRSA-net seal of approval. You could call this our 'hard' approach. The 'soft' approach was that we immediately began to set up a question-and-answer system. The website that was created as part of this project, in both Dutch and German, was a big success (MRSA-net 2020b). All kinds of questions were answered there. The core task of the entire project was setting up networks. And finding out how to ensure that fundamental guidelines in the field of MRSA control are introduced and also observed, both in the Netherlands and in Germany.'

The MRSA-net came about in an unbalanced context. MRSA was a much bigger problem in Germany than in the Netherlands, where a strict policy had long been followed. In addition to this, the hospital landscapes in the two countries look very different. In 2009 there were in Germany almost 2100 hospitals with more than half a million beds (Statista 2020). In the Netherlands there were in 2009 only 85 independent general hospitals and eight university medical centres, with a total number of beds less than a tenth of that in Germany (NZa 2010; De Staat van Volksgezondheid en Zorg 2020). Besides this, in Germany there is the phenomenon of 'resident doctors', which scarcely exists in the Netherlands.

## Difficult Beginnings

Karin Reismann, a member of the CDU party, is Mayor of the City of Münster and is responsible for the city's health policy. Since 1999 she has been a member of the EUREGIO council. 'Basically I found the MRSA-net an interesting project. But in the beginning I was against it, because the Dutch had told me that they didn't need the project and wouldn't give it any money either. They didn't have these germs in Dutch hospitals. And if we in Germany wanted to keep our hospitals germ-free, then that wasn't a EUREGIO project. Professor Friedrich at the hygiene institute in

Münster convinced me that it is important to collaborate across borders in the area of healthcare. I wanted to bring about a situation where Germans could be treated in Dutch hospitals without further ado. I know a married couple: he's German, she's Dutch. The couple went to the Netherlands for a family visit. He fell down the stairs and broke his leg. Then, of course, in the hospital they sent him through this 'sluice gate'.[5] He got terribly agitated about this, and said that at home he would have been treated immediately. I then spoke to the Dutch – not in the EUREGIO council, but at the University of Twente in Enschede. They all told me that this procedure isn't so bad. Just imagine: Dutch people are admitted and treated in Germany. If they have an accident they receive treatment, without any problem. So perhaps it's very important to test patients for MRSA in German hospitals as well – so that the Dutch person who has an accident in Germany, and is treated and cared for there, doesn't subsequently come back to a Dutch hospital for follow-up treatment MRSA-positive. In the course of many, many talks it became increasingly clear that the EurSafety Health-Net project would have to be set in motion. Basically it all started here, in Münster. This town hall is the project's birthplace'.

Jörg Hermann, Director of the Institute for Hospital Hygiene in Oldenburg, remembers that in the beginning EurSafety Health-Net was a kind of one-way street. 'After the successes of MRSA-net, the German side decided that it might be a good idea to extend the Münster, Twente and Enschede project along the entire border. The Germans didn't need to be convinced of this. It was much harder to persuade the Dutch to get involved in a project in an area where they had seen no problems to date. And this has been a challenge throughout the entire project. Only now is this changing, because in the shape of ESBL we have a topic that is a burning issue on both sides'.

For a long time, Robin Köck was on the staff of the Institute of Medical Microbiology at the University of Münster, and since 2018 he is working as leader of the institute for Hygiene of the four hospitals of the DRK Kliniken in Berlin.[6] 'In the projects we carried out as part of EurSafety Health-Net, the focus was often on "one health". We worked in close collaboration with the University of Groningen. We carried out research into the prevalence of antibiotic-resistant pathogens in livestock farming, on both the German and Dutch sides of the border. And we observed how often these gram-negative pathogens can be detected in patients. And what proportion of the pathogens we find in patients come from livestock farming, the genetic fingerprint of the bacteria reveals this. It is a very important issue. We certainly compiled good data showing that, for specific pathogens, the problem is ultimately the same on both sides of the border. This applies, for example, to *E. coli.*

---

[5]By 'sluice gate' Reismann means that, as a patient in the German health system, her friend was first tested in the Dutch hospital as a potential carrier of MRSA, and isolated until the result of the testing was known.

[6]As part of the EUREGIO MRSA-net and MRE-network North-west projects, he is working to form regional networks to promote the prevention of MRSA and other multiresistant pathogens. In addition he is coordinating the MedVet-Staph research association, which is shedding light on the zoonotic components of *S. aureus*/MRSA infections.

In the case of Klebsiellas, we continue to see a certain border between the two countries in those areas where there has been little exchange between the hospitals in both regions to date. That means that the Klebsiellas are obviously circulating in institutions, whereas the *E. coli* are spreading amongst the general public. As far as ESBL-positive *E. coli* are concerned we've basically become one region. That's occurring at the same level in the border region, both in hospitals and amongst the general public. The subtypes of the pathogens in circulation on both sides of the border are actually the same. We also see that food and livestock farming might not be the only sources. These sources explain about 20 to 30 per cent of cases, because here we actually find pathogens in people and animals that are genetically identical. The remaining 70 per cent obviously stem from other sources, which ultimately we haven't really identified yet. In wastewater, by spreading manure on plants – all those are possible routes'.

Lisette van Gemert-Pijnen is proud of the results of the EurSafety Health-Net. 'The Euregional network of hospitals, senior care facilities, nursing homes and public health services that we have built up is now firmly established, and it works. A kind of commitment has developed, and I personally consider that major progress. It was an important aim of this project to create a structure that would also be sustainable in future. Improved collaboration between the universities in Münster, Oldenburg, Twente and Groningen has also come about as a result of the project. In this way we've created fertile soil for further consolidating the collaboration. Everyone has worked together—sometimes it's still *alongside* one another but not always *together with* one another, but the togetherness has been constantly increasing. In the future we'll be collaborating even more closely'.

## MRSA First

'In the beginning', says Alex Friedrich, 'the first priority was to fight MRSA together. But we very soon noticed that you can't adopt the Dutch approach in Germany just like that. There are many more hospitals there, the patients leave the hospitals and switch to outpatient treatment, and they never come back again. It wasn't possible simply to copy the Dutch, that just didn't fit in with the existing treatment structure. We had to revise the Dutch methods and adapt them to the situation in Germany. And that took time. In 2003 I met Ron Hendrix, in 2005 we began setting up the MRSA-net, in 2006 we got the resident doctors on board, and finally from 2008 onwards the MRSA-net was ready to go. And just at that moment, the funding ran out. But we had achieved an incredibly large number of positive things: we'd set up a helpdesk, and every month 300 patients called, who were given direct access to the experts. That was new. There were also more and more people who worked on the help desk. We gave presentations everywhere, and the network was constantly expanding. The idea of a regional network spread, and was adopted everywhere in Germany. But it took until 2013 before we were able to publish genuine results. The first effects already began to appear in 2008 and 2009, but we still had to wait a considerable time before we could report, in an article in

*Eurosurveillance*, that we had achieved a reduction of MRSA prevalence by 40 per cent in the hospitals taking part'. The MRSA-net was so successful that project partners Hendrix and Friedrich asked themselves whether they might not be able to take it further. Not just in Twente and the Münsterland, but also in other places along the Dutch-German border. 'In Lower Saxony Matthias Pulz, the President of the state health authority, was very keen to join us', recalls Friedrich. 'He saw the need to do something to counteract MRSA, and wanted to grasp the opportunity to learn something from the MRSA-net. The Münsterland was a kind of exceptional case. Things were working well there, not least because of the collaboration with the Netherlands. He wanted the same thing'. Matthias Pulz confirms this. 'The successful strategies in the Netherlands have of course very much come under the spotlight. Eur-Safety Health-net has enabled us to learn from the other partner and derive goals from this that release energies and foster motivation. I believe that we give each other reciprocal stimuli. The important thing is that we don't adopt everything on a one-to-one basis. We have totally different structures. The resident doctors, the many hospitals—you can't just say, "we'll copy everything". There are structural differences, but adopting each other's positive features and integrating them in your own system already affords a great opportunity. The professional clarity and rigour with which the Dutch approach things—I think that's the essential feature here, as well as running a patient-focused system of infection prevention and hygiene. I think it was certainly very novel for the Dutch as well to see our federal structures and municipal public health services. In the Netherlands they have these large central structures such as the RIVM and the GGDs (health authorities). The fact that it's also important to anchor such structures locally might perhaps have an educational effect on the Dutch. EurSafety has now focused its attention quite specifically on multiresistant germs and several projects related to patient safety. But there are also many other aspects of hygiene, such as the preparation of medicinal products. I think these are also areas in which the Dutch could still learn something from Germany. Like the rigorous way we act in this field'.

Professor Karsten Becker, who moved from Münster of the University Hospital of Greifswald also sees ways in which the Netherlands and Germany can each profit from the knowledge of the other partner. 'It's important that both countries have gained insights into the different ways in which health systems can work, the influence this has on our work as medical professionals, the impact this has on the fight against infections, and how we can learn from one another. It's particularly important for Germany that we have been able to learn how to keep multiresistant pathogens in check and keep them to a low level. If we look at the trend in Germany, and particularly in the Münster region, then we see that this can be done. Even if there has been a higher level of multiresistant pathogens, particularly MRSA, during the interim. It's been possible to turn this trend around. In my opinion that's the crucial issue for Germany. For the Netherlands, perhaps, it's to see how you can bring a high level down again. At the present time, both countries are facing new challenges. It's no longer just about MRSA, but also about multiresistant gram-negative pathogens, which have other mechanisms of formation and proliferation'.

When the EurSafety Health-Net project began on 19 November 2009, it resulted in a considerable expansion of the areas in which the Dutch and the Germans collaborated. The collaboration was extended to almost the entire Dutch–German border area, which stretches from the mouth of the Ems and the Dollart in the north to Central Limburg in the south. In the southernmost part of the border area—the Maas-Rhine Euregion, which also includes the Belgian border area—a close collaboration came about between the EurSafety Health-Net and the euPrevent-EMR project.

When you hear the mention of the 'Maas-Rhine Euregion', this actually means 'Professor Jacques Scheres'. He was born in 1946 in the border town of Heerlen in south Limburg, and has lived in this border region for the greater part of his life. Professor Scheres is a biologist and medical geneticist. In addition to numerous scientific positions—for example at the university medical centres of Rotterdam, Nijmegen, Maastricht and Utrecht—he has already been active in the field of European health policy for over 25 years. In 1985 Scheres became medical director of the Provincial Council for Health in the province of Limburg, which lies between Germany and Belgium. It was there that in 1990—almost two years before the historic summit in the provincial capital of Maastricht—the initiative to create a cross-border health policy was introduced.[7] Scheres was involved in it right from the start. In addition to this, he was also coordinator of a Euregional health project involving five (teaching) hospitals and ten health insurance providers and health funds, devoted to the topic of antibiotic resistance as a danger for patient mobility inside Europe. Jacques Scheres was Chair of the EurSafety Health-Net steering committee, and represented the European Parliament in the supervisory body of the ECDC in Stockholm. Scheres was already involved in the start-up phase of EurSafety Health-Net. At this time there were regular meetings in the five Euregions. Here experiences were discussed and ideas exchanged. At one of these sessions Scheres got to know Alex Friedrich, who was working in Münster. 'I believe that was just before the MRSA-net was launched in the Twente-Münsterland Euregion. We understood each other at once, and met together more frequently from then on'.

On the day before I spoke to Scheres, the last working meeting of EurSafety had just been held. The lifespan of the INTERREG project had come to an end on 30 June 2015. Since 2015, therefore, EurSafety has been a foundation (non-profit fund), in order to safeguard the sustainability of the structures created. 'In the beginning we were only able to get approval for the project with a great deal of difficulty. At one particular time things looked very bad, but ultimately the project was implemented all the same. And it then developed very quickly and splendidly'. Friedrich and Scheres visited potential new participants for the project. 'We always made it clear to those who took part in the project in the new regions that they

---

[7]It was during the summit in Maastricht that the member states of the European Community concluded the Maastricht Treaty. This was concerned with the further development of the European Union and the formation of the European Monetary Union (EMU). The EMU formed the basis for the common currency. The euro was introduced in twelve countries in 2002. Since then it has been introduced in 19 EU member states (EC 1992).

themselves could best judge what the possibilities of their region were', says Scheres.

'This resulted in many successful initiatives, which also drew attention in political circles. In an extensive project of this kind you should make as few top-down decisions as possible, although unfortunately this can't entirely be avoided. In order to obtain funding, something has to be decided upon first. Here EurSafety had found a kind of middle way, and made optimum use of its possibilities. Cross-border projects in which the people doing the work meet regularly achieve far better results than when ideas are exchanged between the capital cities only. In the border area the doctors, health authorities and universities come together and try to solve problems collectively. Projects are successful if they are carried out by passionate people who are sometimes also prepared to fight against all resistance, like some kind of Don Quixote. Everyone who works in healthcare has their work cut out fulfilling their duties well at their own hospital or in their own region. That makes cross-border projects very difficult, but also at the same time very exciting processes. Once you've found allies who share your goals, the whole thing turns into some kind of task force asking questions like: "How can we implement this, how can we justify it?" That was very distinctly visible in the case of EurSafety. People who found this topic area fascinating, and reciprocally motivated one another. Our work ranged from developing apps to implementing financing for MRSA tests in German hospitals through health funds. A whole series of people were working together with us on this, ranging from molecular biologists and social scientists to political decision-makers'.

Brigitte van der Zanden heads up the secretariat of the patient organisation EPECS.[8] She was involved in the EurSafety Health-Net right from the start. 'Our goal was to incorporate patients and the general public in the project', she says. Van der Zanden was born in Twente, only a few kilometres from the German border. Today she lives in Maastricht, close to both the Belgian and the German border. More than 30 years ago, when she was a child, Van der Zanden's sister often had to have operations on her legs. 'For this she had to go to Nijmegen, even though Münster was much nearer'. She also mentions the case of another patient from Twente who lives practically on the German border. He had to go to Zwolle to receive treatment for a heart condition. There he was placed on a 6-month waiting list for his ablation.[9] 'The patient asked whether he could also go to Münster for his operation, which was much closer to where he lived. His health insurer was prepared to do something about the waiting list and sent him to Antwerp. There he was able to receive treatment almost immediately. This was to the insurer's financial advantage, since in Antwerp only the medical intervention has to be paid for and not, as in the

---

[8]European Patient Empowerment for Customised Solutions.

[9]An ablation is an intervention for the treatment of cardiac arrhythmia. With cardiac arrhythmia, electrical impulses in the heart occur in the wrong places. During an ablation, the doctor destroys the heart tissue in these places to a certain extent. The resultant scars block transmission of the unwanted electrical signals (Mayo Clinic 2020).

Dutch system, the capital costs for the building and all the other costs not directly related to medical treatment'.

Andrea Ammon, Acting Director of the ECDC since May 2015 and its Director since March 2017, is an enthusiastic advocate of the EurSafety Health-Net and similar projects. 'Infections can spread across borders more and more easily. There are increasing numbers of patients from the Netherlands who cross the border to be treated in Germany, and vice versa. The same applies between Belgium and the Netherlands. And, of course, to the border regions between other countries. It is therefore very useful and sensible to approach the question of infection prevention and control together. The collaboration within the EurSafety project works. We were able to prove that. At the beginning there were only a few enthusiasts, until the others realised that it worked. It is obvious that, in this field, you need to collaborate. EurSafety is a model of how collaboration of this kind can be organised across borders'.

## The Project

Around 13 million people live in the region where the EurSafety Health-Net and euPrevent-EMR projects are being carried out. The EurSafety Health-Net has considerably expanded the tried and tested structure of the successful MRSA-net with the addition of hundreds of activities and events. A budget of more than eight million euros was made available for the six-year project. EurSafety Health-Net includes four subprojects and 19 so-called 'work packages', which all have their own agenda and pursue their own goals (Van Gemert-Pijnen 2011). Euregional health networks have been set up in all the Euregions taking part. The establishment of competence centres for specialised topics ensured collaboration between the available expertise throughout the entire project area. The topic-oriented competence centres provided common platforms and ensured collaboration in the entire region. In addition there was collaboration with patients' interest groups—e.g. the EPECS patient organisation mentioned above—regarding issues of cross-border patient treatment, in order to maintain comparable quality standards for patient protection.

People travel, and bacteria do not stop at borders. A German can become a patient in Belgium or the Netherlands just as quickly as the other way round. There are similar problems on both sides of the border. The ageing of the population is just as big an issue in Germany as it is in Belgium or the Netherlands. The same applies to cost controls in healthcare. Multiresistant Gram-negative bacteria are becoming an increasing problem in all three countries—and not just there. The growing number of elderly and chronically sick people goes hand in hand with an increase in the number of healthcare-associated infections. There is therefore a mutual interest in minimising these problems on both sides of the border, and avoiding them if possible: for health reasons, but also for economic ones. Healthcare-associated infections are costly. The report on the period 2009–2011 by the EurSafety Health-Net contains calculations of the economic benefits that arise from avoiding MRSA infections. 'A decline in the MRSA rate on the German and Belgium side, from an average of 25 per cent to the Dutch level of around one to three per cent, would avoid huge treatment costs and loss of working days. If the national Dutch level of MRSA prevalence were transferred to the entire EUREGIO border region, there would be approximately 10,000 fewer MRSA colonisations and 2500 fewer MRSA infections per year. In this way it would be possible to avoid annual costs of approximately 45 million euros, and there would be a gain of around 21,250 working days, the equivalent of creating 89 full-time jobs. These calculations only refer to the MRSA pathogen. If the protective measures were applied to other pathogens and infections, we would expect there to be additional cost savings' (Van Gemert-Pijnen 2011). For those taking part, internal cooperation between the MRSA-net and its successor project EurSafety Health-Net became part of everyday routine. If proof was still needed that a regional approach to infection prevention makes sense, the scientists working under the umbrella of the EurSafety Health-net have provided it (Ciccolini et al. 2013).[10] The healthcare regions must play a key role in this. For example, if there is a lot of patient movement between Oldenburg and Groningen, or Enschede and Gronau, then these become connected health regions, regardless of the fact that these cities are located in different countries.

In the Maas-Rhine Euregion, this also became clear through the international cooperation projects. Henriëtte ter Waarbeek is a medical specialist for infectious diseases at the South Limburg Health Authority, and the project partner of Karl-Heinz Feldhoff, Head of the Health Authority in Heinsberg near Aachen. Ter Waarbeek is one of the coordinators of EMRIC (Maas-Rhine Euregion Intervention in Crises), a partnership organisation for crisis management in the Dutch province of Limburg, the Belgian provinces of Limburg and Liege, and parts of North Rhine-Westphalia. She relates how EMRIC began to develop reciprocal contacts. 'We wanted to set up a consultation structure, but it quickly developed into a project group. Then we compiled a telephone directory, including contact numbers outside office hours, and a list of notifiable infectious diseases'. This was followed by meetings and workshops. 'We pooled our expertise, and decided to keep one another reciprocally informed of what each of us was currently up to. And we began to create protocols specifying exactly when we had to pass on information, and by which means. And how we would manage an outbreak. Sometimes it's possible to do that locally, sometimes you have to react on a cross-border level and, if necessary, a cross-border outbreak management team must be set up. To facilitate this cooperation, our health authority in South Limburg has set up a digital information platform in collaboration with the health authority in the Aachen urban region, which tells us what is happening on both sides of the borders (Ter Waarbeek et al. 2011). The health authorities of North Limburg and Euskirchen are also participating in this information platform. It can tell you, for example, that here in South Limburg we have several cases of whooping cough. Or that there's been an outbreak of Legionnaires' disease in Aachen. Unfortunately the Belgians were not yet ready for this. As a result of our cooperation we have realised that, in the early stages, we

---

[10]See also Chap. 5, *A thin layer of faeces on everything you touch.*

often didn't inform our colleagues on the other side of the border when we should have done. For example, think of the many children in South Limburg who go to school in Belgium'. These examples make it all too clear why infection prevention in the border regions must not stop at administrative boundaries drawn up by chance. Take for instance the EHEC outbreak that plagued Germany in spring 2011. Or the two cases of splenic fever (anthrax) amongst intravenous heroin users in Aachen (RKI 2010). In both these cases there was a connection with 119 infections in Scottish heroin consumers. Anthrax is a zoonosis. Ter Waarbeek also mentioned a mumps outbreak that raged in a number of Dutch university towns in 2011 and 2012 among students that were in large majority vaccinated. This outbreak spread to Kempen in Flanders.[11]

In 2013 there was a measles outbreak in the Netherlands, among an orthodox protestant religious community that refused vaccinations. Some of the measles cases occurred in the Zeelandic Flanders' region near the Belgian border. In 2012 there was an EHEC outbreak in Flemish Limburg caused by infected tartar. Many Dutch people like to go shopping in the big supermarkets just across the Belgian border. The information on an EHEC outbreak just across the border was therefore very important for the Dutch health authorities. These examples are all good reasons for cross-border cooperation.

## Expanding the MRSA-Net

'Where MRSA infections are concerned, the difference between Germany and the Netherlands is huge', says Jacques Scheres, 'but where other problems are concerned there are no such differences, and we can learn from and with one other. In the beginning I actually sensed a certain resistance on the part of insurance companies, patients and even doctors. I no longer feel this resistance now, except perhaps amongst patients who go from the Netherlands to Germany or Belgium for treatment, and ask whether it's safe there as far as MRSA is concerned'. In Moers, Dr. Rüdiger Rau, who worked together with Andreas Voss from Nijmegen, was won over by the first successes.[12] Voss is a Professor of Infection Prevention at the Radboud University Medical Centre and a medical specialist in clinical microbiology at the Canisius-Wilhelmina Hospital, both in Nijmegen. 'The good thing about the EurSafety project is that it has also given us the opportunity to do other things. For example, we were able to set up the 'Vuile Freddy/Schmuddel Fritze' project.[13] This health education project is aimed at schools, and tries to actively involve

---

[11]Kempen is the region enclosed by the Dutch towns of Tilburg, Breda, Eindhoven and Weert to the north and east, by Antwerp to the west, and by Genk and Hasselt in Flanders to the south.

[12]Dr. Rüdiger Rau was responsible for the area of public health at the Department of Health—formerly District Health Authority—of the Wesel district, particularly the Office of the Municipal Health Conference (KGK). Since 2017, he is working for the public health office (*Gesundheitsamt*) in Lauterbach, in the federal state of Hessen.

[13]Stop Dirty Freddy.

children in infection prevention and teach them basic hygiene rules. The focus is on influenza. Voss still regrets that the Schmuddel Fritze project did not become established, because the funding stopped. 'Particularly this year it could be really useful', he says.[14] 'Look how the norovirus is spreading. We're dealing with a nasty subtype here. We could achieve some really fantastic results with Schmuddel Fritze right now'. But what applies to 'Stop Schmuddel Fritze!' actually applies to another project that was close to Voss' heart as well. A network of senior care facilities and nursing homes was set up in the Nijmegen region, which collaborated in the field of infection prevention. As part of the EurSafety project, this network developed a seal of quality for proper care in the area of infection prevention. 'The senior care facilities and nursing homes were still uncharted territory for us in the Netherlands too', recalls Voss. 'There was a lot still to do here. We copied everything that was good about the MRSA-net and introduced it here. Then we transferred the whole thing to Germany. We could count on enthusiastic acceptance there. Our own regional network now includes approximately 40 institutions that are interested in a quality seal.[15] That is not such a bad number either, but meanwhile on the other side of the border they have clocked up around 300 institutions that already have a seal of quality and thousands who are working to achieve one. 'In Inka Daniels-Haardt's view, 'These seals of quality really are a major driver for the project. Their influence extends beyond purely clinical hygiene staff to hospital administration and business management. So then it also involves economic interests. The fact that you can show the outside world 'we're doing our bit'. This also makes us very attractive for patients. Perhaps this success has something to do with the German mentality. Quality, with a certificate and seal. Perhaps we need that so that we can say we are doing it right. You can also see from the photos how excited everyone is when they receive their seal. That motivates people and, as I said, it is also viewed this way by the hospitals' business management.'

## Seals

Peter Bergen is a hygiene specialist for the regional health authority in Lower Saxony. He is responsible for hygiene in outpatient and inpatient care facilities. 'The seals form part of a quality campaign. In the regional districts you have different levels of hygiene in these homes. There are homes that belong to big chains. In those cases the whole thing is very tightly controlled from the centre, including the quality management side. But there are also smaller facilities which, in plain and simple language, so far haven't got round to it. We go to these people and show them how in one year they could achieve so much that they themselves, the health authority and even the residents would be satisfied with it. We do this by

---

[14]This interview with Andreas Voss took place in mid-December 2014, when a large number of healthcare institutions still had their work cut out dealing with the norovirus.

[15]See also Chap. 11, 'A bottomless well, and other solutions'.

means of a relatively simple programme. They are given specific tasks, and there's also a certain pressure to implement these tasks. In addition there's help, work materials and text components for the guidelines. It's a unique opportunity to achieve something that they've always wanted to do. Those who have got everything well organised can also show this to the outside world. I also drop by, I look after things, and at the end everything's checked. In principle this is a very worthwhile experience for all those involved'.

Andreas Voss understands very well why the enthusiasm for the seal is greater on the other side of the border. He was born in Germany and grew up there, but for over 20 years he has been working in the Netherlands. 'In Germany, something like that is carried out via the authorities. A public health official is given the responsibility for it, and then it's carried out'. This is not so easily accepted in the Netherlands, explains Andreas Voss.

'Imagine the health authority popping in and telling the hospital what they have to do. That doesn't work here. In Germany the health authorities have a dual role: they fulfil both the role of our Health Care Inspectorate, and that of our health authorities'.

## Health Inspectorate

Inka Daniels-Haardt shares the vision of Voss: 'In the Netherlands the inspectorate carries out the checks in the hospitals. For us, that's the job of the regional health authority. That's a big difference. We were very impressed by the weighty authority of the Dutch Health Care Inspectorate. It appeared that it was feared, and also effective. Our problem in Germany is that the health authorities are so closely linked to the hospitals. The officials know one another, sometimes even in private life. When it's a question of municipally sponsored hospitals, where the city or district has an interest in whether the hospital performs well economically, then hospital surveillance can look rather as though the public health official is meeting the head physician for a coffee. They talk for a bit, and then everything's all right. It is now becoming apparent to everyone that the problems with nosocomial infections and media attention are somewhat bigger. Perhaps we are now moving more towards genuine surveillance. But certainly things are not yet as they should be, where you have really good standards and make consistent demands. For example, we carried out a survey to find out how often fines are imposed. According to infection prevention law, we can impose fines of up to 25,000 euros if, for example, clusters of nosocomial infections are not reported. In North Rhine-Westphalia this hasn't occurred on a single occasion, even though many things haven't been reported. These are outbreaks that are made known through the media. The health officials often know this, but they just tell the hospitals to do things better in future. The idea of transferring surveillance responsibilities to a higher level, so that there's more distance between the monitor and the monitored, is being considered. Just like in the Netherlands', says Daniels-Haardt. Robin Köck expresses a similarly critical view. 'In the Netherlands they also have unannounced hospital visits, whose findings are published on the internet. In Germany we have health officials who make one pre-announced visit to hospitals per year. This was an issue that we tackled in the EurSafety project through the seals of quality. These made surveillance data visible, showing the public health service how often certain antibiotic-resistant pathogens occurred in the hospitals. Before the project such insights weren't available. General resistance statistics showing, for example the percentage of MRSA in all *Staphylococcus aureus,* already existed before this. But to know, in truly concrete terms, how many patients are being treated in hospitals as a result here and now – that's new. These are data that have now been comprehensively gathered for the first time'.

'Despite all the things you can criticise about the inspectorate in the Netherlands', says Voss, 'I'm still glad we have it. As a means of exerting pressure. If you approach this with mutual professionalism and use suitable indicators, it works well. Sometimes it's gone wrong because we experts have drawn up the guidelines, but not given any indicators that could be used to monitor compliance with these guidelines. We have often left this to people whose ability to establish the right indicators was questionable'.

## Uniform Procedures

Voss is confident that the senior care facilities and nursing homes in his region have a positive attitude towards EurSafety. 'They were confronted with it for the first time when the supervisory authorities came to them and demanded they do everything possible in the field of infection prevention. That was the perfect moment for us to strike. And that was also absolutely necessary, because senior care facilities and nursing homes did not carry out any infection prevention measures. Andrea Eikelenboom, one of our hygienists, has concentrated entirely on infection prevention in senior care facilities and nursing homes, and at the moment is working for several of these institutions on a part-time basis. During the early years this was part-financed by EurSafety Health-Net. In this way we were able to put our project ideas into practice'. Similar initiatives were taken in the region around Breda, in the south of the Netherlands. Infection prevention specialists of the Amphia Hospital in Breda were hired on a part-time basis by senior care institutions to help implement a better hygiene and infection prevention policy. During the corona-pandemic in 2020 this resulted in less contaminations, less ill elderly and less deaths in these facilities compared to institutions where no infection prevention specialists had been deployed.

According to Voss the collaboration with the Germans went well from the start, although initially the project was a one-way street. In the Rhine-Waal Euregion, Rüdiger Rau made a big contribution towards changing this. He worked at the health authority in the Wesel district of around 470,000 inhabitants, which included the towns of Dinslaken, Moers and Wesel. In 2008, MRSA and other hospital bacteria were a hot topic at the regional healthcare conference in the Wesel district. 'We had decided to develop this idea on a district-wide basis, because we knew that in the Netherlands their "search and destroy" strategy had kept tighter control of the MRSA problem for years already', recalls Rüdiger Rau. Hygiene officials from the eight regional hospitals, representatives of health insurance companies and resident doctors formed a working group together. 'Together with these eight hospitals, we then decided that we needed uniform procedures', recalls Rau. 'Patients should be screened according to the same rules in all eight hospitals, MRSA identified early, and MRSA patients or carriers isolated. That was in 2009. In early summer 2009, Andreas Voss called us because he was looking for a twin partner for EurSafety'. Since then, and until his departure to Lautersbach in 2017, Rau has been collaborating closely with Andreas Voss and his colleague Andrea Eikelenboom. 'For me as a public health medic, that's something really new'. Rau gives two concrete examples to illustrate his enthusiasm for the project. Through his Dutch project partner, he has had access to specialist knowledge about microbiological epidemiology, a subject of which he had little prior knowledge. And he is enthusiastic about the 'seal of quality' model.

Two more seals of quality were developed after the initial seal for MRSA prevention in hospitals. The second seal of quality includes other multiresistant pathogens such as VRE, ESBL and CRE, and rational antibiotic therapy. The third seal was for setting up functioning structures and training specialised staff for infection prevention and hygiene. According to the latest available data (in the course of 2019) in total 119 German and 4 Dutch hospitals had at least one of the three existing quality-seals.[16] Among the 360 senior care facilities and nursing homes that received the first seal during the active period of the project until 2015, only 28 were Dutch. The other 332 are German institutions, almost half of them also obtained the second quality-seal.[17] The seals of quality normally remain valid for two years, after which the institution is reappraised to determine if it can retain the seal.

Andreas Voss appears to be very satisfied with the work he did with his German colleague. The Wesel district and Nijmegen have set several things in motion. 'Rüdiger Rau has also started up all kinds of activities himself', relates Voss. 'Perhaps he's told you about what I somewhat irreverently refer to as the "small cross-border enterprise", the STI[18] project'. Rau—who has since moved to south Germany—certainly does remember this, very well. 'That was a prevalence study on the Dutch model that we carried out as part of a job-shadowing exercise at the health authority in Nijmegen. A colleague from Duisburg gave us a lot of help with this. We did a kind of intervention study there on sexually transmitted diseases in prostitutes. And we were also able to publish it nationally in the *Bulletin* of the Robert Koch Institute. This represented a new milestone for us. This wouldn't have been possible without the EurSafety Health-Net or Andreas Voss and his laboratory'. 'The project was successful to the extent that we carefully worked out how healthcare provision

---

[16]Twenty German hospitals had one quality-seal, 66 had two seals and 37 had three seals of quality. The four Dutch hospitals all had one seal (EurSafety Health-net 2019a).

[17]A total of 180 German and 28 Dutch senior care facilities obtained one quality-seal and 152 German institutions also acquired the second one (EurSafety Health-net 2019b).

[18]STI = sexually transmitted infections.

for prostitutes should be organised in collaboration with the health authority', says Voss. And we could see that it was somewhat less well organised on the German side. Because if more than 20 per cent of the women have STIs, then you can certainly end up getting more than you paid for'.

In October 2011 and March 2012, 228 female prostitutes in Duisburg and Wesel were tested for gonorrhoea and chlamydia. The majority (59 per cent) were between 20 and 29 years old. More than 90 per cent of the women had a history of migration. A total of 22 per cent of the woman tested positive for either or both of the STIs in question. Sixteen per cent tested positive for chlamydia, six per cent for gonorrhoea and four per cent of the tested women were positive for both. The authors of the article in the epidemiological bulletin of the Robert Koch Institute underscored the importance of Dutch–German cooperation on this issue: 'The popularity of clubs etc. in rural areas of Germany with Dutch men makes heightened collaboration with the public health service (GGD) in the Netherlands a necessity' (Rau et al. 2014).

Alex Friedrich calls the STI project in the Rhine-Waal Euregion a nice example of how cross-border collaboration can be configured in practice. 'You can see why it was a success', he says. 'Just do what you're good at, but do it in conjunction with your partner on the other side of the border. That's the pioneering innovation. You might think that something like this is perfectly normal, but that's not the case. Around the world everyone is working with every possible kind of partner, but it doesn't take place so often with partners just across the border. For that you have to find a shared topic of concern with a partner met "by chance". The public health service in Nijmegen said that they could not collaborate with the German public health service (ÖGD) because they had not this role of a supervisory authority. But where sexually transmitted diseases were concerned they were able to collaborate, because this is a problem that involves both countries. Infectious diseases and antibiotic resistance are topics that definitely lend themselves to cross-border collaboration, which means anybody can cooperate with anybody else. In this way we can help one another. That was the formula for success. The idea behind EurSafety is a network of experts and interested parties, motivated people who are open-minded and share everything both across the border and along it. It is a loose network structure centred around a common idea: patient safety and avoidance of antibiotic resistance along and across the common border. And the great thing about this is you have a kind of experimental zone with additional financial support, so that you can try out things which wouldn't be possible so easily in Germany or the Netherlands. Because there they've thought about everything already and regulated it according to fixed structures, or because no money is being made available for specific activities. That's the great thing about border regions: you have the opportunity to carry out a natural cohort study, one cohort in the German border region and the other in the Dutch one. In Germany patients who are colonised by specific microorganisms are not isolated. In the Netherlands they most certainly are. That means you can carry out comparative studies in the border region and see which of these makes more sense. That makes it possible to do a kind of comparative epidemiology, which affords a wealth of opportunities for research. Border regions are very innovative, because you can create knowledge there that you don't find anywhere else. Because there are two natural cohorts there. For example, the disinfection efforts that used to be made everywhere in German hospitals have slowly been reduced, except in special cases. That's because we could see that no comparable efforts were being made in the Netherlands, and yet nothing happened. There are several other examples of this, and this has led to the publication of more than 20 scientific articles arising out of the EurSafety project. These articles are primarily about patient safety, infection prevention, genotyping, antibiotics advice and network analysis or behavioural changes in the field of infection prevention (for example: Eikelenboom-Boskamp et al. 2011; Jurke et al. 2013; Ciccolini et al. 2013; Friedrich et al. 2013; Müller et al. 2015; Berger et al. 2016; Jurke et al. 2019). In addition we provide a lot of information by other means. Ron Hendrix and his group, who have set up the MRSA-net database with Lisette van Gemert-Pijnen, receive thousands of questions online every month. With its "frequently asked questions" and helpdesk, MRSA-net has contributed a lot to education and training of specialist staff as well'.

Jörg Hermann regards the cross-border collaboration as a gigantic leap forward. 'We now have a committed group who understand one another extremely well, and who also speak about problems that nobody spoke about before. For example about the difficulties that exist – perhaps also political and financial ones – or outbreaks, which we discuss and assess with one another. And the Dutch have learned a great deal about what it's like to have a germ problem of this kind. They are going to profit from this now where ESBL and CRE are concerned. Previously, the awareness did not exist at all in this form. The Dutch are now discovering that they have a similar situation with ESBL to what the Germans have with MRSA. Forming regional networks is now the issue of the day in the Netherlands as well.'

## The Crucial Role of Border Regions

Friedrich once again underscores the important role that border regions play. 'It's not the case that something was discovered in the Netherlands, adopted in the EU, and implemented in Germany. No: the border regions collaborated, and since it func-tioned in the Münsterland, it ought to function in Berlin as well. In 2011 it was adopted in the whole of Germany. So you've actually got a completely different kind of European cooperation. Once you've implemented the Dutch methods in the border region and adapted them to the medical structures there, and it also works, then you can adopt them. It has to grow organically, and that's what's happening in the border regions. Perhaps that's an important lesson for the whole of Europe. Innovative border regions can make a change in Europe. The EU is needed to enable such joint projects in border regions. I'm not saying you don't need the classic Europe of capital cities. But there's another Europe, the Europe of border regions. And in those we can learn a lot from one another'.

## The Importance of Experts Present at the Site

Since the success of MRSA-net and EurSafety Health-Net, the Germans have become infected by the idea of cross-border regional collaboration, says Professor Martin Mielke. He is Head of the Department of Infectious Diseases at the Robert Koch Institute, and a former member of the steering group and advisory commission of MRSA-net. 'In Germany we have many neighbours with different forms of healthcare provision. This initiative that has been launched between the Netherlands and the neighbouring North Rhine-Westphalia region is a very, very interesting project. Particularly in connection with antibiotic-resistant bacteria. Exactly comparing the recommendations in both countries, recording the differences in the way the problem is perceived by nursing staff at the sickbed—for these purposes we have carried out tasks which could not have been performed without the network, and which have provided a considerable stimulus for mutual learning'. Mielke regards the availability of financial means for clearly defined goals, which must be fulfilled, as decisive for the success of a project. 'If such projects are not expressly promoted, these activities often get lost in everyday routine. The creation of sustainable materials is unquestionably promoted if you stipulate that money will also be spent on it. That makes it possible for a few people to give their attention to it more or less permanently, and then something emerges from it as well. For example, the FAQ section of the MRSA Helpdesk is very helpful and very well designed (MRSA-net 2020b). The internet site is also very well configured. It provided the opportunity to mutually agree the answers. We have an intensive exchange of ideas, which is made possible through the network. For example, in December 2013 we had a very good EurSafety symposium in Nijmegen to exchange information on our procedures for dealing with gram-negative, multi-drug resistant intestinal bacteria (Müller et al. 2015), during which we formulated the decisive questions for the future. In this field we have the same problems. Possibly the Dutch have somewhat higher rates of intestinal colonisation by these pathogens. But we have different mentalities. In Germany we talk a lot about regulations and pass laws. In the Netherlands a lot of weight is placed on the direct understanding of the experts affected. Just becoming aware of such differences in mentality is already interesting in itself'.

At the end of February 2015, German and Dutch EurSafety Health-Net researchers published a study in *Antimicrobial Resistance and Infection Control*, in which they compared the German and Dutch guidelines on multiresistant Gram-negative bacteria with one another (Müller et al. 2015). The study clearly identified two major differences in the countries' approaches. The Dutch guideline prescribes testing multiresistant Gram-negative microorganisms for a series of resistance-causing genetic mechanisms. The German guideline stipulates using a new type of classification based on phenotypic characterisation. And in Dutch hospitals, special hygiene measures apply to all patients with ESBL-producing *Enterobacteriaceae*. In Germany such measures are only prescribed if the ESBL-producing *Enterobacteriaceae* are also resistant to ciprofloxacin (3MRGN).

'The high number of microbiologists in the Netherlands', says Professor Mielke, 'is of course exemplary for us, because you can only achieve anything at the local level if experts are present on-site. Ultimately, the situation in any country is the sum of its activities in each location. The communication culture is also different in the Netherlands. Partly more open, the discussions are directed towards a consensus and, once this has been reached—or at least, this is my perception—the matters on which there is a consensus are implemented very consistently. We have to look at the national and regional aspects in parallel. The healthcare system is mainly nationally organised. Even within a country, however, there are regional differences. In Germany we now have comprehensive regional networks as well, not just in the border regions, but also across the entire Federal Republic (RKI 2019). This idea was actually launched by EurSafety, and an article has been published about it (Ciccolini et al. 2013). Since 2005 we have worked intensively to disseminate this idea of regionally networking healthcare institutions that exchange patients. These are the relevant units where transmissions occur: the university medical centres with their associated hospitals, care institutions and rehab clinics. That is the concrete reality, and not just in the border regions, but in the whole of Germany and other countries as well. There are networks like this in all the federal states in Germany, and they are defined by their referral structures'.

## Dutch–Flemish Euregion

It is not just in Germany that MRSA-net and EurSafety Health-Net have excited interest. In March 2017 a cross-border INTERREG, i-4-1-Health, was launched along the Dutch-Belgian border (INTERREG 2020). In addition to the province of Limburg, the Dutch part of this region also includes the province of North Brabant, which has an extremely high livestock population and high population density. In 2007 Brabant made the headlines with the largest outbreak of Q fever anywhere in the world to date (Schneeberger et al. 2014). By 2010, at least 25 people had died from the disease, thousands had become sick, and hundreds were seriously ill. In November 2020 the number of deaths of the four-year Q-fever outbreak reached 95, and approximately 1300 people were still suffering from the consequences of the disease (RIVM 2020). This epidemic greatly boosted awareness of the dangers of zoonoses and stimulated the development of the 'one health' idea. While there was still a great deal of mutual distrust to begin with, human and veterinary medics are now working together better. The province of North Brabant is very intensively involved. And as if this outbreak was not enough, ESBL then came along to finish the job off. Studies carried out at the time by Jan Kluijtmans' group at the Amphia Hospital showed that meat offered for sale in Dutch supermarkets—and above all chicken meat—was contaminated with ESBL bacteria (Overdevest et al. 2011). The presence of ESBL in the food chain attracted a great deal of attention. The NOS broadcaster gave the topic a lot of exposure.[19] The Dutch–Flemish Euregion project launched in 2017 focused on the following main topics:

- Surveillance and control of antimicrobial resistance in humans and animals in healthcare institutions, childcare institutions and livestock farming in the Dutch–Flemish border region.
- Creating insights into and knowledge about factors, whether linked to individuals or to institutions, that may contribute to the control of antimicrobial resistance in healthcare institutions, childcare institutions and livestock farming.

The i-4-1 Health project consists of different working packages, three of which aim to form networks and share knowledge within the healthcare system (hospitals), in public healthcare (nursing homes, childcare institutions such as day care) and livestock farming (pig and chicken farms). A fourth working package has developed a digital instrument for scanning for the risk of infections (see below), and finally a fifth working package is developing a platform for whole genome sequencing (WGS) of resistant microbes.

Jan Kluijtmans is heading up the project on the Dutch side. 'Over here, Q fever and ESBL provided a high level of motivation to launch a project. Because of Q fever and the whole resistance problem, the province was really keen to take part. Some people from the livestock industry were severely affected, and a movement was formed that brought the project into being. After that we also awakened interest in Belgium.' A meeting on 21 February 2014, in Ulvenhout near Breda, was an important step in this process. Roughly 40 enthusiastic pioneers came together with the aim of fleshing out the project idea. More than a quarter of them came from Flanders. There were microbiologists, experts on infection prevention, doctors from the public healthcare service, specialist physicians for infectious diseases, veterinarians, biologists and advisors from various relevant sectors. Their common goal was collaborating in infection prevention and the fight against infectious diseases across national borders and, because of the high density of the animal population, with a focus on the connections between people and animals.

## Bottom-Up

During the meeting in Ulvenhout, Alex Friedrich explained that the bottom-up approach was the key to the success of EurSafety, because this facilitated the involvement and support of all relevant institutions, persons and authorities. And this automatically leads to further expansion of the project. Moreover, the Dutch–Flemish region has a major advantage compared with the Dutch–German border region. The same language is spoken on both sides of the border. Kluijtmans mentioned the fact that there was hardly any contact or cooperation between

---

[19]Dutch Broadcasting Foundation. The author works for the NOS broadcasting service.

Dutch and Belgian experts in the two countries' health services. 'Because the resistance problem in the two countries is so different, it's very hard to exchange patients or doctors and nurses. There are real barriers that restrict the European idea, and therefore constitute very good grounds for projects of this sort. In our country, a patient coming from a Belgian hospital is isolated because of the heightened risk that they are carrying all sorts of resistant bacteria with them. That is an especially undesirable situation. To make exchanges of staff and patients easier, we must dismantle the differences. I know staff in my own hospital who have also worked in a Belgian hospital, and who gave up their job there to come and work over here. There are already Belgian hospitals that use the Dutch methods, and they have far fewer resistance problems. We would be able to implement this approach far more comprehensively in a network of this kind. Hospitals are part of a treatment network'.

The Antwerp University Hospital in Wilrijk, where Herman Goossens heads the Department of Medical Microbiology, has already been pursuing the Dutch approach for years. 'And they've had only minor problems with MRSA there', tells Kluijtmans. 'But Goossens has had to isolate more patients than us, because many of his patients came from hospitals that were not so strict, and therefore had far more problems with MRSA. If everybody adheres to a strict policy, then the prospects for abolishing the differences quickly are actually pretty favourable. In the senior care facilities and nursing homes in Belgium and the Netherlands, the problems are also increasing fast. Here a lot more still has to be done in order to balance the care situation on both sides of the border'.

The hospitals on both sides of the border are not dissatisfied with the barriers that still exist, since they protect them from losses of revenue. On the other hand, there is also still insufficient interest in treating patients who come from the other side of the border. According to Kluijtmans, this is also connected with the fact that the costs of treating complications are only partly reimbursed, or not at all. 'Therefore at our clinic we're not so interested in patients who go to Belgium to have treatment. As soon as they have complications over there, they want to come back to the Netherlands. And then we get a patient who is carrying all sorts of resistant bacteria'. Kluijtmans mentions the example of a Dutch patient who underwent a bariatric operation in Flanders, during which severe complications arose. His family had to travel 160 km every day to visit him. 'The man eventually ended up in our intensive care unit in Breda, in a pitiful state. He was actually a kind of timebomb that threatened to infect our ICU. For us this was a very difficult matter to discuss, since the patient himself had made the decision to have his operation in Belgium. We did not at all want to have a conversation of this kind. Therefore we must harmonise the policy on both sides of the border'.

'I think', says Kluijtmans, 'that the health systems can learn from one another, and that an optimal blend can be achieved. Resistance is of course only part of the whole problem—a constantly increasing part. However, access to medical care in Belgium is, for example, considerably better than in the Netherlands. Of course this gives rise to yet further problems, for example regarding the provision of medical treatment when opinions differ as to whether it is necessary. A border cannot solve these problems. If we break through this border we will have some difficulties to resolve, but in the end this will help us on our way. For us it's a question of how to align the Dutch and Belgian health systems so that it's possible to guarantee optimum levels of quality and access, so that both countries and, above all, the patients can profit from this'.

## Healthcare on Two Sides of the Border

Kluijtmans' partner in setting up the project on the Flemish side is Bart Gordts. He is a microbiologist and medical coordinator for hospital hygiene in the Antwerp Hospital Network, which comprises three general hospitals and six specialist clinics of the public health service. At the meeting in Ulvenhout he presented a neat example of the reciprocal relationship between the two countries' health systems. It involved a couple from Poppel in Belgium. The husband was insured in Belgium, his wife in the Netherlands. This was because of her work. Their GP was in Poppel. The husband went to the clinic in Turnhout, but to the dentist in the Netherlands. The wife had asthma and was treated for it by a doctor in the Netherlands. Gordt's example perfectly illustrates practice in a border region.

'It is interesting for us to investigate the differences of approach between our hospitals and our countries, to see what is better on the other side of the border and call our own practice into question. However, there are clear cultural differences. Many things that are allowed in Belgium are absolutely impossible in the Netherlands, and this sometimes makes my work in Belgium difficult. If I have to convince doctors to change their normal working procedures, for example by prescribing fewer broad-spectrum antibiotics, it's much more difficult in Belgium than in the Netherlands. Doctors in the Netherlands are more easily convinced that they can't resist measures taken in the public interest. In Belgium, "public interest" is a very relative concept. Besides the cultural differences there are also budgetary ones. The specific budgets for infection prevention and microbiology laboratories are much lower. Therefore it's also much more difficult for Belgian laboratories to introduce new methods of investigating resistance or new diagnostic tests. For thirty years now, laboratories in Belgium have been financed according to a lump-sum system that is hardly ever readjusted. That means the budget gets smaller every year. It's the same in private hospitals. In comparison with the Netherlands, we have a bigger problem and a smaller budget. On top of this, Belgian hospitals are suffering from a chronic shortage of nursing staff. In the Netherlands, hospital departments are closed if the staffing level does not reach the minimum. In our case we just soldier on. The staff have no time for training and informative events. There is a lack of nursing staff, and for financial reasons hospitals only engage the legally prescribed number of employees. My own team of hygiene specialists comprises 3.8 full-time positions, but if one of my colleagues is absent for a year on maternity leave I can't replace her. There are also similarities between our two countries. It isn't just in Belgium that changing existing habits is extremely difficult, but in the Netherlands as well. To convince an operating team that it has to change its working practices for hygienic reasons requires just as great an effort in the Netherlands as it does here. In this project, we must mutually and systematically exchange information on the prevalence and extent of the problems and the various approaches across the border. How is a specific problem handled in the Netherlands, and how certain are people there that the chosen solution makes sense? Or vice versa: What do they do in Belgium? What is the best solution?'

## IRIS

Since the launch of i-4-1-Health, the nine hospitals, seven universities, seven public health institutions and three enterprises participating in this project have started a series of initiatives to map the antimicrobial resistance problems in both the Belgian and Dutch hospitals, other healthcare institutions and livestock sectors in the border region. Several innovations are being developed for this purpose, such as a 'track and trace' system for resistant microbes and IRIS, an instrument to scan for the risk of infections (Willemsen and Klijtmans 2016). Ina Willemsen, an infection prevention consultant at the Amphia Hospital in Breda—a Dutch town near the Belgian border—is the driving force behind IRIS. She was interviewed about it by the internal TV channel at the 2018 European Congress of Clinical Microbiology and Infectious Diseases in Madrid. 'IRIS is a method of measuring the quality of your infection prevention programme', Willemsen explains. 'It provides you with transparency about risk factors in your hospital, antimicrobial use and antimicrobial resistance. It's like normal infection control, but it's bundled. It bundles all the auditing and surveillance operations in a hospital or nursing home, and carries them out all in one go. Then we try to visualise the results in a way that's easy to read: a spider plot'.

This specific method of visualising the results of the infection risk scan is the main difference between IRIS and other available tools. 'I wanted to make something that was easy to read for someone who is not an infection control nurse', says Willemsen. 'To build a bridge between infection control and people on the wards. So it had to fit on one piece of paper—and that's when I came up with the idea of the spider plot. And every time you access the plot, it presents the results of one audit'. The plot is displayed in three colours: green, amber and red, just like a traffic light. The more room for improvement an audit reveals, the larger the figure will be. 'And the more you will find yourself in the red zone', Ina Willemsen adds (ECCMID 2018). By the end of 2016, IRIS had been carried out in five hospital departments, a rehabilitation clinic and 19 nursing homes. Two years later—when she presented her research at the ECCMID 2018 in Madrid—six Dutch Hospitals, three Belgian hospitals, 60 long-term care facilities on both sides of the border, and ten other healthcare institutions, had implemented IRIS (Willemsen and Kluytmans 2018).

The implementation of IRIS is probably the most concrete result of i-4-1-Health so far. More fruits of the project are in the pipeline. 'One of the first cautious conclusions that this first year of the project permits us to draw', says Jan Kluijtmans, the project leader on the Dutch side of the border, 'is that the high level of antimicrobial resistance in Belgian hospitals compared with Dutch ones seems to be more a consequence of the large number of antibiotics prescribed by Belgian GPs than of the usage in hospitals themselves'.

There are several examples of European initiatives in the field of infection prevention. Professor Evelina Tacconelli is a medical expert on infectious diseases. Since 2013 she has been head of the infectious diseases division of the Department of Internal Medicine at the University Hospital Tübingen and a full professor at the University of Tübingen. In 2017 she has also been appointed a full professor of infectious diseases at the University of Verona in Italy. Professor Tacconelli is 'Professional Affair Officer' for infectious diseases for the ESCMID (European Society of Clinical Microbiology and Infectious Diseases), and is an advisor on antibiotic-resistant infections for several international organisations. Moreover, she is also editor of *The Lancet Infectious Diseases, Clinical Microbiology and Infection* and the *Journal of Antimicrobial Chemotherapy*. 'Some years ago I started a project to define a minimum programme of measures that each country must carry out in order to stop the spread of resistant bacteria throughout the whole of Europe. That is our most important task. Resistance is spread by people. But in the EU we don't have a uniform approach towards infection prevention'. Tacconelli has set up a steering committee in the ESCMID that is meant to bring off this feat. Its members now include experts from Sweden, Germany, the Netherlands, the United Kingdom, Switzerland, Spain, Italy, Greece and France. 'This minimum programme differs depending on the situation and the bacterium involved. Once the proposal is ready, the European Commission must then start looking at it. These sorts of standards cannot be implemented without political support'.

## It Is Not Easy

Bringing about a minimum programme of uniform infection prevention measures is not easy. It takes years. 'About a year ago the ESCMID committee took its first steps on the long path we have to follow', Professor Tacconelli explained to me by phone from Verona at the beginning of December 2018. She has moved from Tübingen in Germany back to Italy, where she now runs the Department of Medical Microbiology at the University Hospital of Verona. She is extremely busy controlling an outbreak at her hospital.

'We have chosen to start with education: a European master's programme in infection control. It is a unique idea: students from all over Europe come to universities that are performing outstandingly well in this specific subject. This leads to a constant exchange between the north of Europe and the south. We learn from each other. In the Scandinavian countries for example, they are very strong in the field of gram-negative outbreaks on a theoretical level. But they are lacking in experience of how to deal with such outbreaks. So we in the south can teach the Nordic countries how to control an outbreak of gram-negative microbes, and they can teach us how to prevent such outbreaks. Since we started we have trained 40 infection prevention specialists. What's nice about this is that they've started a network where they share their knowledge and carry out research projects together.

They're also reviewing existing guidelines, with the aim of trying to establish new European guidelines for infection prevention. These 40 experts are young, enthusiastic doctors, nurses and scientists who are now collecting evidence from a range of different European countries. They are producing a great deal, and asking a lot of questions. I'm expecting them to come up with European guidelines in another 12 months or so'.

Tacconelli has started another key project called *Stop Negatives*. It started out as an international survey focusing on the limitations of infection prevention measures in different countries owing to political and cultural differences. 'The legislation you need in the Netherlands, for instance, is completely different from what you need in Italy or Spain', says Tacconelli. 'In the Netherlands you can require patients carrying CRE to be isolated in a single room. In Italy or Spain this law would not be implemented very successfully—perhaps in up to 20% of cases—simply because there are not enough rooms in the hospitals. So the regulators should take these differences into account when they make new rules or regulations'.

The differences in approach between various countries are remarkable, says Tacconelli. 'But I think these differences may possibly be very practical. We need guidelines tailored to local needs. But we are lacking a common path. We need to achieve agreement on a minimum programme of infection prevention measures that countries have to adhere to. If they don't, this could lead to sanctions. Ten years ago, Europe proceeded in precisely this way on the question of air pollution. If your emissions are too high, you have to pay a fine. Doctors from all European countries agree that we need this minimum programme, and that sanctions should be applied to countries that do not adhere to it. This is the only way to force countries to follow the programme'.

After years of work, Tacconelli now has the impression that things are starting to work out. 'In the beginning there was a certain amount of suspicion: we were asking people to do more work, without providing something for them to do. Now we realise that we have to do the two things together. Unfortunately, political awareness is lacking in the southern part of Europe. Italy and Greece, respectively, have the highest and second highest numbers of deaths from infections caused by multiresistant bacteria (Cassini et al. 2018; Tacconelli and Pezzani 2018). And this despite all the efforts of doctors and nurses. The medical profession is certainly aware of these problems. What we need now is increased political awareness. We have to establish contact with politicians'.

In Italy, says Tacconelli, contact with politicians has merely been getting worse since the end of 2018. The Five Star Movement/League government is busy with immigration and social measures for which they have no money.[20] 'Better healthcare

---

[20]The Five Star Movement/League government was in office from 1 June 2018 until 20 August 2019. Prime minister Giuseppe Conte remained as leader of a new coalition government, this time without the League and with participation of the Partido Democratico. Conte had to resign on 26 January 2021 as the small party Italia Viva led by former prime minister Renzi left the governement. Since 13 February 2021 Mario Draghi, former president of the European Central Bank, is the new Italian prime minister.

could be a very interesting topic for populist parties, but it requires serious funding. The Five Star Movement/League government has made many promises, but it lacks funds and its budget has run into problems with the EU. So there is no scope for promises on healthcare. Let me give you just one example. In November 2017, the Italian government came up with an antibiotic resistance plan for the first time (PNCAR 2017). The last item on a long list of measures to be carried out stated that there was no budget for them. It was a fake plan. There is no budget for doing what it asks us to do, and there is no system to control whether it gets done or not. So this plan is not working'.

## Groningen-Heraklion Collaboration

In Greece too, just as in Italy, it is difficult to start up new projects or realise new plans. In 2014, the University Medical Centre Groningen (UMCG) began a scientific collaboration in the field of carbapenem-resistant microorganisms with the University of Heraklion, on the Greek island of Crete. The collaboration has two aims: to train the Greek staff in the treatment of infections by carbapenem-resistant *Enterobacteriaceae* (CRE), and to analyse the CRE of the Cretan patients using the latest laboratory techniques. 'In the process we're learning something about the proliferation dynamic', says Alex Friedrich, 'and we can develop quick tests which we can use here in Groningen to rapidly identify imported cases and make them available to our colleagues at the four hospitals on Crete. Our aim is to make Crete CRE-free, and to keep Groningen free from infections by CRE'. Greece has been struggling for years with *Klebsiella pneumoniae* with the KPC-2 enzyme, which makes the bacterium resistant to carbapenem antibiotics. In such cases, only a few reserve medicines are still left to treat infections, which are often less effective or have more side effects. If the outbreak of KPC-2 *Klebsiella pneumoniae* in Greece cannot successfully be brought under control, there will be more and more pan-resistant bacteria that do not respond to any antibiotic. In Crete, the rate has risen from 9 per cent in 2010 to 30 per cent in 2014. Since then basically nothing has changed. As a result of tourism to Crete, Greece in general and other countries with a high prevalence of CRE, the probability of this pan-resistant strain spreading across the whole of Europe is very high.

Athanasios Tsakris is Professor of Medical Microbiology, Head of the Department of Microbiology at the Medical School of the University of Athens, and senior editor of the *Journal of Antimicrobial Therapy* (JAC). 'A lot of hard work is being done as part of the Procrustes programme', he says. 'We gather a lot of information about the type of problems we have with multiresistant bugs, and where they're located. These data trigger reactions in the field of infection prevention. We're seeing a slow decrease in the number of carbapenem-resistant *Klebsiella pneumoniae*, but there is still a long way to go' (WHONET Greece 2020).

One of the ideas currently being discussed in Greece is that of a 'living laboratory'. 'Could we take stricter infection prevention measures in an isolated area, such as Crete for instance? If this led to fewer problems with multiresistant microbes and infections that are very hard to treat, it might have a positive effect in the sense that it could be considered as an example of best practice. Hospitals in other regions might copy such an approach. So I'm convinced this is the way to go. But to perform such an experiment, we need money. Money and a lot of hard work'.

The lack of finance is a huge problem. The financial crisis that has hit Greece so hard has also left its mark on the healthcare system. 'For example, we don't have enough infection prevention doctors and nurses to carry out cohort nursing of our patients carrying multiresistant microbes or becoming infected by them. We don't have enough money for it. But the crisis also had an advantage: we used fewer antibiotics to save costs, or often because we didn't have them. Frequently they weren't delivered to us because there was no money to pay for them'.

Tsakris stresses that it is high time to intervene decisively in Greece's current problems with antimicrobial resistance. 'Although things are gradually getting a little better, many people are still too scared to go to a Greek hospital. They refuse to go because they are afraid of becoming infected by a multiresistant bug'. One of the initiatives taken to improve the safety situation in Greek hospitals is training more professionals who are able to implement the proper infection prevention measures. But hospital budgets are low, and this is a handicap. 'Nevertheless we have organised training programmes in Athens and on Crete, where doctors can get a diploma in infection prevention. These courses have been very popular among Greek doctors. So the awareness is there'.

Athanasios Tsakris is a member of the scientific advisory board of EurHealth-1Health. At first sight, this may seem odd. Coming as he does from a country where antibiotics use and antimicrobial resistance are far bigger problems than in almost any other country, what role could he have as an advisor for a project in two northern countries where such issues are far less urgent? 'It is a two-way street. In this project, I have learned how to think outside the box. How to look at infection prevention in a different way—for example, by considering the role of health networks. And how to find ways to implement these ideas on infection prevention in a situation that is culturally and sociologically different. And it's not just about implementing guidelines or other ideas. It's also about how to explain them to people, and convince them that they're useful'.

Tsakris stresses that, even in a very small area such as the Dutch–German border region, there are still considerable differences in the use of antibiotics and the levels of antimicrobial resistance. 'So it is not surprising that there are also differences in this respect between the northern and southern parts of Europe,' he says. 'In southern Europe, the mentality is often that you take an antibiotic for any medical problem you have'. The pressure on doctors is huge. To solve this, we need a cultural change in society. Although there are some barriers, it is still too easy to obtain antibiotics over the counter without a prescription. There is also the problem of overtreatment. As in Spain and Italy, we have an oversupply of GPs and medical specialists in Greece. This creates an oversupply of healthcare, including the use of antibiotics. At the same time we do not have enough infection prevention specialists, and that includes doctors as well as nurses'.

But what can Tsakris teach his colleagues on the EurHealth-1Health project? The Athenian Professor mentions the slow increase in the number of carbapenem-resistant invasive isolates throughout the EU. 'Any knowledge on the measures you can take to deal with these forms of antimicrobial resistance, and what you can do to contain them, is very useful. We in Greece have, unfortunately, a great deal of knowledge of this field. We have developed tests in our lab that not only detect the presence of carbapenemases, but also distinguish their type. That is not only interesting from an epidemiological point of view, but also for infection prevention measures, since it allows us to cohort patients according to the type of carbapenemase that is causing the carbapenem resistance. These tests are used in several countries, but in Greece we lack the money to use them'.

## The New INTERREG Projects in the Dutch–German Border Region

The EurSafety Health-Net project has come to an end in 2015. But EurSafety will continue to exist. A foundation has been established, and the EurSafety brand name has been protected. The new foundation will concentrate on the fight against healthcare-associated infections and antibiotic resistance, in order to promote the quality of healthcare and patients' safety with the aid of the seals of quality already developed. 'In addition to this', says Friedrich, 'we're received adequate funding for two new cross-border INTERREG projects: *health-i-care: Innovations for Safer Healthcare* and *EurHealth-1Health—Euregional Prevention Against Antibiotic Resistance and Infections*. Both projects began on 1 April 2016, and their official public launch took place in November 2016. In these new projects we want to address new questions and challenges, for example the further expansion of the network. And that doesn't just involve hospitals, senior care facilities and nursing homes, but also rehab clinics, rehab hotels and doctors' practices. The network must be further developed, in collaboration with new partners from the healthcare sector, universities and middle-sized enterprises. Another focus is on education. There are far too few people who know how to carry out infection prevention. In the Netherlands we now have a few more than in Germany, but even here there are too few hygiene staff, particularly in senior care facilities and nursing homes. We have to train these together. All of that leads to the development of innovations. Alongside this, we must collaborate with small- and medium-sized enterprises. In a border region there are two markets converging with one another. There are experts in hospitals and other institutions within the network who might become future customers, who can ask questions, and who can create innovations in partnership with companies. Answers to these questions can then be sought in public–private partnerships across borders: national borders, but also—and especially—the borders between private enterprises and public institutions. In this way we can develop good technical solutions, e-health solutions or services, for the questions that people are really concerned about. We can try out these solutions and, if they do not work well, we can simply discard them. In this way, we create a kind of selection pressure on small- and medium-sized enterprises to create the things that people or patients really need. And if these are then used in hospitals during the development phase of this kind of project and launched on the market, you immediately have two markets at your disposal as well: German and Dutch healthcare facilities. We call this the Euregional innovation motor. In healthcare innovation partnerships, the partners from the health and science sectors will generate questions, which companies will then answer in collaboration with their partners from those sectors. We have called this project health-i-care. The innovation partnerships will form a bridge between private enterprises and public institutions.

At the end of November 2017, some of the key figures involved in both EurSafety Health-Net and the new projects health-i-care and EurHealth-1Health published an article explaining the aims of the two new projects in the journal *Umweltmedizin— Hygiene—Arbeitsmedizin.* In the summary of their article, '*Germany—the Netherlands: Health Protection without Borders*', they wrote: 'With the increasing mobility of citizens inside and outside the European Union, the healthcare sector is facing new challenges. Just as with humans, animals and plants, bacteria and other microorganisms also cross frontiers. Thus the organisation of infection prevention should consider this challenge, in order to ensure patient safety. Germans can be hospitalised in the Netherlands just as quickly as Dutch people can become patients in Germany. The Dutch-German border region has been trying to pioneer the process of synchronising important procedures in the healthcare sector for many years. In order to ensure and maintain quality and patient safety in the healthcare sector on both sides of the border, coordinated standards for the prevention of infections should be established by the actors in the healthcare sector across borders between institutions and sectors, or any other borders. This is of utmost importance, owing to the difference in the prevalence of antibiotic-resistant pathogens in both countries. The INTERREG V A projects launched in mid-2016, "EurHealth-1Health— Euregional Prevention against Antibiotic Resistance and Infections" and "health-i-care—Innovations for safer healthcare", both aim at improving networks in the healthcare sector in the Dutch-German border region.[21] Both projects deal with the prevention of infections, in particular those caused by antibiotic-resistant microorganisms. Transcending all borders, including those of science, business and health, both projects have the ultimate aim of improving the health of the population in the Dutch-German Euregion' (Glasner et al. 2017).

The networks along and across the Dutch-German border are essential to understanding and overcoming the differences in the organisation of the health system as a whole, and infection prevention in particular, in both countries. The same applies to the different outcomes for patients. These include, for example the clear difference between MRSA incidence in the Netherlands, where in 2016 1.2% of all invasive *Staphylococcus aureus* isolates tested are MRSA, and Germany, where the figure

---

[21]The INTERREG VA Programme is one of 60 EU funding programmes designed to help overcome the issues arising from the existence of borders. These issues range from access and transport to health and social care services, environmental issues and enterprise development (SEUPB 2020).

was 10.3% (ECDC 2017).[22] The authors in the *Umweltmedizin* article ascribe this difference mainly to the far quicker reaction to the appearance of MRSA in Dutch hospitals than in Germany. In Dutch hospitals a 'search and destroy' policy was implemented. This basically means that all patients potentially at risk of MRSA colonisation (e.g. people who have recently been admitted to a hospital abroad, patients from abroad, pig farmers) are first tested for MRSA, and then kept in isolation. If they are infection-free they are admitted to the hospital as normal. If not, they stay in isolation and are treated there. This 'search and destroy' policy is accompanied by strict antibiotic stewardship. Moreover, hospitals have the necessary human and financial resources to deal with MRSA in this way. These kinds of differences in the way the same problems are tackled on the German and Dutch side of the border are appearing more frequently. The definitions of multiresistant Gram-negative bacteria, for example are different in Germany and the Netherlands. The same applies to the guidelines prescribing how to deal with cases of colonisation or infection of one or more patients by a multidrug-resistant Gram-negative microbe (Müller et al. 2015). Infection prevention specialists and microbiologists from both countries began synchronising these guidelines wherever possible as part of the former cross-border project EurSafety *Health-Net* and its follow-up projects *health-i-care* and *EurHealth-1Health*. This was done as an attempt to halt the further spread of multiresistant Gram-negative bacteria, and to nip any potential outbreaks in the bud. According to the authors of the *Umweltmedizin* article, the cross-border networks provide a perfect platform for interrogating the experiences and results in each country and adopting the best of both. In an ideal scenario this will lead to adjustments in the healthcare systems of both Germany and the Netherlands that will make it easier to cope with patients' increasing cross-border mobility. Particularly in border regions, people cross borders without being all that aware of their existence. Bacteria, multiresistant or otherwise, cross the border along with these people. According to the German and Dutch scientists, this is why cross-border coordination of infection prevention and patient safety cannot be postponed any longer.

The EurHealth-1Health project is designed to achieve cross-border prevention of antimicrobial resistance and healthcare-related infections. In this way it aims to tackle one of the main challenges of healthcare today. It intends to prevent infections by multidrug-resistant organisms and stop the rise of antimicrobial resistance from a 'one health' perspective 'that understands the health of humans and animals as closely related and also influenced by the environment'. Many infectious diseases are communicable from animals to humans. The same is true of multiresistant microbes. The use of antibiotics for humans and animals results in antimicrobials and resistant bacteria being introduced into wastewater and subsequently spreading. The project focuses on the most important (zoonotic) infections and the microbes and infectious diseases that carry the risk of causing the highest societal costs, such as ESBLs, CRE, CRAb (carbapenem-resistant *Acinetobacter baumannii)*, MRSA,

---

[22]By 2019 the MRSA-rate in blood isolates has decreased in Germany to 6.7%, in the Netherlands it hard increased to 1.6% (ECDC 2020).

VRE and Enteroviruses. The zoonotic infections that form the focus of the EurHealth-1Health project include relatively newly discovered ones such as livestock-associated MRSA, which was long regarded as not posing any threat to human health. The mere use of antibiotics for humans and animals leads to the introduction of antibiotics and microbes with antibiotic resistance into the sewerage system and surface water. This makes cooperation across borders between regions and sectors very important. Partners in the project include university hospitals, universities, laboratories for medical microbiology, institutes for public health and an institute for food safety and consumer protection (Eurhealth-1Health 2020).

The health-i-care project aims to achieve innovative solutions for safer healthcare. According to the article 'Germany – the Netherlands: Health Protection without Borders', the Dutch–German border region, with its nine universities and a vast number of small- and medium-sized enterprises (SMEs), is the region with the 'highest concentration of combinations of high-tech and expertise in Europe'. But this alone is not sufficient for business success, since most SMEs fail to find an adequate market for their products. Supply and demand do not yet match one another in the cross-border region—and, according to the authors of the article, this is particularly true for innovations in the prevention and diagnostics of infectious diseases and antibiotic-resistant microbes. Health-i-care is therefore trying to estab-lish a new Euregional market for innovative healthcare-related products. Scientists from the participating universities and university hospitals can cooperate with SMEs in the first phase of research and development. The health-i-care network guarantees access to all the healthcare institutions in the Dutch–German cross-border market.

According to the authors of the article, 'Within the health-i-care network, thirty selected consortia for innovation are developing innovative products, technologies and services in areas such as medical information and training/e-health, diagnostics and prevention, infection prevention, "one health" and medical (e-)technology. Every consortium is composed of an SME plus a university and/or healthcare institution. Moreover the partners within one consortium must come from both sides of the border. The products developed are chosen because there is a need for them. Every 6 months, the progress made by the thirty consortia is discussed by the health-i-care innovation forum, where experts from different backgrounds are invited to discuss the latest professional developments and market trends' (Glasner et al. 2017).

Health-i-care has already achieved some very valuable innovations, says Alex Friedrich. Within the health-i-care project, thirty SMEs are developing products that will facilitate the implementation of improved methods of infection prevention. Some of the project's achievements since it began in April 2016 include developing tests for ESBL and CRE, plus a new serological test for EHEC *E. coli* and a test that makes it possible to differentiate between HUS and atypical HUS, which can be far more dangerous for patients.

The computer model developed by the University Medical Centre Groningen to map patient mobility between hospitals had been converted into a software tool that maps their mobility inside one hospital, and therefore the patient network. 'That makes it possible to find the hubs in your hospital', says Friedrich, 'i.e. the locations in your hospital where there is the greatest risk of spreading infection when you have an outbreak. Sometimes these risks are not what you might expect intuitively. Within health-i-care we democratised this software tool, which until recently had only been available to us at the UMC Groningen'. Some twenty hospitals in various countries now use this software tool and are providing feedback for the producers. Of course, the proof is in the pudding, which means you need an actual outbreak in order to see whether the tool really helps. 'In the spring of 2017 we had an outbreak of two different strains of VRE', says Friedrich. '46 patients were colonised. One strain arrived with a patient from a Dutch hospital. The other came from a German hospital that had forgotten to inform us. So it was only at a later stage that we discovered that this patient was carrying VRE'. Friedrich and his staff tackled the VRE outbreak in the way to which they were accustomed, while at the same time using the newly developed software tool. 'In 80 per cent of cases, both methods led us to the same hospital wards. However the software tool came up with a further 20 per cent of wards to which it saw a link, even though there seemed to be no logical connection in our view'. The next step planned for the project is to map the networks between hospitals. 'But then it is much more difficult to obtain data'.

More highly sophisticated tools are being developed as part of the Health-i-care project. 'My colleague John Rossen is working on a new diagnostic test with a company based in the German town of Münster. The software they use identifies sections of the genome of an outbreak strain. Within three days, they can create a highly specific test solely for this strain. It enables them to screen hundreds of patients in a very short time. And it's cost-effective. Moreover it allows other hospitals in the region to search for this same outbreak strain'.

Both the health-i-care and EurHealth-1Health projects are cooperating with three other INTERREG projects along the Dutch border. The first of these is the i-4-1Health-project on both sides of the Dutch–Belgian border, which has already been mentioned. The second is the MEDUWA-Project, whose aim is to keep water free from residues of human and veterinary medicines and multiresistant microbes (MEDUWA 2018). Twenty seven German and Dutch companies, universities, hospitals and (non-)governmental organisations are taking part in this project, which has a budget of 8.5 million euros over three years. The third project is called Food Protects. This too is a German–Dutch cooperation, and aims to realise sustainable, regional solutions for the production of better-quality foods. The project has a budget of ten million euros over four years (Food Protects 2016).

'Antibiotic resistance and healthcare-associated infections will become topics of even more concern over the next few years', the authors of 'Germany—the Netherlands: Health Protection without Borders' predict. 'Under the increasing influence of migration and demographic changes, the quality of medical care will mainly be measurable by its capacity to protect patients from infections and ensure that unavoidable infections remain treatable. For reasons of pathogenic biology, it is basically not possible to avoid the formation and selection of antibiotic-resistant microorganisms. However, by using a raft of measures—e.g. developing innovative diagnostic procedures, new antibiotics or alternative antimicrobially effective substances—antibiotic-resistant pathogens can be identified, contained and controlled. It is a question of carrying out the necessary on-site measures to protect patients, as far as possible in a regionally coordinated manner, particularly in situations where they are most likely running the risk of developing an infection. This will succeed if, on the one hand, the necessary expertise in preventing, diagnosing and treating infections is available, and on the other hand if a modern, patient-oriented and personalised microbiological diagnostic system is implemented. This requires microbiological and hospital hygiene services that are proactive, organised regionally and in close contact with day-to-day patient care, thus forming part of clinical provision. The German public health service (ÖGD) must develop into a further pillar of antibiotic resistance prevention, that can intervene as a neutral moderator on behalf of players in the regional healthcare system. The link between the ÖGD and the university institutions is of particular importance here, because in this way research can react to the practical needs of the ÖGD in a targeted manner, and the translation of research findings into the practices of public health protection can be guaranteed' (Glasner et al. 2017).

Networks such as those described above may provide the key to this reinforcement of the role of public health organisations in combatting antimicrobial resistance.

## Hospitals Get Their Labs Back

Since the publication of the article in *Umwelt—Hygiene—Arbeitsmedizin* at the end of 2017 considerable progress has been made, says Professor Alex W. Friedrich, head of both the ongoing EurHealth–1Health and health–i–care projects, and the former projects MRSA-net and EurSafety Health–Net. His own hospital, the University Medical Centre Groningen, has signed collaborative agreements with ten German hospitals. 'Two of our medical microbiologists are now working full-time in ten German hospitals in the Dutch-German border region. Every day of the week they go to a different German hospital, where they carry out their work in the way we're used to doing it here in the Netherlands. They start with the intensive care unit, where they give consultations to infection prevention specialists and also train the relevant staff. These ten German hospitals are very satisfied with this approach'.

In the *Klinikum Leer* regional hospital, where Dutch medical microbiologists have been active since March 2015, things have evolved further already. 'In May 2018, *Klinikum Leer* opened a lab for medical microbiology', relates Friedrich (Klinikum Leer 2015, 2019). 'They insourced the lab that had been outsourced many years previously. We make a distinction between classical diagnostics, where time plays a less important role, and diagnostic stewardship. Diagnostic stewardship comprises appropriate diagnostic facilities for the specific type of patients treated in the hospital in question. It focuses on diagnostic stewardship for infection prevention and adequate therapy, and includes rapid detection tests for multidrug-resistant microorganisms, microscopic imaging, blood cultures and resistance determination. Diagnostic stewardship is hospital-specific, quick, and therefore cost-efficient'. Financing has been made independent of productivity. All diagnostics are included in the price for the consultations by the medical microbiologists. 'This is the path we have to follow', says Friedrich. 'From a model that is production-driven to an economic model based on prevention. We stop paying for the water the fire service uses to do its job'.

The changes that *Klinikum Leer* had made to its mode of operation since 2015—with the help of UMC Groningen medical microbiologist Berry Overbeek—were copied by the nine other hospitals that had signed collaborative agreements with the University Medical Centre Groningen. 'Two months after the reopening of the microbiological lab in Leer, the hospitals in Borken and Bocholt also wanted to reopen their labs', recalls Friedrich. 'What we saw, in fact, was the introduction of the Dutch system adapted to German circumstances'. And it is this approach towards tackling antimicrobial resistance that the Dutch government supports, in a letter to parliament written by the new health minister Bruno Bruins—who resigned for health reasons in the mid of the SARS-CoV-2 pandemic in march 2020—at the end of April 2018 (Bruins 2018). 'The government wants us to work in regional networks, to carry out the same approach on the other side of the borders, and to cooperate across borders. That is what we are doing, and it is what Jan Kluijtmans is doing with his INTERREG project in the Dutch-Belgian border region'.

Friedrich explains that it is no longer adequate simply to follow the national guidelines for infection prevention. 'The larger a country is, the more generalised they are. And where they imply increased costs, they tend to become vaguer. That means you can no longer just follow the guidelines. Today you have to do more—especially in border regions. And that's exactly what we're doing. In the EurHealth-1Health project, one of our principal activities is trying to keep our border region free of CRE. Everyone on both sides of the border is participating: hospitals, long-term care facilities, public health authorities, and so on. It's a very clear objective, that's highly relevant and easily measurable'.

## The Tragedy of the Commons

Jochen Mierau is an economist born in the former East Germany. He is a full Professor for Health Economics in the Faculty of Economics and Business at the University of Groningen, and founder and scientific director of the Aletta Jacobs School of Public Health.[23] 'Antibiotic resistance is very interesting from an economic perspective, because it is a classic example of an externality. We are familiar with externalities under various guises—pollution, for instance. We both came here today by car, and while we're driving we don't necessarily take into account the pollution that we're creating by doing so. One of the features these externalities often

---

[23]The School of Public Health is named after Aletta Jacobs, who in 1878 became the first female doctor in the Netherlands. Aletta Jacobs was also an important figure in the feminist movement, which waged a long campaign for the right of women to vote. In 1919, women finally won their voting rights.

possess is that they are not tradable', Mierau explains. 'I cannot buy a protection from your pollution, nor can you buy one from me. So therefore we now have things like the $CO_2$ rights that firms sell and buy from one another. Let's move closer to health matters and consider passive smoking. If I were smoking now, you would be disadvantaged by that because you'd be inhaling the smoke I exhaled. And that disadvantage is a threat to your health. But we can't trade it. You cannot buy from me a situation where I'm not smoking, and I can't buy back from you the impact I have had on you by smoking in your presence. These externalities are very important, because they are one of the reasons why we have market interventions. The major intervention in smoking behaviour was made mainly because of passive smoking. Antimicrobial or antibiotic resistance has the same traits. When I use antibiotics, at that moment I'm mainly thinking of myself. I want to cure the infection I have. What I don't take into account is the fact that every time I use antibiotics, the overall resistance to antibiotics increases a little. And we all do this. But we never take into account the fact that it increases a little bit, a little bit more, and then again another a little bit. And eventually antibiotics lose their effectiveness. But there is no market for this overall concept of resistance, and so we overuse antibiotics. Which should provoke us to implement more regulation'.

This is why Mierau considers antibiotic resistance a very interesting example of an externality. 'At the same time, it is also a classic example of what we call the *tragedy of the commons*. We know that when there are no ownership rights to an object, it's going to be overused. The classic example of a "commons" is a field without an owner. We all send our cattle to graze there, and as a result the field is depleted of grass. If we were to define the ownership of this field, we might have more stewardship over the fact that we need this field both now and in the future. Which brings us to antimicrobial stewardship. As a society, we haven't enshrined the ownership of antibiotic effectiveness or resistance in any way. This is a very important step towards moving forward. We need to pay more attention to the fact that there is a private benefit from antibiotics—using them when you have an infection—and there are costs: the costs of the medicine *per se,* but also the cost in terms of a small reduction of their effectiveness. How do we take that price into consideration at the moment of prescription? In our pollution policy, we now do that by having pollution trading rights. I can buy a unit of $CO_2$ emissions. We can come up with something similar, so that you get a certain quantity of emission rights for resistance, which can be traded. We might think of other ways of dealing with this, but we must be aware of the fact that we have something in common here, which is the effectiveness of the medicine—and every day we use this medicine we also impact on this common, and inflict damage on it. But we don't take these costs into account. It is a classic example of a collision between individual and collective value. We don't consider the impact that we have on each other, and from an economic perspective that makes it very interesting. We know that the existence of externalities can lead to market breakdown. There is no market for antimicrobial resistance—which means that we are going to overuse antibiotics, and they are going to run out. This is an interesting case, because the classic economic theories don't hold here. And of course it is a clear and present public health danger, which we have to solve. I think that the solution is not simply a medical one. Inventing new antibiotics, and eventually perhaps an antibiotic that does not lose its effectiveness—that might happen one day. We could also think of stewardship in terms of the way we use antibiotics—our prescription behaviour, our therapy behaviour. Do we complete our therapies? Are we using the correct dosage? The right targeted antibiotic that only treats the infection, or one with broader applications? Are we overusing, are we underusing? These are all things that are interesting from an economic point of view: the efficient use of limited resources that will run out if we don't stop. There is a certain amount of economic literature on antimicrobial resistance, and the concept of externality is a key topic in it. This is what makes it interesting from an economic perspective. When you think about any other form of medicine, whose effectiveness does not decline or does not depend on how many people use it, it's a different story. But vaccines on the one hand, and antibiotics on the other, share the common property that there is an interrelationship between their effectiveness on a population level and the degree to which they are used. That's why it's interesting to consider these two, because they're slightly different. The literature that considers antimicrobial resistance from an economic perspective focuses on how their usage reduces their effectiveness. If you take this to the extreme, you could say, "We have a resource, and this resource is effectiveness, and this will run out just like any other natural resource you can think of: oil, gas or whatever. So, how are we going to handle this resource so that we have maximum effectiveness for the longest period?" Of course, for the individual doctor, the optimum situation is being able to give antibiotics to the individual patient with an infection that can be treated by them. And the doctor should also do this if the guidelines prescribe it—because we don't want doctors to deviate from the guidelines. But we have to consider the way we structure those guidelines—whether we're paying sufficient attention to the impact doctors' prescription behaviours have on each other. The interesting thing about guideline-based healthcare, such as we have here in the Netherlands, is that the person drawing up the guidelines is obliged to take public health into consideration. Overall, I think that the amount of antibiotics currently prescribed in the Netherlands exceeds what is stipulated by the guidelines'.

Professor Friedrich is an enthusiastic advocate of international cooperation in the field of antibiotic resistance and resistance prevention. He regards borders as irrelevant to healthcare, and seeks ways to create regional healthcare systems that are adapted to the reality on the ground. 'We're now developing *Common Care,* which is actually a healthcare region covering both sides of the border', Friedrich tells me. The University Medical Centre Groningen in the Netherlands, the University Hospital Oldenburg and Leer Hospital in Germany, and the new Ommelander Ziekenhuis in Scheemda in the Netherlands jointly organise some of their treatments. 'At the UMC Groningen, we've recently opened a treatment centre for proton therapy. This doesn't exist in the north of Germany. German patients are coming to us for proton therapy. We have a waiting list for hip replacements. If they want, we send these patients to Oldenburg or Leer for their operation. Afterwards they come back to us, and we discharge them from hospital'. The four hospitals participating in the *Common Care* concept look after the financial aspect. 'So nothing changes for healthcare insurers in Germany or the Netherlands. They just get a bill from one hospital for the entire treatment the patient received'. Friedrich stresses that there is an important and indispensable precondition for an initiative like *Common Care.* 'Patient safety must be equal on both sides of the border. This is an issue we're now starting to address. Patients need this approach. Many people in our regions, including politicians, can see the advantages. We are a site of innovation. It's advantageous to be a border region. At the University of Groningen, we've founded the Aletta Jacobs School of Public Health, headed by Jochen Mierau. There is now a similar institution in Oldenburg. Together, these institutes study and compare the healthcare systems in Germany and the Netherlands. They try to identify lessons that could help us on both sides of the border' (Keep.EU 2020).

Mierau is very enthusiastic about the possibilities offered by both the EurHealth-1Health and the health-i-care projects, as well as those afforded by the mere fact of living and working in a border region. 'As part of our scientific cooperation with the University of Oldenburg', Mierau tells me, 'we're setting up a number of projects, one of which is concerned with antimicrobial resistance. But, antimicrobial resistance apart, this border region provides an interesting case study for understanding all kinds of things. Basically we have here a natural cohort study with a closed experimental set-up, i.e. the border. The healthcare systems on both sides of the border are fundamentally different. The people, however, are pretty much the same in terms of their basic genetic structure or cultural traits. Of course, we can zoom in. But in the bigger picture, I think the northern Netherlands and the north-western part of Germany have a shared history that is longer than the history they share with their respective countries. So this makes it interesting to research things like health, equality and microbial resistance, now that we're trying to move towards prevention-based care and health policies. Because this is not really so much a matter of curing illness as of how we can adjust, change or influence behaviours of individuals with different lifestyles. These individuals are actually quite close to one another in many respects. So it would be interesting to see whether the way we try to foster children's mobility in the Netherlands would be equally effective in Germany. Because in prevention policy we can't do randomised, controlled trials. We have to look for these paired regions, and then implement things in various quantities to better understand why things work. The list of things you can study in a natural laboratory like this is endless. This is the way in which we have to start thinking about regions like ours. They can teach us so much. They are not the ends of Germany and the Netherlands. They are the two halves of a living laboratory from which we can learn many things: how to carry out prevention, how we can think about health and equality, or about antimicrobial resistance. This is certainly possible in many other border regions, but what makes this border region in a certain way unique is the fact that both sides of it are relatively compact—that in the northern Netherlands you have about three million people living there. If you think about it from a knowledge perspective, in my view that is a good size for a healthcare landscape. It is very accessible. You have the UMC Groningen and the University of Groningen as knowledge hubs; there are of couple of polytechnics that provide training; there are two or three top-class clinical hospitals; everybody networks well, and everybody collaborates. Maybe sometimes we emphasise the differences, but in the end we all have the same goal. So this really is a good region to study. And things are more or less the same on the other side of the border, with Oldenburg as the knowledge hub'.

Mierau is convinced of the usefulness and importance of the work carried out by the two health projects in the Dutch–German region. 'Not only can these regions teach us a great deal; at the same time, we must remember that many millions of Europeans live within, say, eighty kilometres of a national border. Furthermore, we have a European directive that says we have the right to enjoy healthcare on the other side of the border. That is very relevant for regions close to the border – because why should we go to Utrecht, almost a two-hour drive away, for certain treatments that we don't have in Groningen? Don't get me wrong here – the University Medical Centre Utrecht has excellent facilities. But why travel so far, when you have excellent healthcare just across the border? For people in Nieuweschans or Delfzijl or Appingedam, people who live practically *on* the border, it really can improve their lives if they can go to a hospital in Germany, especially if they are chronically ill patients who have to go to hospital often. At present, it's still only very few people who are doing this. But if we look forward to what the healthcare landscape will look like in, say, 2030, then in my opinion we should have achieved two things by then. The first is integration of social care and therapeutic care, so that the prevention and therapeutic landscapes become one. And the second is cross-border integration of healthcare systems. People go back and forth for shopping. But they don't do this for healthcare. So if we can achieve this, it will make it clearer to people what the benefit of having good health is. Maybe the language difference will be a problem for some people. Maybe. But let's just see how it goes. People have so many ways of communicating that go beyond language, there are so many interfaces we can think of. And also you can look for differences there, or emphasise the areas in common'.

The Aletta Jacobs School of Public Health at the University of Groningen and the University of Oldenburg have co-founded an institution that has already been mentioned, the Cross-Border Institute of Healthcare Systems and Prevention. The co-operation that takes place within this institute has two main objectives. The institute is planning to study patient flows, the infrastructure of healthcare, and healthcare and welfare policies. A comparative study of this sort between two major healthcare systems should lead to knowledge about best practice. It should also allow to optimise the use of cross-border healthcare. In addition to this, the institute is preparing to work on better use of the healthcare and welfare infrastructures existing on both sides of the border. The institute also aims to become the regional point of contact for the EU cross-border health directive. 'At present you have to contact the offices in The Hague and Bonn for the cross-border health directive', says Mierau. 'That makes no sense. People in those offices are not aware of the situation on the ground in a border region like ours. That simply does not work'.

# References

Berger, P., Rocker, D., Claußen, K., et al. (2016). EurSafety Health-Net: MRSA eradication in nursing homes and home care – A practice report. *Gesundheitswesen, 78*(01), 37–41. https://doi. org/10.1055/s-0035-1548851. Accessed from https://bit.ly/3r5CXp9

Bruins, B. (2018). *Kamerbrief over voortgang aanpak antibioticaresistentie. 132796-175206 PG.* In Dutch. Accessed December 18, 2020, from https://bit.ly/3muQRxx

Cassini, A., Diaz Högberg, L., Plachouras, D., et al. (2018). Attributable deaths and disability-adjusted life-years caused by infections with antibiotic-resistant bacteria in the EU and the European Economic Area in 2015: A population-level modelling analysis. *The Lancet Infectious Diseases, 19*(1), 56–66. https://doi.org/10.1016/S1473-3099(18)30605-4.

Ciccolini, M., Donker, T., Köck, R., et al. (2013). Infection prevention in a connected world: The case for a regional approach. *International Journal of Medical Microbiology, 3030*(6–7), 380–387. https://doi.org/10.1016/j.ijmm.2013.02.003.

De Staat van Volksgezondheid en Zorg. (2020). *Ziekenhuisbedden.* In Dutch. Accessed December 15, 2020, from https://bit.ly/3hVV5xL

EC. (1992). *Council of the European Communities/Commission of the European Communities. Treaty on European Union.* Accessed December 15, 2020, from https://bit.ly/2Wi4Axb

ECCMID. (2018). *IRIS - Infection Risk Scan.* Interview of Ina Willemsen. Accessed December 17, 2020, from https://www.youtube.com/watch?v=w6OsI-GKeMM&t=11s

ECDC (European Centre for Disease Prevention and Control). (2017). *Surveillance of antimicrobial resistance in Europe 2016. Annual Report of the European Antimicrobial Resistance Surveillance Network (EARS-Net).* https://doi.org/10.2900/296939. Accessed December 18, 2020, from https://bit.ly/3nvdWAX

ECDC (European Centre for Disease Prevention and Control). (2020). *Surveillance of antimicrobial resistance in Europe 2019. Annual Report of the European Antimicrobial Resistance Surveillance Network (EARS-Net).* Country summaries. Accessed from https://bit.ly/3nvVIQs

Eikelenboom-Boskamp, A., Haenen, A., Koopmans, R., et al. (2011). EurSafety Health-net: Development of an EURegional infection control quality certificate for nursing homes. *BMC Proceedings, 5*(P164). https://doi.org/10.1186/1753-6561-5-S6-P164.

Eurhealth-1Health. (2020). *Projectpartners.* Accessed December 18, 2020, from https://bit.ly/3ntH5wj

EurSafety Health-net. (2019a). *Qualitätssiegel-Inhaber Krankenhäuser.* In German. Accessed December 16, 2020, from https://bit.ly/2LIRXt5

EurSafety Health-net. (2019b). *Qualitätssiegel-Inhaber Pflegeeinrichtungen.* In German. Accessed December 16, 2020, from https://bit.ly/3oVN6mz

EurSafety Health-net. (2020a). In German. Accessed December 13, 2020, from https://eursafety.eu/aktuelles/

EurSafety Health-net. (2020b). In German. Accessed December 15, 2020, from http://www.mrsa-net.eu/ See tab Projekt.

Food Protects. (2016). *Food Production Technologies.* In German. Accessed December 18, 2020, from https://www.foodprotects.eu/

Friedrich, A. W., Voss, A., Daniels-Haardt, I., et al. (2013). EurSafety Health-net. Grensoverstijgend project voor patientveiligheid in de Nederlandse-Duitse Euregio. *Nederlands Tijdschrift voor Medische Microbiologie, 21*(1), 24–26. Accessed from https://bit.ly/3hVVKiJ

Glasner, C., Rocker, D., Köck, R., et al. (2017). Deutschland – Niederlande: Grenzenloser Schutz der Gesundheit EurHealth-1Health und health-i-care: Grenz- und sektorenüberschreitende Netzwerke zur Infektionsprävention. *Umwelmedizin-Hygiene – Arbeitsmedizin, 22*(6), 313–323 English summary. Accessed from https://bit.ly/34oaGQX

Interreg. (2020). *Vlaanderen-Nederland. I-4-1Health.* In Dutch. Accessed December 16, 2020, from https://bit.ly/3ozdyCI

Jurke, A., Köck, R., Becker, K., et al. (2013). Reduction of the nosocomial meticillin-resistant *Staphylococcus aureus* incidence density by a region-wide search and follow-strategy in forty German hospitals of the EUREGIO, 2009 to 2011. *Eurosurveillance, 18*(36). https://doi.org/10. 2807/1560-7917.ES2013.18.36.20579.

Jurke, A., Daniels-Haardt, I., Silvis, W., et al. (2019). Changing epidemiology of meticillin-resistant *Staphylococcus aureus* in 42 hospitals in the Dutch-German border region, 2012 to 2016: Results of the search-and-follow-policy. *Eurosurveillance, 24*(15), 2–12. https://doi.org/10. 2807/1560-7917.ES.2019.24.15.1800244.

Keep.eu. (2020). *Common care.* Accessed January 9, 2021, from https://bit.ly/3s6LZmp

Klinikum Leer. (2015). *Erfolgreich in der Krankenhaushygiene.* In German. Accessed December 13, 2020, from https://bit.ly/3nAJBRC

Klinikum Leer. (2019). *Zusammenarbeit mit ausgezeichnetem Partner.* Accessed January 9, 2021, from https://bit.ly/3boGGsD

Mayo Clinic. (2020). *Cardiac ablation.* Accessed January 9, 2021, from https://mayocl.in/3ntsZeu

MEDUWA. (2018). *Het Meduwa/Vecht(e) Project.* In Dutch and German. Accessed December 18, 2020, from https://bit.ly/2Xs5xnk

MRSA-net. (2020a). *Definities.* In Dutch. Accessed December 15, 2020, from https://bit.ly/3bn9x0l

MRSA-net. (2020b). *Meestgestelde vragen.* In Dutch. Accessed December 15, 2020, from https://bit.ly/3pXO9CW or in German https://bit.ly/3i5l4D2

Müller, J., Voss, A., Köck, R., et al. (2015). Cross-border comparison of the Dutch and German guidelines on multidrug-resistant Gram-negative microorganisms. *Antimicrobial Resistance and Infection Control, 4*(7). https://doi.org/10.1186/s13756-015-0047-6.

NZa. (2010). *Nederlandse Zorgautoriteit (Dutch Health Authority). Medisch Specialistische Zorg 2010.* In Dutch. Accessed December 15, 2020, from See data on page 9 https://bit.ly/3hVOpzJ

Overdevest, I., Willemsen, I., Rijnsburger, M., et al. (2011). Extended-spectrum β-lactamase genes of *Escherichia coli* in chicken meat and humans, the Netherlands. *Emerging Infectious Diseases, 17*(7), 1216–1222. https://doi.org/10.3201/eid1707.110209.

PNCAR. (2017). *Piano Nazionale di Contrasto dell'Antimicrobico-Resistenza (PNACR) 2017-2020.* In Italian. Accessed December 17, 2020, from https://bit.ly/35GMn1B

Rau, R., Waggeling, H., Altwasser, D., et al. (2014). Untersuchungen auf STI bei Sexarbeiterinnen im Rahmen aufsuchender Arbeit durch den ÖGD 2011/2012. *Epidemiologisches Bulletin,* (9), 75–79. Accessed from https://bit.ly/34fmiph

RIVM. (2020). *Q-koorts.* In Dutch. Accessed December 17, 2020, from https://www.rivm.nl/q-koorts

RKI. (2010). *Robert Koch Institut. Zweiter Fall von Milzbrand bei einem Heroinkonsumenten in Nordrhein-Westfalen.* In German. Accessed December 15, 2020, from https://bit.ly/37mlaSZ

RKI. (2019). *Regionale MRE-Netzwerke.* In German. Accessed December 16, 2020, from https://bit.ly/34jLyLh

Schneeberger, P. M., Wintenberg, C., Van der Hoek, W., et al. (2014). Q fever in the Netherlands – 2007–2010: What we learned from the largest outbreak ever. *Médecine et maladies infectieuses, 44*(8), 339–353. https://doi.org/10.1016/j.medmal.2014.02.006.

SEUPB. (2020). *Special EU Programmes Body.* INTERREG VA Programme Overview. Accessed December 18, 2020, from https://www.seupb.eu/iva-overview

Statista. (2020). *Anzahl der Krankenhäuser in Deutschland in den Jahren 2000 bis 2018.* In German. Accessed December 15, 2020, from https://bit.ly/37kUbak

Tacconelli, E., & Pezzani, M. D. (2018). Public health burden of antimicrobial resistance in Europe. *The Lancet Infectious Diseases, 19*(1), 4–6. https://doi.org/10.1016/S1473-3099(18)30648-0.

Ter Waarbeek, H., Hoebe, C., Freund, H., et al. (2011). Strengthening infectious disease surveillance in a Dutch-German crossborder area using a real-time information exchange system. *Journal of Business Continuity and Emergency Planning, 5*(2), 173–184.

Van Gemert-Pijnen, J. E. W. C. (ed.) (2011). *Eursafety it is your safety: EurSafety Health-net – Euregionaal netwerk voor patiëntveiligheid en bescherming tegen infecties Rapportage over de periode 2009 – 2011.* In Dutch. Accessed December 13, 2020, from https://bit.ly/3gGxQqG

WHONET Greece. (2020, updated every 6 months). *Choose: Cumulative results [select desired period], Klebsiella pneumoniae, blood isolates.* Data available form 1996 until 2020. Accessed November 28, 2020, from http://www.mednet.gr/whonet/

Willemsen, I., & Kluytmans, J. A. J. W. (2016). The infection RIsk scan in clinical practice: Improving infection prevention and antibiotic use through transparency. *Nederlands Tijdschrift voor Geneeskunde, 160,* D518. Accessed from https://bit.ly/3bnashj.

Willemsen, I., & Kluytmans, J. (2018). The infection risk scan (IRIS): Standardization and transparency in infection control and antimicrobial use. *Antimicrobial Resistance and Infection Control, 7,* 38. https://doi.org/10.1186/s13756-018-0319-z.

# A Bottomless Well and Other Solutions    11

*Political leaders organised conference after conference, leading to just as many declarations. For the first time in history, the United Nations addressed the issue of antibiotic resistance in a special meeting during the 2016 General Assembly. With intentions undoubtedly good, these initiatives so far have brought little change. The research and development of antibiotics with a really novel working mechanism has hardly taken off. The new antibiotics on the market are mostly variants of existing ones, so the fear remains that bacteria may become resistant to these antibiotics in a short time. Furthermore, several big pharmaceutical companies have pulled back from the research and development of antibiotics. So, the problem of antibiotic resistance is far from being resolved.*

In many parts of the world, it is now recognised that the battle against antibiotic resistance is an urgent problem. In the second decade of this century, this idea has even begun to gain traction in countries such as India and China. In October 2011, the first global forum on the topic of bacterial infections took place in New Delhi, with 400 participants from 40 countries (Vlieghe 2012). One of the organisers of the conference was Professor Ramanan Laxminarayan. He is an economist, and Director of the Center for Disease Dynamics, Economics & Policy (CDDEP) in Washington, DC and New Delhi. 'The interest and commitment shown both by the Indian participants and the Indian Ministry of Health and Family Welfare lead us to believe that, although their number was small, most people working in this field share these concerns. Organizations such as GARP are necessary because, unfortunately, issues surrounding AMR do not feature on low- and middle-income countries' priority lists' (CDDEP 2020).[1] The CDDEP has set itself the goal of enabling politicians to make better decisions about healthcare with the help of scientific research. Laxminarayan teaches at Princeton University and is Vice Chairman of the Public

---

[1]The Global Antibiotic Resistance Partnership (GARP) is an initiative of the CDDEP. GARP is attempting to establish realistic guidelines for countries with low and low-middle incomes. In 2020, the income in low-income countries amounted to 1036 dollars or less per head of population, and in low middle-income countries between 1036 and 4045 dollars (World Bank 2020).

© The Author(s), under exclusive license to Springer Nature Switzerland AG 2021    261
R. van den Brink, *The End of an Antibiotic Era*,
https://doi.org/10.1007/978-3-030-70723-1_11

Health Foundation of India (PHFI). 'Compared with Europe, little attention is given to issues surrounding AMR. For instance, India does not have a policy on antibiotic use in livestock', says Laxminarayan. 'In human medicine, while some good policies exist, these are seldom updated or well regulated.' Laxminarayan thinks that the negative reporting following the discovery of the NDM-1 carbapenemase had a positive effect.[2] 'In 2010, for example, the government commissioned a working group to develop a national antibiotics guideline. But only one year later, this working group could only look on helplessly as health minister Ghulam Nabi Azad refused to accept the experts' recommendation that the sale of important antibiotics over the counter should be banned. Azad feared that, as a result, a large proportion of the rural population would no longer have access to these medicines' (The Times of India 2011).

The first Global Forum on Bacterial Infections organised by the CDDEP and PHFI in 2011 was followed by a second conference a year later. On 24 August 2012, one day before the second AGM of the Indian Clinical Infectious Diseases Society (CIDS), several Indian medical associations organised the meeting 'A Roadmap to Tackle the Challenge of Antibiotic Resistance' in the south-eastern city of Chennai. Experts from India, the USA, Europe and Oceania took part in the discussions, which centred around reducing the use of antibiotics and combatting antibiotic resistance. There was also some discussion of the necessity of increasing the number of microbiological laboratories in India. The role of medical journals and the public media in disseminating knowledge about antibiotic resistance was discussed, as was the topic of how the sale of antibiotics without prescriptions could be reduced. Professor Herman Goossens from Antwerp was one of the European speakers in Chennai. 'Very hesitantly, something is starting to stir in India', he says. 'But it is extremely difficult to change anything there. The initiatives which, to date, have mainly been launched by the internist Abdul Ghafur, are still very fragile'. However, in Goossens' view, he deserved considerable recognition for successfully organising the conference in Chennai at all (Goossens 2013). After the congress, Ghafur wrote the Chennai Declaration (Ghafur et al. 2013). In 2013, Goossens gave another presentation on the European concept for the control of antibiotic resistance at a congress attended by several thousand Indian doctors. According to Goossens, the Indian healthcare system is entirely geared towards profit. 'On the one hand this makes things difficult, because infection prevention costs money. On the other hand, precisely because of their profit-orientated mentality they have a great fear of resistance, because medical tourism might suffer as a result of it. Perhaps that opens up a few windows of opportunity'.

Ten days after the meeting in Chennai, in a letter to minister Azad, the highest Indian medical authority announced that it would impose sales restrictions on 92 different antibiotics (The Times of India 2012). The new measures were designed to make the sale of antibiotics without prescription impossible. Even before this,

---

[2]Carbapenamases are enzymes that neutralise the effect of carbapenem antibiotics. NDM-1, or New Delhi metallo-beta-lactamase, is one of these.

some antibiotics could only be sold on the presentation of a prescription. Of the 92 medicines, no fewer than 55 were different brands of carbapenems.[3] In neighbouring Pakistan, six different brands of carbapenems are on sale, and in the USA only five. The initiative led to the Indian government passing a law. From 1 March 2014, the sale without a prescription of 24 antibiotics, eleven anti-tuberculosis medicines and eleven other medicines was forbidden (The Times of India 2014).

The problem of sale without prescription, however, is not just confined to India and other developing countries. On 13 November 2014, the WHO regional office in Europe published a research report. Of 53 countries sent questions, 44 replied. In 19 of these European countries, it is legal to sell antibiotics without a prescription. In 12 countries, antibiotics are available on the black market or from veterinarians (WHO Europe 2014).

## In China Too

In China too, awareness of antibiotic resistance and of the use of antibiotics is on the rise. When Dutch health minister Edith Schippers visited China in autumn 2012, this was one of the items on the agenda (Schippers 2012). Paul Huijts, at that time General Director of Public Health at the Dutch health ministry (VWS) and now Secretary-General at the Ministry of Foreign Affairs, accompanied the minister to China. At the beginning of May 2012, he had accompanied her to India as well. 'It is very important to sensitise people to antibiotic resistance and the appropriate use of antibiotics. It is not just the Netherlands that is doing this, but also the EU and the WHO. There's a growing consensus that there's a problem here regarding the use, or abuse, of antibiotics and the development of new antibiotics. In recent years something has started to stir here'. But even if China is now beginning to show an interest in the topic of antibiotic resistance, it actually remains one of the countries where almost any medicine imaginable can be ordered online. Moreover, these medicines are not always of the best quality and often contain too little active ingredient. In the case of antibiotics, not only are they then less effective, but they also aggravate the resistance problem. 'In China, the medicine and pharma industries that supply the active ingredients are vast operations', says Huijts (USCC 2014; SumOfUs 2015). 'A large share of our regular imports come from China and another, not inconsiderable proportion from India. This is also one of the reasons why we are actively involved with these countries. In all kinds of ways, we are trying to help adjust their own quality systems to the same level that we have in Europe. By this means we're trying to ensure that whatever is imported to Europe corresponds to our standards. In addition to this, there's the internet and illegal imports. That's an extremely complicated problem and a challenge for all governments. On the internet

---

[3]There are four different carbapenems: meropenem, imipenem, ertapenem and, newest and most expensive, doripenem.

there's a flourishing market for anything and everything. We rely totally on the quality of the legal imports. The scale of these is still far larger than the import of illegal substances. We want them to fulfil European quality requirements. We therefore exchange information via our inspectors, and carry out joint checks. We try to enable an exchange of ideas, in order to implement a common procedure. It is much more effective to take action early than to track down deliveries that do not fulfil our quality standards in the harbours of Rotterdam'.

## Collaboration

Since 2007, the Chinese Centre for Disease Control (CDC) and the RIVM have been working together. 'The RIVM has made an essential contribution to the development of surveillance expertise in China', says Huijts. 'The RIVM staff worked alongside their Chinese colleagues in the laboratory and exchanged information about techniques and much more. And it's not just the RIVM that's been active in this way in China, but also the WHO'. In autumn 2016, a delegation of researchers from the RIVM returned to China to attend conferences in Beijing and Shanghai. 'The Chinese are very interested in our experience of constructing the EARS net (European Antibiotic Resistance Surveillance Network, RvdB), which collects data on antimicrobial resistance from thirty countries', explains Mariken van der Lubben, one of the RIVM scientists taking part in the cooperation with Chinese counterparts. 'How, for example, do you organise data exchange between so many countries from a technical point of view? It is amazing to see how much the Chinese already know. They have a lot of data at their command'. Van der Lubbens' colleague Tjalling Leenstra does not conceal his enthusiasm for the quality of the Chinese personnel involved in the Sino-Dutch collaboration. 'Their laboratories are highly developed, the level of knowledge is high. We can cooperate on an equal footing. The Chinese are very open to outside ideas. Most of the people we work with have been educated in the United States'. The RIVM helped the Chinese CDC organise a surveillance system for antibiotic resistance. Within a short time, 1400 hospitals began to participate in it. In 2010, there were more than 41,000 hospitals of different categories in China and around 33,000 community health service centres and urban health centres. These last two have often been converted from small urban hospitals (Barber et al. 2014). 'Using the data collected to formulate adequate antibiotic policies will take more time', says Leenstra. 'Just as it did in Europe. It isn't easy to adopt policies in a country as big as China, with all its levels of government'.

The University Medical Centre Groningen is also active in China. Professors Alex Friedrich and Hajo Grundmann organised a workshop on the genetic typing of MRSA strains with the Chinese CDC and set up an exchange programme between students of the universities of Groningen and Beijing.

The Chinese health ministry imposed a number of new requirements, which in 2012 led to the introduction of a management system for antibiotics use in hospitals. For this, minister Chen Zhu had guidelines on antibiotics use in hospitals drawn up and set up three surveillance networks: one for the use of antibiotics, one for the occurrence of antibiotic resistance, and one for responsible handling of medicines. According to Minister Chen Zhu, a survey of 430 hospitals at the end of 2011 already revealed a 'clear improvement in three areas': The control systems in the hospitals were improved. The use of antibiotics inside and outside the hospitals declined, and the doses used were smaller. Preventative use of antibiotics during operations certainly fell, but the use was better targeted. Medicines costs were reduced by 0.5% per year for outpatients and by more than 2% in the inpatient sector.

## Bilateral Agreements

In September 2013, health minister Schippers concluded an agreement with China regarding collaboration in the healthcare field, with particular emphasis on the use of antibiotics and antibiotic resistance. The Chinese are big users of antibiotics, both in livestock farming and in hospitals (Schippers 2013a). Two months later, Schippers concluded a similar agreement with her Russian counterpart in Moscow. A Russo-Dutch commission will develop appropriate plans for a joint course of action to tackle antibiotic resistance (Schippers 2013b). In Geneva at the end of November 2013, Schippers met Margaret Chan, until July 2017 Director-General of the WHO. In their talks, she advocated addressing the topic of antibiotic resistance on five levels (Skipr 2013):

- Infection prevention through improvements in hygiene
- Orderly use of antibiotics
- Joint development of new antibiotics
- Restrictions on the sale of antibiotics without prescription
- Further reduction of the use of antibiotics in the veterinary sector

During a further visit to India at the end of January 2014, minister Schippers also signed an agreement with her host country on developing collaboration in the fight against antibiotic resistance and the use of medicines (Schippers 2014a).

Schippers is not on her own in Europe. German Chancellor Angela Merkel is also devoting a lot of attention to the issue of antibiotic resistance, says Jörg Hermann, Head of the Institute for Hospital Hygiene in Oldenburg.

In October 2015, during the German presidency of the G7, the health ministers of the G7 countries discussed joint measures to tackle antimicrobial resistance. Antibiotics should only be provided on a prescription basis, both in human and in veterinary medicine. Furthermore, the ministers agreed to establish a global network of experts and promote research into new antibiotics (G7 2015). The final report of the German G7 presidency, published in January 2016, also includes a section devoted to antimicrobial resistance (The Federal Government 2016).

The Dutch minister found support in Denmark as well. On 17 January 2014, the *Etiske Råd* (Ethics Council) published a series of recommendations for the Danish government regarding the use of antibiotics. The greatest commotion was caused by the recommendation that doctors should prescribe antibiotics sparingly even when these could help a patient. In the opinion of the Ethics Council, if that were to pose risks for patients, these would have to be accepted. Of course, this gives rise to major ethical questions: in that case, which patients have a right to antibiotic treatment? The Ethics Council also raised the question of how far one should go to prevent an infection by resistant bacteria. What measures are permitted to protect people from carriers of (multi-)resistant bacteria, and for how long? The government should, according to the Ethics Council, do more, both nationally and internationally, to reduce the use of antibiotics and contain antibiotic resistance. The focus should be on compliance with and, if necessary, amendment of the professional guidelines for doctors and veterinary surgeons. First and foremost, the risk of infection by (multi-)resistant bacteria must be reduced by improving general hygiene. The Ethics Council demands that stigmatising, isolating or discriminating against carriers of resistant bacteria should be prevented. Moreover, the Ethics Council wants to secure guarantees from governments that consumers can buy foodstuffs that are produced with fewer antibiotics (The Danish Council of Ethics 2014).

The extent to which the Ethics Council was touching on a sensitive issue here can clearly be seen from the verdict passed on journalists Nils Mulvad and Kjeld Hansen. On 22 May 2014, a Danish court sentenced them to pay fines equivalent to 336 euros each for violating the privacy of several Danish farmers (Investigative Reporting Denmark 2014). On 21 October 2010, Mulvad and Hansen published an article describing how Danish citizens had been colonised by livestock-associated MRSA originating from 12 pig farms, which were named. The strain in question was CC398. They also described the efforts of the health authority, the SST (*Sundhedsstyrelsen*) to keep the facts secret and play down the dangers of livestock-associated MRSA. During the trial, it emerged that four Danes had died from infections with livestock-associated MRSA. Even these deaths were hushed up (Investigative Reporting Denmark 2010). The High Court confirmed the court's sentence, but in January 2016 the Supreme Court ruled in favour of the journalists: they were entitled to publish the names of the MRSA-infected farms (Council of Europe 2017).

The CC398 MRSA strain has meanwhile become widespread in Denmark. In 2009, CC398 was confirmed in 13% of Danish pigs. By the end of 2015, two-thirds of all pig herds in Denmark tested positive for CC398. The number of people colonised by this MRSA strain in Denmark increased from 12 in 2007 to 1173 in 2015. In 39% of all 2973 MRSA cases, the strain involved was CC398 (Statens Serum Institut 2016). In 2019, the total number of MRSA isolates had reached the level of 3657 cases, of which 1163 were CC398 MRSA (32%). Altogether 2233 people contracted an MRSA bacteremia in Denmark in 2019. The total number of new MRSA cases recorded in 2019 was in line with the previous years (which is more than four times the 2008 level (853 cases)). CC398 cases constituted roughly a third of the new MRSA cases, of which 97% belonged to the LA-MRSA (Statens Serum Institut 2020).

## A Huge Leak

It is hard to overestimate the significance of the increasing awareness in China and India that antibiotic resistance is a major problem. Because of the size of their populations, the abuse of antibiotics in these countries has consequences of global proportions. On 3 October 2012, at the close of a conference of ministers in Amsterdam, the former EU Commissioner for Health, David Byrne, summed it up in these words: 'If there's a leak anywhere in the world, that leak affects the whole world'. And if it happens in a country where a fifth or sixth of the world's population live, then you've got a huge leak. At the ministerial conference on rational use of medicines, Dutch health minister Edith Schippers underscored the crucial impor-tance of international cooperation. 'Particularly with antibiotics, it's very important to develop strict international guidelines. We are dealing with a genuinely global problem here. Irresponsible use of antibiotics is not just wasteful but also, and most importantly, it puts people's health at risk. What are we going to do if the available antibiotics become ineffective, and no new ones are developed? I therefore ask all of you to only use the recently developed "last-reserve" antibiotics in cases where there's no other option. This is crucial for our future safety'. Schippers stressed that the problem of antibiotic resistance can only be solved in collaboration with scientists and industry (Government of the Netherlands 2012).

The European Union has already guided us a few steps along the way. On 17 November 2011, the European Commission published an 'Action plan against the rising threats from antimicrobial resistance'. The plan includes 12 measures that equally affect the human and veterinary sectors. The two most important of these are the restriction on the use of antibiotics in livestock production, and the reduction and optimisation of their use in human medicine. The Commission would also like to see heightened prevention and control of infections in healthcare institutions, in order to prevent them from spreading as far as is possible. In addition to this, systematic surveillance of antibiotics use and the emergence of resistance should be introduced. The ease with which antibiotic resistance is spread by people's travelling habits and the transport of goods demands international cooperation. Moreover, stimuli must be provided for the development of new antibiotics or alternative treatments, both for the human and veterinary sectors. This could, for example, be achieved by collabo-ration between governments, industry and business, but also by creating incentives for research and development (EC 2011).

## The Copenhagen Recommendations

The European Commission's action plan is based on earlier initiatives mainly carried out in the Scandinavian countries. In September 1998, Denmark organised the first summit on antibiotics use and resistance. The conference led to the creation of the 'Copenhagen Recommendations', which are still highly topical, and essentially identical to those of the European Commission's 2011 action plan (Rosdahl and Pedersen 1998):

- The European Union and member states must recognise that antimicrobial resistance is a major European and global problem.
- Pharmaceutical companies should be encouraged to develop new antimicrobial agents, but these will not solve the problem in the near future.
- The European Union and member states should set up a European antimicrobial resistance surveillance system.
- The European Union and member states need to collect data on the supply and consumption of antimicrobial agents.
- The European Union and member states should encourage the adoption of a wide range of measures to promote the prudent use of antimicrobial agents.
- The European Union, member states, and national research councils should make coordinated research on antimicrobial resistance a high priority.
- A way should be found to review progress with these recommendations and proposals.

Slovenia, France and the Czech Republic also engaged with the issue of antibiotic resistance during their EU presidencies, following Denmark. In the second half of 2001, the Belgian presidency led to a European recommendation on responsible use of antibiotics in human medicine and the creation of a European network for surveillance of antibiotics use. Professor Herman Goossens made a substantial contribution to this. He is now the coordinator of the 'European Surveillance of Antimicrobial Consumption' (ESAC) project. Goossens is an enthusiastic champion of the EU. 'Why did we begin with the campaign in Belgium in 2000, and why did Frank Vandenbroucke[4] give us money for it? Because he had seen the European figures. He saw that between three and five times as many antibiotics were prescribed in Belgium as in the Netherlands. And why did Kouchner[5] do the same thing two years later? Because he too had seen the figures, and it annoyed him that France was using far more antibiotics than neighbouring countries. That's why I believe that the system in Europe actually functions quite well. Thanks to the approach of the European Commission and the rotating presidency, experts can play a very important role. That works in countries where there's very close cooperation with the government. You can see that in the UK, but now also in France, Sweden, Denmark and the Netherlands. For example, I've invested a lot of time in Belgium. Why aren't

---

[4]Social Democrat Frank Vandenbroucke (1955–) was Minister of Social Affairs and Pensions, Foreign Minister, and Minister of Employment, Teaching and Education. Before and after this he was for many years a senator, member of parliament and councillor. After his political career he became a Minister of State and Professor at the universities of Leuven and Amsterdam. On 1 October 2020, he made an unexpected return in politics. Vandenbroucke was appointed Minster of Health and Social Affairs and also became vice-prime minister. Vandenbroucke is responsible for managing the coronacrisis in Belgium.

[5]Bernard Kouchner was Health Minister in 2001 and 2002. He also held this post in 1988 (State Secretary) and 1992. Kouchner is one of the founders of Médecins Sans Frontières (MSF). From 2007 to 2010, he was Foreign Minister. Since 2015, he is helping Ukraïne to build up a healthcare system.

things going so well in Italy? Because there—and this also applies to other southern European countries such as Greece, Spain and Portugal—the connections between doctors and the pharmaceutical industry are closer than in central and northern Europe. Doctors there are less inclined to collaborate with the government in order to start a campaign aimed at reducing the use of antibiotics—even though the rates of antibiotics use in these countries are the highest. And another group of colleagues is sitting in the laboratory doing their work without really bothering about clinical practice. Now and again they discover a resistance gene and publish papers about it in interesting journals'.

## Special Medicines

On 1 July 2009, Sweden took over the presidency of the European Union. They made antibiotic resistance a priority of their presidency. On 17 September 2009, the 'Innovative Incentives for Effective Antibacterials' conference was held in Stockholm. Experts from science, industry and governments discussed how industry could be encouraged to produce new antibiotics. The attendees came from Europe—above all Scandinavia, the Netherlands and the UK—and the US. 'For several decades new classes of effective antibiotics were regularly being developed', states the document produced at the end of the meeting. 'But in the last 40 years, only two new classes have been launched on the market. The main cause for this is a failure of the market, because less profit is made with antibacterial medicines than with medicines for other indications' (Swedish EU-Presidency 2009). In December 2009, the health minister's council decided to call upon the European Commission to develop an action plan that would promote the development of new antibiotics.[6] 'At this conference in Stockholm, the member states were politically united in their view that something must be done', relates a senior official who was intimately familiar with the negotiations, and who wishes to remain anonymous. 'But a number of countries, including France, wanted to prevent this giving rise to additional costs at any price. Some finance ministers were of the opinion that too much money was being poured into the health sector already. They did not want even more money to pour into this sector as a result of an antibiotics action plan. Headed by France, they wanted this condition to be included in the final declaration of the council meeting at all costs. But demanding a solution for the problem which can manage without extra costs is demanding the unachievable. In the end it was set down in writing in such a way that there was still some scope for additional expenditure'.

---

[6]This is the plan mentioned above that was presented on 17 November 2011.

## Bad Business Model

Antibiotics are developed to be used as little as possible. The less a new effective antibiotic is used, the longer it is before resistance to it develops. For industry, this prospect holds little attraction: years of research that costs hundreds of millions for a medicine which is then only rarely used. And the antibiotic cures the patient's illness after a short course of treatment. That offers far fewer opportunities to make a profit than is the case with medicines for chronic illnesses. Of the 15 biggest pharma companies in the world, only a minority are active in antibiotics research.

'There is actually less research into the development of antibiotics than there was 10 or 20 years ago', explained Paul Miller at the end of June 2010. At the time, Miller was Head of Antibiotics Research at Pfizer.[7] 'But despite extensive research efforts in the industry, the pipeline for new antibiotics is not very full. They generate less profit than many other medicines, and it also takes them much longer. Therefore there aren't really many new molecules being developed. Recently, because of the problems with increasingly multiresistant bacteria—e.g. ESBL—the industry's interest has begun growing again', says Miller.[8] 'As a company you normally work on the assumption that you can sell a medicine anywhere a couple of years after it has been approved. But with antibiotics it's different. In the beginning we only sell very little, because the new antibiotic is a reserve medicine. After a certain time, the resistance to other medicines increases to such an extent that doctors start prescribing the new one. The sales figures for the new medicine then rise. If that happens before the patent expires and generics appear on the market, you can perhaps still earn something. But that's a quite different business model from what you find with other medicines. Not all companies can, or want to wait for their profits'. The relatively low sales price of antibiotics does not offer any extra incentive to boost investment in their development either. 'Antibiotics should be allowed to become more expensive. The importance of antibiotics for society should be reflected in their price'.

The senior European official quoted above shares Miller's opinion. 'The price of antibiotics bears no relation to their importance and effectiveness', he says. 'I think that even pharma businesses are truly concerned, and conscious of their ethical responsibility. They also see that regulatory requirements and the mechanisms of the sector themselves make solutions more difficult. But medicines manufacturers will only continue their research, or start researching again, if they have a clear long-term outlook. We must offer them this, and then they'll assume their responsibilities'.

---

[7]Paul Miller is since 2019 Chief Scientific Officer at Artizan Biosciences after working in similar positions at AstraZeneca and Synlogic.

[8]Extended spectrum beta-lactamases (ESBL) are enzymes produced by bacteria that make them resistant to beta-lactam antibiotics.

## Good Price

John Rex, until the end of 2016 Vice-president and Head of Antimicrobial Research at AstraZeneca, entirely agrees with Miller.[9] 'We're convinced that it's possible to set a good price for antibiotics, and promote responsible handling of them, if their true value is recognised. Then companies can achieve appropriate gains, and will want to become involved in this sector again. Antibiotics provide cures, they save lives, they give you your life back and give you many more productive years of it'.

Rex quotes a few figures from a study by Brad Spellberg et al. that appeared in a supplement of *Clinical Infectious Diseases* in 2008 (IDSA 2008). The research that provided the basis for it was financed by AstraZeneca and other pharma companies. Antibiotics reduce the mortality of pneumonia patients under 30 from 12% to 1%. Amongst 30- to 59-year-old pneumonia patients antibiotics reduce mortality from 32% to 5%, and amongst over 60s there is still a reduction from 62% to 17% (Spellberg et al. 2008). 'And all that is achieved by a short treatment', says Rex. 'It is important to recognise that pharma companies cannot be forced to develop antibiotics. You have to make sure that they want to do it. Innovations should therefore be rewarded, and this should take place as early as possible—for example by applying the same rules to research and development of antibiotics as are used for orphan drugs.[10] Furthermore, we should consider extending patents, providing tax breaks or loans under favourable conditions, and promoting research'. Some of Rex's suggestions are taken from a report that scholars at the London School of Economics produced for the Swedish EU presidency (Mossialos et al. 2010).

According to Rex, if the pharma industry does not develop new antibiotics quickly, the future looks bleak. 'I hope that we'll never have to experience this future, because it's not the sort any of us would wish to live in. Without effective antibiotics you won't be able to get a new hip, look after premature babies, or carry out any cancer treatments. If it gets to the point where our present antibiotics become even less effective than they are now, then we enter a very complex situation. I don't want to experience that'. When I spoke to him in summer 2010, AstraZeneca's leading researcher at the time was not very optimistic. 'In the case of some patients we have so few options left that we have to fall back on old medicines with serious side effects. Nobody wants to be treated with those. In recent years a survey was

---

[9]By the end of 2016, John Rex joined the biotech firm F2G as Chief Medical Officer. He is one of the two Industry-based cofounders of the Innovative Medicines Initiative's New Drugs for Bad Bugs (ND4BB) and member of the US Presidential Advisory Council on Combating Antibiotic-Resistant Bacteria.

[10]Orphan drugs are medicines for rare diseases. Special conditions apply to clinical trials using these drugs, because there are only very few patients worldwide. Randomised and double-blind studies are almost always excluded because potentially effective medicines cannot be withheld from patients.

carried out in the European Union.[11] It was concerned with thousands of deaths per year as a result of multiresistant bacterial infections'. Rex receives approbation from Margaret Chan, Head of the WHO. At the 'Combatting Antimicrobial Resistance' conference that took place in Copenhagen in April 2012, during the Danish EU presidency, she warned the world of a future post-antibiotic era in which modern medicine would disappear, and people would once again die of sore throats or urinary tract infections (Chan 2012).

## Complicated Conditions

In our conversation, Rex named three factors that explained why so few new antibiotics are being developed. 'First, finding something that kills bacteria and doesn't harm humans is very complicated. Only cancer medicines are similar in this respect. If you're trying to find new antibiotics, you look for chemicals with quite specific characteristics. The second factor relates to the legal requirements. With antibiotics, we can't carry out any placebo-controlled studies. It isn't ethical to allow patients with an infection to take part in a study in which they're given a placebo—or a medicine we believe to be ineffective. In this case you have to administer the new medicine and, as alternative, another medicine you also believe to be effective. This leads to a vicious circle: the only patients we can test are patients with bacteria that respond very well to antibiotics. Paradoxically, we can't allow the patients with resistant bacteria—the ones we actually want to test—to take part in one of the usual clinical trials on patients. This is a very big problem, which we have to solve in collaboration with health authorities all over the world. The third factor is of an economic nature. Since patients only use antibiotics for a short period, and antibiotics cure a disease, companies usually make less profit from them than from other medicines. It is very expensive to develop antibiotics. Developing a new medicine takes 10 to 15 years, and can cost up to a billion dollars. The profit that it yields is lower than you think, and perhaps doesn't even cover the costs of development'.

In Oldenburg, Jörg Hermann seems to be not unsympathetic to the arguments put forward by Miller and Rex. 'It's clear that pharma firms aren't interested in producing antibiotics. Today, if you produce a new antibiotic such as linezolid[12] and launch it on the market, then all the experts say: "That's fantastic—but let's not make the old mistake of using it for a whole crowd of patients, otherwise in two or three years

---

[11]It emerged from an ECDC study from 2009 that at least 25,000 people die every year from antibiotic-resistant bacteria. The annual costs caused by antibiotic resistances in the EU are estimated to be at least 1.5 billion euros (ECDC/EMEA 2009). In November 2018, a study published in *The Lancet* provided a new estimate of 33,000 deaths due to infections by antibiotic-resistant bacteria (Cassini et al. 2019).

[12]Linezolid is a synthetic antibiotic from the group of oxazolidinones. It is a reserve medicine for infections caused by vancomycin-resistant bacteria. Linezolid inhibits the protein synthesis of bacteria, which stops them from growing.

we'll have no end of resistance to this medicine". And so it gets locked away. Here at our clinic, the rule is that even head physicians can only prescribe linezolid after they've discussed with me whether it's sensible or not. So we try hard to use as little of this fantastic new antibiotic as possible. Of course, the company has invested millions in order to manufacture this new antibiotic, and they want to sell it. That's why research into antibiotics and manufacture of new antibiotics have become an international public responsibility. This means we must set up funds to which all the countries of the world contribute. We can then offer companies the opportunity to apply for money from the fund in order to develop a new antibiotic. In this way the costs for research and development are borne by the public purse, and the company can develop a new product without any anxieties. If as a result something really successful is produced, which sells well and earns the company a profit, then we can obligate them to pay back a specified percentage of the investment they received—so that the public doesn't have to bear the costs and the company runs away with the proceeds afterwards. But the risk that developments possibly might not work has to be borne by the public purse. We can't leave this to individual firms any more. Even today we see that there are hardly any firms investing in antibiotics development anymore'.

## Stimulating the Market

Karsten Becker was for over 20 years a Professor at the Institute for Medical Microbiology of the University of Münster in Westphalia.[13] He does not consider the end of antibiotics to be an immediate threat. 'We're a long way from understanding the diversity of biological mechanisms that lead to resistance, but we don't know everything about those that overcome resistance or damage microorganisms either. From a scientific or epistemological point of view, I'd basically says that we needn't worry. Certainly there are still a vast number of mechanisms that we haven't yet identified. And there are many that we know already, but haven't yet used. The question is whether we're in a position to keep pace with the development of resistance. And on that point I incline towards pessimism, because we see the pharma industry withdrawing from antibiotics research, at least as far as the big firms are concerned. There's a whole lot of small firms that are still active in this field, but don't have the necessary financial means. Society must decide what it wants. If it wants to promote the development of new antibiotics, then you have to pour money in and create regulations that make it attractive for firms. We're now living in a world where profit is decisive for industry. We—in other words, those who elect our politicians—must exercise pressure. We must demand that the market be regulated in such a way that it pays off to invest money in anti-infectives— whether they be vaccines or antibiotics. And we also need to draw up regulations for

---

[13]Karsten Becker currently works at the Friedrich Loeffler-Institute of Medical Microbiology, University Medicine Greifswald.

other things that have paid off to date—regulations that make them less financially rewarding. And then industry will invest its funds wherever they earn the most profit. That's the way it works everywhere. The market is out there—it's just not so lucrative at the moment. That means it has to be stimulated. If we can spend billions on farming subsidies, then billions could also be spent on research into anti-infectives. It isn't just important to feed people—they also need to be kept healthy'.

According to a report by Transparency Market Research, the size of the antibiotics market in 2019 is expected to be 45 billion US dollars, compared to 43.5 billion in 2012 (CenterWatch 2014). According to a report published in October 2016 by Grand View Research, the antibiotics market may increase to 57 billion US dollars by 2024. The higher prevalence of infectious diseases, especially in the developing world, is expected to contribute to this growth (Grand View 2016).

Paul Huijts agrees with the former top researchers at Pfizer and AstraZeneca even more than Becker. 'New antibiotics are developed just so that they can be kept on the shelf for as long as possible. That's an economic prospect you can't sell to the shareholders. You may find that unethical, but in the real world this kind of argument makes sense'. Huijts favours a pragmatic approach. 'With the current state of the market, you can't blame companies for not developing any antibiotics. A kind of collective problem is gradually developing. We all want something, and there's a need for a collective product. So then you have to look for new ways of ensuring that it happens. And then very soon you wind up with the EU'.

## Swedish Pioneers

The first steps along this new path were already taken in September 2009 in Stockholm, during the 'Innovative Incentives for Effective Antibacterials' conference, referred to previously. Exactly 1 year later, further steps were taken in Uppsala. Scientists, doctors, high-ranking representatives of the pharma industry, delegates from international organisations and senior officials from several dozen countries converged on Sweden. The meeting was organised at the Swedish government's request by the independent international network 'ReAct—Action on Antibiotic Resistance'. The ReAct head office is located at Uppsala University. After three days the experts—totalling nearly 200—presented a declaration. Governments should support the pharma industry financially in the development of new antibiotics. But manufacturing new antibiotics is not enough. Responsible use of the available medicines is at least equally important. The experts did not propose giving the pharma companies hundreds of millions of dollars to finance the search for new antibiotics. The financial support should be comprised of a mix of fiscal measures, research funds and incentive payments for the development of a new medicine. Forms of sales guarantees—governments concluding agreements to buy a new antibiotic—might also play some part. The key message of the plan is that the industry should not be dependent on the sales of antibiotics for the amortisation of their development costs. This would only promote unnecessary use or abuse of antibiotics. Up to now, the industry has been trying to earn money from antibiotics as quickly as possible. Or at least, until resistance to a medicine arises to a major extent—because then the medicine loses its value. This process is accompanied by a quite aggressive marketing campaign for antibiotics, particularly in less developed countries (Cars et al. 2011). A similar model as proposed at the meeting in Uppsala was employed very successfully for the development of new medicines against malaria and HIV.[14]

## Commercial Enterprises

Professor Inge Gyssens, professor at the Radboud University Medical Centre in Nimwegen and emeritus professor at the university in Hasselt in Belgium and specialist for infectious diseases at the Jessa Hospital there, was present in Uppsala. She had already proposed an approach of this kind in 2008, in *Clinical Microbiology and Infection* (Gyssens 2008). 'If you could develop a model that financially rewards industry for developing an expensive antibiotic for the right indications, things would be completely different. But to do this you have to put money on the table, and all stakeholders must agree to collaborate. This topic has to be right at the top of the agenda'. Industry would then see opportunities to earn money from antibiotics again. 'This is the way it works: commercial enterprises decide whether these kinds of medicines should be developed'. Gyssens believes that thinking patterns will have to change. 'Effective antibiotics are a common good. You could compare it with the right to clean water. In exactly the same way, there also needs to be a right to antibiotics. In the past, everyone used to think that environmental pollution was part of our society. Until public opinion changed, and regarded it as no longer acceptable. It's high time that a similar change of mentality occurred with regard to antibiotics. Changes have already started occurring, but the question is whether it's happening fast enough'.

In recent years, a series of new initiatives that help boost sensitivity to antibiotic resistance has been launched. In April 2012, the World Alliance Against Antibiotic Resistance was founded in France. The membership of the WAAAR now includes hundreds of doctors and scientists, and dozens of scientific associations from the human and veterinary medical sectors of several countries. The WAAAR scientific council comprises 80 leading medical specialists from 41 countries. And already the first patients' and consumers' organisations have also joined. The members of WAAAR try to convince the health authorities and politicians in their countries that stricter measures to control antibiotic resistance are urgently needed. Antibiotics should be given a special status that equips them with the relevant regulatory requirements. Governments should facilitate research into new antibiotics. More

---

[14]In Millennium Goal no. 6, it was agreed that the spread of malaria and HIV would be stopped by 2015. One of the outcomes was that two new medicines against malaria could be launched on the market. Thanks to the Stop TB Partnership and the international campaign against tuberculosis, more the 20 million people were cured of tuberculosis worldwide (WHO 2011).

must be done to prevent infection, above all by improving the hand hygiene of doctors and nursing staff, but also through education and training programmes for healthcare staff and the general public (Carlet et al. 2012).

Mid-November 2012, 25 American medical organisations published a joint statement on antibiotic resistance with similar content (CDDEP 2012). On 23 June 2014, the WAAAR published a new appeal for a global initiative aimed at maintaining the provision of effective antibiotics for infected patients (Carlet 2014). The WAAAR's new declaration was published on the eve of 'Joining Forces for Future Health', an international meeting of ministers to discuss antibiotic resistance at the Peace Palace in The Hague. Here, on the 25th and 26th of June 2014, ministers, state secretaries and senior officials from 30 countries met with the leaders of a range of international organisations. In her opening speech on 25 June, Dutch health minister Edith Schippers did not beat about the bush. 'Let us ensure that we do not become the generation of politicians who are made responsible for the fact that we no longer have effective antibiotics', she said. 'In the last century, antibiotics saved the lives of millions of people. They increased our life expectancy by around 20 years. If we lose these precious medicines, the lives of millions of people will be in danger' (Schippers 2014b).

## A Simple Urinary Tract Infection

After her opening speech, Schippers gave the floor to former top model Daphne Deckers, who came to the lectern wearing a short dress and high-heeled shoes, which made her quite an appearance compared to the dark suits most of the distinguished guest were wearing. Deckers now works as a writer, columnist and TV host. She did not offer polite pleasantries but instead came straight to the point. 'Last year, around this time, I started to feel ill', Deckers related. Her doctor diagnosed cystitis and gave her an antibiotic, which she took as prescribed. 'But the pain and the tiredness never left. So after a while I went back to the doctor, got some more antibiotics, and ignored the fact that, even after that, the symptoms never really went away'. Deckers described how she persuaded herself that she was just tired and needed a holiday. After all, she had taken antibiotics. 'This is what we have come to believe: antibiotics are strong, they cure all, and they make you better. Until they don't'. A couple of months after the cystitis had been confirmed, Deckers literally broke down. Immediately after she had hosted a live TV broadcast, her whole body began to tremble. She was hospitalised for 5 days and given an infusion containing yet another antibiotic. But this also turned out to be ineffective. At Christmas 2013, she was hospitalised again. 'And this was the first time the urologist said to me, "Your bacteria [are] multi-drug resistant." She told me that there are eight antibiotics that can be used against E. coli. "But in your case, seven of these eight do not work anymore," the urologist said. So, I'm on number eight now. And it works. So far. But,' said Deckers, 'what will happen if this bacterium learns how to defend itself against number eight?' Deckers' urologist always scheduled her appointments with her at the end of her consultation hours, because everything had to be disinfected afterwards. For the first time, this made Deckers aware that she was not just a patient, but also a potential infection risk for her surroundings—and, therefore, also for her husband and children. 'Thankfully, nobody else around me got sick. But my urologist told me that more and more young children come into the hospital with bacterial infections which turn out to be multi-drug resistant'. Deckers ended her impressive speech with an appeal. 'With the huge amount of antibiotics going around, it is time we start asking ourselves: Are we on the right track here? We should not be defeated by bacteria. But we should definitely not be defeated by our own passive attitude' (Deckers 2014).

For the rest of that conference day, Deckers was constantly approached by people who saw her as an ideal ambassador for the fight against antibiotic resistance. These included for example Margaret Chan, and also the Indonesian health minister Nafsiah Mboi. 'It was very good to hear that here, because it is the story of personal experience, and told by such a beautiful young woman with two children. It touches one's heart. That was an eye-opener, because it gives antibiotic resistance a human face. We must do something! It's still possible now. If no antibiotics work anymore, what then? So: no more words, it's time for action'. The Indonesian minister got to work at once. While she was still at the conference, she went to see the Dutch state secretary for agriculture, Sharon Dijksma. In her speech, she had reported on the drastic reduction of antibiotics use in Dutch livestock farming. 'She asked me whether we could collaborate', recalled Dijksma. 'Whether we could help Indonesia to reduce the use of antibiotics in livestock farming, as we've done here in the Netherlands. Indonesia is a large country with a lot of livestock farming and a high use of antibiotics. I said to her at once: We will help' (Dijksma 2014).

## Action Plans

The concluding statement at the conference in The Hague included a list of priorities for a global WHO action plan. At the very top of the list are reducing the use of antibiotics, developing new medicines, and creating and implementing national and global guidelines and standards for infection prevention. It is also necessary to proceed carefully, so that all countries—including developing countries—can achieve progress in improving antibiotics use and reducing antibiotic resistance. Further key points are: establishing innovative models for the development of new antibiotics (e.g. public–private partnerships); sensitising medical and veterinary professionals and the wider public to the dangers of antibiotic resistance; and carrying out economic analyses of the costs of antibiotic resistance, and the costs and benefits of strategies for responsible use of antibiotics in human medicine and the veterinary sector (Joining Forces for Global Health 2014).

Less than a year later, the Global Action Plan Against Antimicrobial Resistance actually became reality. In May 2015, the 68th World Health Assembly decided on the general outlines of a plan whose aim was 'to ensure, for as long as possible, continuity of successful treatment and prevention of infectious diseases with effective and safe medicines that are quality-assured, used in a responsible way, and accessible to all who need them'. The action plan mentions 'five strategic objectives':

- To improve awareness and understanding of antimicrobial resistance
- To strengthen knowledge through surveillance and research
- To reduce the incidence of infection
- To optimise the use of microbial agents.
- To develop the economic case for sustainable investment that takes into account the needs of all countries, and increase investment in new medicines, diagnostic tools, vaccines and other interventions (WHO 2015).

## The O'Neill Commission

But before the WHO's global action plan was drawn up, the struggle against antibiotic resistance was given an important boost. In 2014, David Cameron, at the time UK prime minister, commissioned the independent 'Review on Antimicrobial Resistance', chaired by macroeconomist Jim O'Neill. Cameron asked the review to study the threat of antimicrobial resistance from a purely economic point of view and recommend solutions. The O'Neill commission published nine reports between December 2014 and May 2016: eight on different aspects of problems related to antimicrobial resistance, and a final report entitled *Tackling drug-resistant infections globally: final report and recommendations*.

This last report summarises the findings of the previous eight studies and proposes a series of measures to be taken (O'Neill 2016). O'Neill's 'Review on Antimicrobial Resistance' has been creating a stir ever since its first publication in December 2014 (O'Neill 2014). Every year 700,000 people die worldwide from the consequences of antimicrobial resistance. Without targeted policies to tackle the problem of antibiotic resistance, the report estimates that by 2050 antimicrobial resistance would cause 10 million deaths every year, more than the annual mortality rate by cancer (WHO 2018a). Most of the deaths would occur in Asia (4.73 million) and Africa (4.15 million), but also in Latin-America (392,000). The mortality figures for Europe (390,000) and North America (317,000) would also be considerable. In Oceania, the number of deaths would be relatively limited (22,000).

'This is truly shocking', writes Jim O'Neill in the foreword to his final report. 'As well as these tragic human costs, AMR also has a very real economic cost, which will continue to grow if resistance is not tackled. The cost in terms of lost global production between now and 2050 would be enormous—100 trillion USD—if we do not take action'. During its work, the O'Neill Commission was confronted with newly emerging problems 'such as the highly disturbing discovery of transferable colistin resistance, reported in late 2015' (O'Neill 2016).

## Criticism

The O'Neill report's predicted figure of ten million deaths annually due to antimicrobial resistance by 2050, if no targeted action is undertaken, has met with severe criticism. In late November 2016 Marieke de Kraker, Andrew Stewardson and Stephen Harbarth published an analysis of the O'Neill report in *PLOS Medicine*, entitled 'Will 10 million people die a year due to antimicrobial resistance by 2050?'. In it, they blame the authors of the document for a lack of scientific scrutiny: 'When estimates of the burden of AMR are provided, they should be accompanied by clear acknowledgement of the associated uncertainties regarding the incidence of infections, the prevalence of resistance, and the attributable mortality'.

De Kraker, Stewardson and Harbarth insist that 'predictions always require assumptions, but modelling future scenarios using unreliable contemporary estimates is of questionable utility'. After detailed criticism of the methods applied in the O'Neill report, the three authors of the *PLOS Medicine* article delineate an approach that would, in their view, be more helpful. 'Clearly, there is a need for more reliable AMR burden estimates, including uncertainty boundaries, and more careful modelling of future scenarios, including sensitivity analyses. The key prerequisite for this is more comprehensive antimicrobial resistance surveillance data, especially for low- and middle-income countries and, in particular, for community-acquired infections. The next step would be to provide AMR-related morbidity and mortality data through these population-based surveillance networks. Demographic data would also enable age- and gender-specific estimates to be made, making detailed results available on which to build the most effective AMR control measures. Until these types of data are available, global AMR burden estimates are not reliable and will not be able to inform meaningful action. As a bare minimum, these estimates should be reported with more transparency and be interpreted with caution' (De Kraker et al. 2016).

The question of the reliability of the O'Neill reports predictions was also raised at a conference on antimicrobial resistance at the UMC Utrecht. Not one of the several hundred microbiologists, infectiologists, infection-prevention nurses or other medical staff present believed that O'Neill's prediction could ever become reality. But a large majority of them considered the report to be 'a useful instrument for positioning antimicrobial resistance high on the global political agenda'.

## 10-Point Plan

Some of the recommendations O'Neill and his colleagues made in their reports were adopted by the various actors. In February 2015, the commission suggested that 'a dramatic boost in surveillance was needed to track resistance, especially in the emerging world'. The British government founded the Fleming Fund and donated 375 million USD to do precisely this in low- and middle-income countries. Similarly, a recommendation that there should be 'more funding to kick-start early research into new antimicrobials and diagnostics' led to both the UK and China contributing 72 million USD each to a new Global Innovation Fund. When compared with the immense costs of doing nothing, writes O'Neill in the foreword of the final report, 'our recommended interventions are extremely good value for money'. But much more remains to be done, concludes the commission, which put forward a 10-point plan to tackle antimicrobial resistance:

- A massive global public awareness campaign, 'so that patients and farmers do not demand, and clinicians and veterinarians do not prescribe, antibiotics when they are not needed, and so that policy makers ensure that policies to tackle AMR are taken forward now'.
- Improvements in hygiene and prevention of the spread of infection. 'Improving hygiene and sanitation was essential in the 19th century to counter infectious diseases. Two centuries later, this is still true and is also crucial to reducing the rise in drug resistance: the less people get infected, the less they need to take medicines such as antibiotics, and the less drug resistance arises'.
- Reduction of the unnecessary use of antimicrobials in agriculture and their dissemination into the environment. O'Neill proposes three steps: 10-year targets to reduce unnecessary antibiotic use in agriculture, restrictions on the use of certain types of antibiotics that are highly critical for human health and, finally, improved transparency on the part of food producers regarding the antibiotics used to raise the meat we eat.
- Improvements in global surveillance of drug resistance and antimicrobial consumption in humans and animals. 'Surveillance is one of the cornerstones of infectious disease management', says the O'Neill report, 'yet has until recently been often ignored and remains under-resourced in the fight against AMR'.
- Promotion of new, rapid diagnostics to reduce the unnecessary use of antibiotics. 'Rapid diagnostics could transform the way we use antimicrobials in humans and animals: reducing unnecessary use, slowing AMR and so making existing drugs last longer'. The O'Neill report calls upon rich countries to impose legislation by 2020 stipulating that 'the prescription of antibiotics will need to be informed by data and testing technology, wherever available and effective in informing the doctor's judgement to prescribe. This will spur investment by giving diagnostics developers the assurance that effective tests will be used. Our proposed Global Innovation Fund for AMR would support early-stage research in this area. In low- and middle-income countries where access and affordability are the main barriers, a diagnostic market stimulus would provide top-up payments when diagnostics are purchased, in a similar way that setting up Gavi, the Vaccine Alliance, in the early 2000s revolutionised global vaccine coverage in what was one of the best returns on investment to support economic development and wellbeing'.
- Promotion of development and use of vaccines and alternatives. Preventing infections is an important method of reducing the use of antimicrobials and thereby the level of antimicrobial resistance. The same is true for the alternatives to antibiotics that are being studied, such as phage therapy. In this field, O'Neill recommends that we 'use existing vaccines and alternatives more widely in

humans and animals; renew impetus for early-stage research; [and] sustain a viable market for vaccines and alternatives'.

- Improvements in the numbers, salaries and prestige of people working with infectious diseases. In the US infectious disease doctors are the lowest paid of the 25 medical fields O'Neill analysed, leading to a lack of candidates to fill vacancies. 'A similar story applies to other professions relevant to tackling AMR, from nurses and pharmacists in hospitals trained to improve stewardship, to microbiologists and other laboratory scientists carrying out surveillance, diagnostic testing and R&D in academia, governments, public sector organisations or companies: focusing on AMR-related specialties is often less rewarding financially and in terms of prestige than other areas of science and medicine. To change this we need an urgent rethink and more funding to improve career paths and rewards in these fields'.

These first seven recommendations aim to reduce the use of antibiotics. Recommendations eight and nine aim 'to increase the number of effective antimicrobial drugs to defeat infections that have become resistant to existing medicines'.

- Establishment of a Global Innovation Fund for early-stage and non-commercial research. O'Neill wants the proposed fund to dispose of 2 billion US dollars over 5 years. 'Exciting progress has already taken place during the lifetime of this Review, including the UK and China's nascent Innovation Fund focused on AMR, improved efforts in the US via the Biomedical Advanced Research and Development Authority (BARDA), and in Europe via the Innovative Medicines Initiative (IMI) and Joint Programming Initiative for AMR (JPI-AMR) programmes. The spirit of the Global Innovation Fund we envisage could be achieved by linking up and increasing the size of these initiatives. It is crucial however that it becomes more than the sum of its parts: funding both early-stage "blue sky" science, and R&D that may not be regarded scientifically as "cutting-edge", and which lacks a commercial imperative, in a way that breaks down barriers to entry and makes funding available in countries and for organisations that would not have had access to funding previously'.
Better incentives to promote investment for new drugs and improving existing ones. The report states very clearly why most pharmaceutical companies are not inclined to develop new antibiotics. 'For antibiotics, the commercial return on R&D investment looks unattractive until widespread resistance has emerged against previous generations of drugs, by which time the new antibiotic may no longer have patent protection or may soon lose it. The total market for antibiotics is relatively large: about 40 billion USD of sales a year, but with only about 4.7 billion USD of this total from sales of patented antibiotics (that is about the same as yearly sales for one top-selling cancer drug). So it is no wonder that firms are not investing in antibiotics despite the pressing medical needs. This will not change until we better align the public health needs with the commercial incentives. Governments must change this at the national level by considering possible adjustments to their purchase and distribution systems for antibiotics, to

find ways to support better rewards for innovation while helping to avoid overuse of a new product. This can be partly achieved through adjustments to national purchasing and distribution systems, to reflect the diversity of health systems around the world. At the same time, for the drugs that are most needed globally and for which global stewardship and global access are important, we need new ways to reward innovation while reducing the link between profit and volume of sales and ensuring that developers provide access and promote stewardship globally. We have proposed a system of market entry rewards of around one billion USD per drug for effective treatments, whether they are based on new or old drugs, that work against resistant pathogens in areas of most urgent need. As an example, tuberculosis, gonorrhoea, so-called "Gram-negative" pathogens and some fungal indications are all recognised to represent a high area of need that is currently ill-served by antimicrobial development. Finally, harmonised regulations and clinical trial networks can play an important role in this area to lower drug development costs'.

## Costs

Finally, the O'Neill Report stresses that none of its recommendations will become reality without the tenth proposal, 'building a global coalition on AMR' through the G20 and UN. 'AMR is not a problem that can be solved by any one country, or even any one region. We live in a connected world where people, animals and food travel, and microbes travel with them. Global action is therefore essential to make meaningful progress over the long-term. We call on the G20 and the UN to focus on this issue in 2016, and to take action on both the supply and demand of antimicrobials, sparking a step-change in the fight against AMR'. O'Neill and his colleagues estimate that 'the cost of taking global action on AMR is up to 40 billion USD over a 10-year period. [. . .] Our costs are modelled on achieving 15 new antibiotics a decade, of which at least four would be breakthrough products targeting the bacterial species of greatest concern. [. . .] So in total, we estimate that the world can avert the worst of AMR by investing three to four billion USD a year to take global action. This is tiny in comparison to the cost of inaction. It is also a very small fraction of what the G20 countries spend on healthcare today: about 0.05 percent'. O'Neill estimates that in case of inaction the costs of AMR will increase to 100 trillion US dollars by 2050. 'Governments can afford to cover the cost of addressing AMR by allocating resources from existing health and economic development budgets: committing funds to AMR now will reduce the amount it costs later when it develops into an even bigger crisis, which will inevitably fall to governments' (O'Neill 2016).

## EU Presidency

During the first 6 months of 2016, the Netherlands held the EU presidency. The Minister of Health, Edith Schippers, chose three priorities for her 6-month term: timely access to affordable medicines for patients, improvements in foodstuffs, and fighting antibiotic resistance (Schippers 2016). Ms. Schippers organised the One Health conference in Amsterdam, where for the first time in history health and agriculture ministers met to discuss how to tackle the problem of antibiotic resistance. In Brussels in June 2016, the Council of Ministers of Health adopted a plan making national One Health action plans mandatory for all EU member states. In addition, an EU network for One Health was established. The European Commission and member states were urged to increase their ambitions regarding the regulation of antibiotics use in veterinary medicine. They were also asked to do more to stimulate European research into the development of new antibiotics and alternatives to antibiotics. Ms. Schippers considered it one of the major achievements of her presidency that the United Nations decided to table a discussion of antibiotic resistance on the General Assembly agenda (Koenders 2016).

The special meeting on antimicrobial resistance during the UN General Assembly, bringing together world leaders on this issue, was in itself unprecedented. Never before had antimicrobial resistance been discussed at this global political level. It was only the fourth time in the history of the UN that a health topic had been discussed during the General Assembly. The other three were concerned with HIV/AIDS, non-communicable diseases and Ebola (UN News 2016). The political declaration agreed on by the UN member states can be considered an important signal to the world that the growing problem of antimicrobial resistance needs to be addressed, but it includes only a few recommendations for concrete action, and these are not necessarily new. Member states are requested to develop national action plans on antimicrobial resistance and to find the money to realise those plans. The Global Action Plan of the World Health Organisation, and its One Health approach, should serve as the model for these national action plans. Member states should 'support a multisectoral One Health approach to address antimicrobial resistance, including through public health-driven capacity-building activities and innovative public-private partnerships and incentives and funding initiatives, together with relevant stakeholders in civil society, industry, small- and medium-sized enterprises, research institutes and academia, to promote access to quality, safe, efficacious and affordable new medicines and vaccines, especially antibiotics, as well as alternative therapies and medicines to treatment with antimicrobials, and other combined therapies, vaccines and diagnostic tests'. Furthermore, member states should 'call upon the World Health Organisation, together with the Food and Agriculture Organisation of the United Nations and the World Organisation for Animal Health, to finalise a global development and stewardship framework, as requested by the World Health Assembly in its resolution 68. Member states should support the development, control, distribution and appropriate use of new antimicrobial medicines, diagnostic tools, vaccines and other interventions, while preserving existing antimicrobial medicines Finally UN-members should promote affordable access to existing and new antimicrobial medicines and diagnostic tools, taking into account the needs of all countries and in line with the global action plan on antimicrobial resistance' (UN 2016).

## Roadmap

During the same UN General Assembly, 13 large pharmaceutical companies published the *Industry Roadmap for Progress on Combatting Antimicrobial Resistance* (IFPMA 2016). The companies belong to a larger group of over 100 pharmaceutical companies who have signed the Davos Declaration on Antimicrobial Resistance since its publication in January 2016 (Davos Declaration 2016). Some of the promises made by the companies in the Declaration include 'to work to reduce the development of antimicrobial resistance', 'to invest in R&D to meet public health needs with new innovative diagnostics and treatments' and 'to improve access to high-quality antibiotics and ensure that new ones are available to all'. In the September 2016 Roadmap, the rather general goals of the Davos Declaration are given a more concrete form. For example, the general support for measures to reduce environmental pollution from antibiotics expressed in the Declaration is translated into four concrete actions in the Roadmap:

- 'Review our own manufacturing and supply chains to assess good practice in controlling releases of antibiotics into the environment.
- Establish a common framework for managing antibiotic discharge, building on existing work such as the Pharmaceutical Supply Chain Initiative (PSCI 2020), and start to apply it across our own manufacturing and supply chain by 2018.
- Work with stakeholders to develop a practical mechanism to transparently demonstrate that our supply chains meet the standards in the framework.
- Work with independent technical experts to establish science-driven, risk-based targets for discharge concentrations for antibiotics, and good practice methods to reduce environmental impact of manufacturing discharges, by 2020'.

Similarly, the companies formulate concrete actions regarding

- Antibiotic stewardship: 'By the end of 2017, [we will] examine our promotional activities to ensure they align with the goal of advancing stewardship and eliminate those that do not, to protect the utility of antibiotics by encouraging their correct use'
- Access to existing and future antibiotics: '[We will] work with international bodies, governments and other stakeholders to identify and address specific access, market sustainability and supply bottlenecks for existing antibiotics, diagnostics and vaccines, and develop innovative financing and procurement mechanisms to resolve them'

- The development of new antibiotics and other antimicrobials: '[We will] engage with stakeholders, including the new GARDP[15] initiative, to facilitate data exchange on old antibiotics to try and fill specific gaps in the global pipeline (DNDi 2016)'.

## Benchmark

On 18 January 2018, the AMR Industry Alliance—comprising the companies involved in the Davos Declaration and the Industry Road Map for Progress on Combatting Antimicrobial resistance—published 'Tracking Progress to Address Antimicrobial Resistance', an initial progress report on their efforts, compiled by the consultancy firm SustainAbility. During 2016, 22 of the companies invested at least two billion dollars in R&D of products related to antimicrobial resistance, e.g. new product classes, 10 antibiotics in late-stage clinical development, 13 clinical bacterial vaccine candidates, 18 diagnostic products, and other preventative therapies. 'Two out of three' of the companies with relevant products on the market had 'strategies, policies or plans in place to improve access to their products' (AMR Industry Alliance 2018). Only days after the publication of this report, another report was published on the same issue. On 23 January 2018, during the World Economic Forum in Davos, Switzerland, the Access to Medicine Foundation published the Antimicrobial Resistance Benchmark 2018. The Foundation, a non-profit organisation, has had 10 years' experience of reporting on the behaviour of pharmaceutical companies regarding the accessibility and affordability of their medicines in low-income countries. This has led to the publication of the biannual *Index of Access to Medicine* (Access to Medicine 2020a). In 2017, the organisation published its first *Access to Vaccines Index* (Access to Medicine 2017), followed by the first *Antimicrobial Resistance Benchmark 2018,* which was itself followed by a 'white paper' on the vulnerable antibiotics supply chain, which leads to 'shortages, stockouts and scarcity' (Acces to Medicine 2018, 2020b).

The *Benchmark* compares the relevant actions taken against antimicrobial resistance by eight large research-based pharmaceutical companies, 10 manufacturers of generic medicine and 12 biopharmaceutical companies with R&D projects for priority pathogens. These 30 companies were chosen because they were the best-performing of those that signed either the Davos Declaration or the Industry Road Map for Progress on Combatting Antimicrobial Resistance. Regarded in that light the results of this analysis are, not surprisingly, rather disappointing. As the Access to Medicine Foundation researchers put it (somewhat mildly) in their conclusions: 'The pharmaceutical companies' actions to address AMR priorities evaluated here only represent a start. Overall, there is more that all the companies in question can do. It is likely that this is also true for other pharmaceutical companies active in antimicrobials, but not analysed by the *Benchmark.* Important products are being

---

[15]Global Antibiotic Research and Development Partnership.

developed, yet they are too few to replace the antimicrobials that are now losing their effectiveness. The pipeline needs to be strengthened more. Once candidates reach the late stages of clinical development, they must be supported by concrete plans to ensure that they will be accessible, yet used responsibly when they reach the market. For products already on the market, the *Benchmark* finds some examples of companies addressing both access and stewardship. All companies should look at how they can expand these practices, particularly for antibiotics that fall into the WHO's "Access", "Watch" and "Reserve" groups. As companies review their strategies for improving access and stewardship, such products must take priority. Governments and other funders must act to ensure the antimicrobial market can offer sufficient commercial incentive to keep pharmaceutical companies active in this space, for example by acting on commitments to develop additional and robust market-shaping mechanisms that support access objectives, stewardship, global supply and quality. Governments and NGOs can forge partnerships with pharmaceutical companies to ensure antimicrobial supplies are sufficient to meet demand, with reliable supply chains, and support pharmaceutical companies in managing the access and stewardship of antimicrobials'.

The 'white paper' on the antibiotics supply chain maintains that shortages of antibiotics used intensively around the world, such as benzathine penicillin, result from the fact that only very few producers of active ingredients for antibiotics are left. Sometimes there is only one. Most of these factories are based in China or India. Almost always, technical incidents at production facilities automatically lead to shortages under such circumstances. But commercial decisions to discontinue production of certain antibiotics also play a part here. As the Access to Medicine Foundation authors write: 'Few pharmaceutical companies are willing or able to invest in rebuilding supply chains. Antibiotics offer slim margins, R&D is risky and expensive, and growth in demand comes mainly from the poorest. [...] Multiple players at critical links in the chain are needed to rebuild a healthy antibiotic market. Success will depend on the development of stronger incentives for pharmaceutical companies to enter and stay in the market'.

The 2020 *Antimicrobial Resistance Benchmark* evaluate the same thirty companies as the first edition did. 'There are signs of improvement since 2018 in how pharmaceutical companies are tackling AMR', write the authors, 'particularly when it comes to stewardship. Examples of good or even best practice can be found in many areas. Nevertheless, the pace of change does not match the scale of the AMR challenge. A few companies deserve recognition for continuing to step up their efforts across multiple areas, yet others have rolled back good practice since 2018 or taken steps to leave the market. In most areas of R&D, the bulk of the activity is carried out by just a few companies. This concentration puts important candidates at risk should more companies withdraw from this space. The Benchmark finds that companies are more likely to take action in response to clear priorities or external incentives, offered by, for example, civil society or public health agencies. Leading generic medicine manufacturers continue to expand beyond their conventional role as major producers, with at least one investing in R&D against priority pathogens. Meanwhile, research grants and other "push" incentives for R&D have stimulated SMEs to become leaders in developing innovative antibacterial and antifungal medicines, but lack of sufficient returns from the market is putting some at risk of bankruptcy'. The findings of the Benchmark on the pipeline of antibacterials and antifungals are not very optimistic. 'The 2020 AMR Benchmark assessed R&D projects that target the bacteria and fungi that pose the biggest threats from AMR. Since 2018, 40 have dropped out of the pipeline and 49 have been added. Of the 138 R&D projects in the pipeline, ten are for 'novel' medicine candidates. Most of the novel clinical stage projects are being developed by SMEs. Overall, Enterobacteriaceae are targeted most, followed by Mycobacterium tuberculosis, Staphylococcus aureus and Pseudomonas aeruginosa'. The Benchmark presents four key findings.

- 'The clinical pipeline of antibiotics for priority infections remains small, but companies have plans for access and stewardship in place for more of them than in 2018. Eight out of 32 key candidate antibiotics (25%) have such plans, up from 2 out of 28 (7%) in 2018. However, such advance planning is so far benefitting only a few diseases.
- Companies are missing opportunities to make antibiotics available, by not seeking to register new antibiotics in countries where the need is greatest and by not widely supplying to low- and middle-income countries older antibiotics that are still clinically useful.
- There is progress in responsible promotional practices that address the overselling of antibiotics. By decoupling bonuses from sales volumes, or not using any sales staff at all, companies mitigate against overselling antibiotics and driving resistance. Ten companies now take such steps. That compares with five companies taking such action in 2018.
- More companies are supporting or running AMR surveillance programmes that track the rise and spread of resistance, and most publish the results. Pfizer has become the first company to share the raw data, publishing it on an open-access AMR online register.' (Acces to Medicine 2020b).

## Best Practice

The idea behind the *Antimicrobial Resistance Benchmark*—and also behind the *Index of Access to Medicine* and the *Access to Vaccines Index*—is to present best practice so as to encourage pharmaceutical companies to follow suit. In 2018 as well as 2020 GlaxoSmithKline was the best-performing large pharmaceutical company, with the biggest pipeline for antibiotics, and with programmes to ensure access to and proper use of new and existing antibiotics. GSK's strategy for amoxicillin/ clavulanic acid (Augmentin)—an off-patent first-line antibiotic also produced by a number of other manufacturers—is one of the examples of best practice described in the 2018 *Benchmark* report. Amoxicillin/clavulanic acid is placed in the 'Access' category of the 2017 WHO List of Essential Medicines (WHO 2020). This means 'that it should be widely available, affordable and quality assured as a first- and second-line treatment for many infectious diseases'. Since its ready availability makes it one of the most widely prescribed drugs. many pathogens such as *Klebsiella spp.* or *Streptococcus pneumoniae* achieve high rates of resistance to it in different countries around the world. This makes antibiotic stewardship as least as important as access to this drug. GSK registered its version of amoxicillin/clavulanic acid in 71 out of 106 low- and middle-income countries where access to the drug is likely to be limited. Prices are decided according to an equitable pricing strategy based on GDP, the burden of disease, and health system financing. Nevertheless, there are quite a few generic versions of amoxicillin/clavulanic acid on the market that cost less than GSK's version. According to the 2018 *Benchmark,* GSK runs stewardship programmes, including continuing medical education programmes and surveillance activities, to encourage the proper use of its drug. In its marketing materials, the company includes information on AMR trends. Moreover, sales staff no longer earn more if they sell more. GSK had already severed the link between sales volumes and sales agents' bonuses in 2013. The Japanese company Shionogi is the only other company investigated in the *Benchmark* that had decoupled the two in this way. Pfizer is starting a pilot scheme in 2018, and Novartis adapted their incentives by decreasing the percentage of the bonuses linked to sales volumes.

## Bedaquiline

Johnson & Johnson does not deploy any sales organisations to market its anti-tuberculosis drug bedaquiline (Sirturo), which after an accelerated procedure was approved by the FDA in 2012. Bedaquiline 'is provided solely through national tuberculosis programmes and therefore does not require any marketing materials'. The bedaquiline case is the second example of best practice described in the 2018 *Benchmark* report. Bedaquiline not only has a new mode of operation but is also the first new drug against tuberculosis in roughly 40 years. Bedaquiline is only available for patients with multiresistant or extensively resistant tuberculosis (MDR-TB or XDR-TB), and only when these patients fulfil the restrictive access conditions formulated in an interim WHO guideline on the use, monitoring and pharmacovigilance of the drug (WHO 2013).

Access to the drug is only provided through national action programmes, and is funded by donations from the StopTB Partnership (StopTB 2020). Johnson & Johnson had registered in 2018 bedaquiline in 23 countries where access is likely to pose problems. The company is also involved in training and education programmes on antimicrobial resistance and the treatment of tuberculosis for healthcare professionals. Furthermore, it runs the DREAM (Drug Resistance Emergence Assessment in MDR-TB) surveillance programme in association with the WHO and National Tuberculosis Programmes.

The third example of best practice given in the *Antimicrobial Resistance Benchmark 2018* is the work of Cipla, an India-based generic manufacturer with a broad antimicrobial portfolio, which 'is distinguished by its outstanding stewardship practices'. Cipla has 25 antimicrobials on the market, of which 23 are on the

WHO 'Emergency' list. The company has a presence in 80 countries, and 43 production facilities worldwide. Its business model is low-cost and high-volume. Once the patents on antibiotics expire, and prices decrease thanks to the appearance of generic versions of these off-patent medicines on the market, access to these drugs increases. 'Yet', says the *Benchmark,* this 'is seemingly at odds with the need to reduce the overuse of antibiotics. Looking ahead, generic manufacturers have a clear responsibility to market their antibiotics appropriately'. Cipla—and the American company Mylan, the best-performing of ten generic manufacturers evaluated—are the only two companies out of these ten that have an equitable pricing strategy based on the per capita GDP of the countries where they sell their products. Cipla is the only generic manufacturer assessed in the *Benchmark* that is involved in multiple stewardship activities, such as the education of healthcare professionals on antibiotic stewardship, the adaptation of packaging to support rational use, and the surveillance of AMR. Cipla performs less well in manufacturing and production and lags behind Mylan in environmental risk management (Access to Medicine 2018).

Although a few companies have been intensifying their efforts since the publication of the 2018 Benchmark, the threat from drug resistance is still not sufficiently impacted, the authors of the most recent *Benchmark* conclude (Access to Medicine 2020b). The progress made in limiting the spread of antimicrobial resistance is the work of only a small group of pharmaceutical companies. Even if it is true that more companies are joining this group—with some promising ideas for dealing with the most resistant pathogens, improving the surveillance of resistant microbes and safeguarding the efficacy of existing antibiotics and antifungals—other major players are leaving the pharmaceutical market of anti-infectives. Increasing the reliance on only a few companies for the supply of these life-saving medicines. In an article published in The Pharmaceutical Journal in August 2020, two researchers of the Access to Medicine Foundation draw the conclusion that the antibiotics market is failing. At the same time, they advance some proposals to solve that problem. 'The need for strict stewardship measures means that high-volume, high-return markets are unlikely to emerge for antibiotics. Pharmaceutical companies therefore have little commercial incentive to commit to the antibiotic market. Our report shows that this is leaving the world precariously reliant on just a handful of pharmaceutical companies to develop and manufacture antibiotics. Pharmaceutical companies need to stay in the game, invest, develop new medicines, make them accessible and ensure they are produced and promoted responsibly. To do this, these companies need commercial market incentives—also called 'push' and 'pull' incentives—to drive antimicrobial R&D that targets diseases predominantly affecting vulnerable populations in resource-limited countries. Push incentives subsidize new antibiotic development, while pull incentives financially support and reward companies (post-market) for successfully bringing in new antibiotics to market. Alongside pharmaceutical companies, there is a critical role for all to prevent and control the spread of resistance. While investing in R&D is key, it is also critical to ensure the appropriate use and disposal of medicines, contribute to surveillance, and to strengthen the policies, programmes and implementation of infection prevention and control measures' (Hellamand and Rafiqi 2020).

Two researchers of the PEW Chartible Trusts came to similar conclusions in an analysis they published in January 2021. 'The Pew Charitable Trusts's analysis of antibiotics in clinical development demonstrates that both the number and diversity of drugs in the pipeline is inadequate. The majority of antibiotics in development today are derived from existing classes of drugs. And while such drugs may offer some clinical improvements in combating resistant pathogens, the truly innovative and novel antibiotics that are needed to overcome resistance must be prioritised' (Lepore and Kim 2021).

Developing an effective and safe antibiotic is scientifically difficult, resource intensive and time-consuming, requiring 10–15 years and costing as much as $1.3 billion. Once successful, companies continue to face challenges even after bringing the drugs to market. In 2019 alone, two small antibiotics companies with newly approved antibiotics—Achaogen and Melinta Therapeutics—filed for bankruptcy. Another company, Tetraphase, was recently acquired for a small fraction of its valuation of only a few years ago (Rex 2020).

'There are several reasons for this. Since antibiotic prices are relatively low and physicians are asked to use new antibiotics sparingly to delay the onset of resistance for as long as possible, sales do not sustain commercialisation. So, companies that create a drug that is important for public health actually lose money. Compare this to oncology, where from 2014 to 2016 drug companies generated more than $8 billion in profits on cancer drugs, antibiotics companies incurred a net loss of $100 million during the same period' (Lepore and Kim 2021).

The authors see some 'promising solutions' to overcome these problems. 'Developments in 2020 offer hope to turn the tide, including a private sector fund to encourage antibiotic innovation, the introduction of legislation in the US Congress to establish government incentives for new antibiotics, and a promising payment pilot in the United Kingdom's National Health Service (NHS)'.

The AMR (antimicrobial resistance) Action Fund is a partnership of more than 20 pharmaceutical companies with the goal of bringing two to four new antibiotics to the market by 2030. The initiative plans to invest more than $1 billion for late-stage clinical development in smaller biotech companies that currently dominate the clinical pipeline. However, its founders recognise that a fundamental market failure cannot be solved by a single cash infusion. Global governments need to change the way antibiotics are valued and reimbursed if they are to create a viable market (AMR Action Fund 2020).

Developing novel antibiotics that treat multidrug resistant pathogens must be the highest priority, but we also need to adjust reimbursement policy to better value new antibiotics that provide incremental improvements. The proposed Developing an Innovative Strategy for Antimicrobial Resistant Microorganisms (DISARM) Act in Congress (DISARM Act 2019) would allow for antibiotics to be reimbursed outside of existing payment structures, paired with strong stewardship provisions designed to help preserve the effectiveness of these drugs by reducing inappropriate use. Removing price as a consideration in a hospital's decision to use new, potentially more expensive antibiotics for patients would enable appropriate patient access to these antibiotics (Lepore and Kim 2021).

## Reservoir of Resistance

Johan Mouton worked as a clinical microbiologist and Professor of Pharmacokinetics and Pharmacodynamics of Antimicrobial Medicines at the Radboud University Medical Centre in Nimwegen. Since December 2013 he also worked for the Erasmus University Medical Centre in Rotterdam as Head of Research and Development in the Department for Medical Microbiology and Infectious Diseases.[16] Mouton led one of the working groups at the conference in Uppsala in 2010. 'One of the speakers in Uppsala warned of regressing to the medicine of the Middle Ages. That's a doomsday scenario. But even now we regularly find ourselves unable to give patients with immunodeficiency optimum treatment anymore, because they are suffering from infections by multiresistant bacteria. This also applies to premature babies and patients who have received a transplant or artificial hip. That's why it's so important to develop new antibiotics, and to do everything we can to preserve the efficacy of the antibiotics we currently have for as long as possible'. Mouton explained that the patients who are difficult to treat are very often patients from nursing homes, for whom intravenous treatment with antibiotics is impossible. 'Then the disease can persist for a very long time. Sometimes it spontaneously heals itself, sometimes not at all'. Mouton's colleague Andreas Voss, who works as a Professor at Radboud, is familiar with this problem. 'Nursing homes are a well-known source of resistant bacteria', he says. 'With urinary infections, it is only when the second or third course of antibiotics has been ineffective that they carry out a culture of the germs. Cultures are regarded as too expensive'. The rate of infection by resistant bacteria in senior care facilities and nursing homes in the Netherlands is around 10%. Half of these are urinary tract infections, often caused by ESBL-producing bacteria. Many residents of senior care facilities and nursing homes are incontinent. 'The quality of the incontinence materials used, and the frequency with which they are changed, play an important role in the formation or prevention of infection', says Voss. 'Often records are well kept and there is a lot of good will, but sometimes incontinence underwear is simply used incorrectly, or for too long. And now ESBL has become a big therapeutic problem in senior care and nursing homes'. If the infections are caused by ESBL-producing bacteria, then the patients can only still be treated using intravenously administered antibiotics. 'For this, the patients must go to hospital', explains Voss. 'That gives rise to extra costs and an additional risk of transferring the resistant bacteria to other patients. We now have teams who can give patients intravenous antibiotics at home. This should also be introduced in senior care and nursing homes'.

---

[16]Professor Johan Mouton (1956) died on 7 July 2019. He played a major role not only in the Dutch microbiology world, but also internationally.

## Lowering the Costs of Trials

Developing an antibiotic takes an average of 15 years, Mouton explained. The lion's share of the costs is incurred during the last 4 years, when clinical trials have to be carried out. In a phase 1 study, the drug is tested on healthy volunteers to see how the medicine behaves in the human body, whether it is toxic and, if so, to what extent. In a phase 2 study, the correct dosage is established. The phase 3 study has to confirm the effectiveness of the drug on large groups of patients. These studies usually take place in various countries and hospitals, and they are expensive. 'This procedure could perhaps be shortened if the relationship between dosage and effectiveness were tested on mice. Then with our present state of knowledge we could predict how it would work on humans, and phases 2 and 3 of the studies on human beings could be combined together. This speeds up the process and makes it more cost-effective, because fewer patients are needed. After that you could grant a company a conditional approval to launch the medicine on the market. Of course this would only be on the condition that the toxicity of the new medicine, and the emergence of resistance, were closely monitored during the first two years'. Ex-Pfizer researcher Paul Miller also stresses the importance of transparent and pragmatic rules for clinical trials. 'Sometimes requirements change when a study is already in progress. The good news is that constructive talks with the authorities are now taking place. The rules for the studies are becoming somewhat more flexible. This is very important for the industry'. The Swedish medical microbiologist Andreas Heddini was one of the organisers of the conference in Uppsala, and at the time was Director of ReAct. 'All over the world doctors are prescribing vast amounts of antibiotics, even when it's totally unnecessary. They often choose broad-spectrum antibiotics, which can best be compared to treatment with a shotgun or barrage fire. If an antibiotic is necessary, they should choose targeted treatment with a narrow-spectrum antibiotic that attacks precisely those bacteria that are causing the disease symptoms. The problem arises because doctors mostly prescribe drugs empirically, i.e. on the basis of their experience. We usually treat what we think the patients have, without investigating whether they actually have it', says Heddini.

## Responsible Use

One of the working groups at the conference in Uppsala drew up proposals for the responsible use of presently available antibiotics. In other words, only when it is necessary according to the guidelines, and only on prescription. And not without prescription through drugstores or pharmacies—which in countries such as Spain and Greece is considered the most natural thing in the world, even though it is actually forbidden by the EU guidelines. Professor Jesús Rodriguez Baño of the Virgen Macarena University Hospital in Seville criticises the medical curriculum at Spanish universities. 'Our education places insufficient emphasis on avoiding the unnecessary use of antibiotics. There's also a lack of awareness of those cases where it is possible to react by waiting. Giving antibiotics immediately is a defensive form of practising our profession. Perhaps the doctors who are active in basic care, in my country and also some others, are under too much pressure. And the patients' expectations of antibiotics are far too high. The general public knows far too little about them. For example, patients often don't know that antibiotics cannot help against viral infections'. The major financial crisis, which has also affected Spain, does not make things any easier. Rodriguez Baño fears further savings measures, as a result of which more microbiological laboratories in hospitals could disappear than have already done so, and that there could be a further reduction of medical and nursing staff in hospitals. He also fears further cuts in the scientific budget[17] and delays in the introduction of better diagnostic techniques, which are important for selecting the right antibiotics. The Spanish professor supports a multidisciplinary approach, ranging from control and restriction of antibiotics use in livestock farming to active surveillance and mandatory reporting of multiresistant microorganisms and improvements to water and foodstuffs safety. In addition to this, he wants antibiotics advice to be introduced in basic medical care, in hospitals and in long-term nursing homes. 'And we need more professional staff, and higher standards for infection prevention'.

## Greek Dramas

Rodriguez Baño's Greek colleague Olympia Zarkotou is a microbiologist at the Tzaneio Hospital in Piraeus. The Greek problem is of a similar nature to that in Spain, but much bigger. And this applies both to the financial crisis and to the resistance problems. 'First of all', says Zarkotou, 'we should concentrate on surveillance, in order to gain a good overview of the situation. In addition, an obligation to report infections by resistant bacteria must be introduced. And we need a uniform, centrally administered approach to surveillance, infection prevention and the treatment of patients with infections caused by multiresistant bacteria'. The Greek figures on multiresistant Klebsiellas are, as mentioned earlier,[18] dramatic.

The good news is that motivation in Greek clinics to tackle the problem is somewhat on the increase. 'Voluntary participation of hospitals in the Action Plan was surprisingly good. 85 per cent of all public hospitals participated, plus the largest military and private hospitals', Flora Kontopidou informed me in an e-mail of July 2014. She is Head of the Office for Antibiotic Resistance at the Hellenic Centre for Disease Control and Prevention (HCDCP). Earlier attempts to do something to counter increasing antibiotic resistance had collapsed owing to a lack of political support. But now the HCDCP was picking up speed. In August 2013 it developed a new strategy for the health ministry, with the emphasis on infection prevention programmes for every hospital. In 2014, this led to a new law obliging hospital administrations to report at regular intervals on the organisation of infection

---

[17] According to Rodriguez Baño, these had already been reduced by a quarter.

[18] See Chap. 7 *The end in sight*.

prevention, the record-keeping systems used, and the results of the measures introduced. 'The most important of these were: compliance with infection control measures (hand hygiene and contact precautions), incidence of blood stream infections (BSIs) due to multidrug-resistant organisms (MDROs) (gram-positive and -negative), antimicrobial resistance, and antibiotic consumption rates', Kontopidou wrote. The commissions for infection control in hospitals have been given more powers. These allow them to decide for themselves how to check the infection prevention measures. They also play an important role in the mandatory training programmes that the HCDCP organises for staff in hospitals. In addition to this, an antibiotics advice service has been introduced in all hospitals. On account of the extensive spread of highly resistant bacteria in Greek hospitals, Zarkotou supports a policy similar to that practised in the Netherlands towards MRSA. At her own hospital, she tests patients in risk groups on admission to find out whether they are carrying multiresistant Klebsiellas. In practice, this means that all patients coming from nursing homes, other Greek hospitals or foreign countries are tested. This has led to a decrease in infections by Klebsiellas.

## Different Consequences

Professor Ramanan Laxminarayan of the Global Antibiotic Resistance Partnership also stresses how important responsible use of antibiotics is.[19] But the problems with this responsible use have completely different consequences in poor countries from those they have in, for example, Greece or Italy. According to Laxminarayan, excessive use of antibiotics is taking place in hospitals as a result of incorrect and irrational dosages of medicine and excessively frequent prescriptions, and because of incorrect lengths of treatment. Laxminarayan is of the opinion that various measures are necessary to restrict the free sale of antibiotics, above all those of the latest generation. These include compiling a list of the most important medicines, information campaigns for the general public, increased use of diagnostic tests before an antibiotic is prescribed, and setting up the appropriate infrastructure required for this in hospitals. He also regards the education of pharmacists as equally important, so that they can ensure that first-line antibiotics are used correctly and that new generation antibiotics are not handed out without prescription. 'Lack of access to antibiotics', says Laxminarayan. 'is indicative of a greater problem: the lack of access to affordable healthcare facilities. Socio-economic factors and distance from the nearest healthcare facility, in addition to the availability of medical practitioners, limit patients in seeking the help they require'. Laxminarayan also has a couple of suggestions. 'A decrease in out-of-pocket expenditures—in India, 80% is out-of-pocket and 20% is government. Ensure pharmacies are fully stocked with the drugs

---

[19]Laxminarayan is a health economist and an outstanding specialist in this field. He is intensively involved in interdisciplinary research into improper and excessive use of antibiotics.

from the essential drug list (WHO 2020). Subsidise medication to make it affordable'.

For the Director of GARP, affordability of antibiotics and other medicines, and therefore access to medical care, is a key issue. 'This is evident from the millions of children dying every year from pneumonia. In hospitals all around the world, and in some communities too, there are problems both of overuse and of resistance. Although having to deal with resistance may seem to be a luxury, when so many don't have access to antibiotics, this is not exactly correct. Unless we take action against resistance, we will lose these drugs without having had the opportunity to treat the millions of patients who need them. Moreover the poor are the first to suffer from resistance, since they are least able to afford expensive second-line drugs'.

Although the Netherlands has an excellent reputation and record on the moderate use of antibiotics, they are handled incorrectly there as well. Ina Willemsen, expert on infection prevention at the Amphia Hospital in Breda, earned her doctorate from VU University Medical Centre with an investigation into improving antibiotics use, carried out in 18 hospitals. She discovered that almost 5% of all patients in Dutch hospitals received antibiotics without any justification. In the worst-ranking hospital, the figure was as high as 30%. In hospitals that use antibiotics more responsibly, there are fewer resistant bacteria. Willemsen was also able to prove that training, clear guidelines and a restrained antibiotics policy influence antibiotics use and the development of resistance (Willemsen 2010).

## Increase Availability of Antimicrobials

The European Commission used the results of the 2010 Uppsala conference to form an important component of its November 2011 action plan for combatting antibiotic resistance. TATFAR, the Euro-American Transatlantic Task Force on Antimicrobial Resistance founded in 2009, also adopted the proposals. In 2011, TATFAR published 17 recommendations (TATFAR 2011). One of their most interesting suggestions concerned simplifying market approval of new antibiotics. This could be achieved by harmonising the relevant American and European regulations for clinical trials. In this way, a single research programme could provide access to both the European and American markets. The European Federation of Pharmaceutical Industries and Associations (EFPIA) is an important partner for the European Commission in implementing its 'Action plan against the rising threats from antimicrobial resistance', presented in Brussels on 17 November 2011 (EC 2011).

On 29 June 2017, the European Commission published an updated version of its 2011 action plan, a 'European One Health Action Plan against Antimicrobial Resistance' (AMR) (EC 2017a, b). The new action plan largely builds on the initial plan for the period 2011–16. According to the European Commission, 'the new action plan sets out a comprehensive framework for more extensive action to reduce the emergence and spread of AMR and to increase the development and availability of new effective antimicrobials inside and outside the EU. It focuses on activities with a clear EU added value and, where possible, on measurable and concrete outcomes. Whilst ensuring the continuation of EU actions that are still needed, the new action plan will enhance its support to help EU countries deliver innovative, effective and sustainable responses to AMR. For example, it aims to scale up collaboration and surveillance efforts to reduce data gaps and to create more synergies and coherence between different policies according to the One Health approach' (EC 2017a, b).

## Inadequate Market

Richard Bergström, up to September 2016 Director of the EFPIA, who was previously with the Swedish pharma industry association LIF, was one of the speakers when the first plan was presented on 17 November 2011. 'To say that there are only a few medicines in the pipeline is accurate', Bergström said. 'The problem for us was that the market was not functioning adequately. Commercially speaking, it was no longer attractive to develop antibiotics. The solution is complicated, but part of that solution can be seen in the European Commission's plans'. Bergström explained that better chances of market approval would of course reduce business risks considerably. In addition, he announced a special initiative. 'There are large numbers of bacteria that are resistant', he said. 'Individual companies can't do much about this. In the initial phase of research projects—and therefore long before a medicine might possibly enter the market—we must pool our knowledge. We must share our research findings and develop joint projects, and we must also carry out the phase 2 and phase 3 studies together.[20] In this way we can also share the common risks. If the European Commission co-finances our research, then the general public must also share any potential revenues. We must ensure that a new pipeline is constructed and that it's kept filled for decades—because bacteria will also continue to develop resistance'. This model of bringing together the various pharma companies' expertise and infrastructure in order to develop new antibiotics is the idea of EFPIA President Sir Andrew Witty, the 'big boss' of GlaxoSmithKline (The Guardian 2016).[21]

During a lecture organised by the EFPIA, Bergström spoke out again. 'The pipeline is almost empty and that has led us, just a few weeks ago, to launch a new public-private partnership in conjunction with the European Commission, where we will collaborate in *a way you have never seen before*. Companies would pool everything they have, receive co-funding for clinical trials, and so on. There would probably be more areas where there is not enough research going on because the private sector has left them'. According to Bergström, the pharma companies' crisis 'is that we pay too much per molecule; that is what the investors say. Divide

---

[20]In a phase 2 study, tests are carried out to see whether a medicine is effective and what dose is required. In a phase 3 study the effectiveness of a new medicine on patients is compared with an existing standard treatment or placebo. Phase 4 studies are not carried out until after a medicine is approved, in order to investigate the safety and effectiveness of a medicine in large patient groups.

[21]Andrew Witty retired from his post as CEO of GSK on 1 March 2017. His successor is Emma Walmsley, until then head of Glaxo's consumer health division.

€100 billion in research spent by the number of molecules and you can work out for yourself that it is too expensive per capita' (Bergström 2011). At the end of January 2014 the *Wall Street Journal* reported that, for the first time in years, pharma companies had started to look for new antibiotics again. Only to a limited extent—but at least they had started. The state support that comes from both the US government and the European Union seems to play an important role here (The Wall Street Journal 2014).

'The exchange of knowledge is very important', says Michel Dutrée of Nefarma.[22] 'Even for developing antibiotics that have a quite different working mechanism—for example, a mechanism that ensures that a bacterium which changes when it absorbs a resistance mechanism automatically self-destructs. One could also envisage developing bacteriophages—i.e. viruses that kill bacteria.[23] The problem with this is that you never know how a virus will mutate, and therefore you also don't know whether you can keep the virus under control'.

## Joint Development

Jacques Scheres is a Professor of Genetics and has already been interested in phages for years. 'The first living creatures all appeared in the sea. Then there was a period of more than two billion years during which bacteria and viruses that attacked bacteria—i.e. phages—developed alongside one another in the sea, and deployed every possible mechanism of reciprocal attack or defence. These processes are still going on. A large part of our genome is based on bacterial principles. We have simply brought these along with us in the course of our evolution from one-cell to multiple-cell organisms. For example, if we take a closer look at mitochondria,[24] we find that these are probably bacteria that were adopted by one-cell organisms to regulate their energy balance. A kind of symbiosis arose, and as a result these bacteria were incorporated. There is not one single organism with which we humans have lived through our development more closely than with bacteria. Every one of us has between one and a half and two kilos of benign bacteria inside their body, and we need them. Without them we'd die. Before there was life on land, there was only life in the oceans. Every millilitre of sea water contains a million bacteria and ten million phages. Most of the bacteria you find in the sea—around 60–70 per cent—are infected with bacteriophages. That's a kind of biological balancing mechanism. The bacteria are killed by a bacteriophage. This phage penetrates the bacterium's body like a virus and alters its metabolism in such a way that, from this point on, the bacterium produces only phages. After about 20 min the bacterium explodes and releases a couple of hundred phages. Each of these can infect a new bacterium again, and so it goes on'.

---

[22]Since 2016 known as Association Innovative Medicines. Mr. Dutrée left the organisation on 1 August 2015.

[23]This has been going on for many years in Georgia, for example.

[24]Mitochondria function as power stations in the cells.

## Phage Therapies

Bacteriophage therapies for infections were introduced after the First World War. In those days there were still no antibiotics. 'These phage therapies were used to combat typhus and cholera epidemics', explains Scheres. 'Back then there was a dysentery epidemic in India. The specialists who advocated phage therapy carried out an experiment. In one village all the children were administered phages for prophylaxis and treatment, and in another village they were not. In the villages where the phages were used, the epidemic was very quickly over (Fruciano and Bourne 2007). Over the course of time bacteria become resistant to the phages, but the phages in turn immediately make themselves virulent for the bacteria again'.

Félix d'Hérelle, a French-Canadian microbiologist, was one of the discoverers of bacteriophages in 1917. He worked at the Institut Pasteur in Paris, where he taught students that came to him from all over the world (Sulakvelidze et al. 2001). The work of D'Hérelle was internationally recognised. In 1924, he received an honorary doctorate of the Leiden University in the Netherlands and, more important, was awarded the Leeuwenhoek Medal, a reward that the Royal Netherlands Academy of Arts and Sciences (KNAW) only grants every 10 years to the scientist that is considered to have made the most significant contribution to microbiology during the preceding 10 years. D'Hérelle shares this honour with Louis Pasteur who got the first Leeuwenhoek Medal in 1895. Many countries sent their best microbiologists to d'Hérelle, so that they could learn from him how bacteriophages could be used to combat infections. One of these students was the Georgian microbiologist Georgyi Eliava. After a while, he returned to Tbilisi convinced that phages had medical applications, and some years later he founded an institute there—now the Eliava Institute for Bacteriophages, Microbiology and Virology. Furious that the Institut Pasteur had refused to give him more funds for his increasingly expanding research and education activities, in 1933 d'Hérelle moved to Tbilisi at Stalin's invitation and collaborated with his former student there. In 1937, in the period of Stalin's terror, Eliava was arrested and executed as an 'enemy of the people'. Anecdotical sources give different explanations for the tragic execution of Eliava. Some say the mere fact he was an intellectual was sufficient reason for his execution. Others pretend that the real reason for Eliava's execution is the fact that he fell in love with a woman desired by Lavrenti Beria, the head of Stalin's feared secret service NKVD, the predecessor of the KGB. D'Hérelle decided shortly after the killing of Eliava to return to France where he died in 1949.

## The Cold War

'Not long after that the Second World War broke out', relates Jacques Scheres. 'The West had already discovered antibiotics and started producing them. A split then developed between East and West, and bacteriophage therapy continued to be used in Eastern Europe. During the war following the Russian invasion of Afghanistan too, the Russian soldiers were treated with phages (Encyclopeadia Brittanica (2020).

The ostbloc was primarily a military block. Everything related to healthcare and research was under military control. This also explains why only one hospital in the West—the Queen Astrid Military Hospital in Brussels—carried out research into the use of phages in infection control. This hospital could talk to the Russians about phage research via its military contacts'.

Scheres continues: 'Phages cannot be administered to human beings as a medicine against infection without further ado. Clinical trials to determine the safety of the phages have to be carried out first. For example, in 2011 two phages that killed EHEC O104 were identified within a week. But it was not possible to treat any patients with them, because studies first had to be carried out to investigate whether the phages were safe for humans. Those who support the use of phages are now collectively attempting to draw up criteria for their safe use. They have documented which safety criteria are used, and are now trying to create uniform rules. The problem is that existing regulations are entirely adapted to the markets, patents and safety of medicines that are manufactured from chemical substances. A biological system, such as that represented by bacteriophages, does not fit this structure at all, even though it is much more efficient from an evolutionary point of view. I do not think we can afford to ignore this system, which was already effective before antibiotics existed. It is by no means as well researched and documented as we would wish. Most of the available material was published in Russian, and in Russia, there are fewer regulatory requirements than here. But that must not stop us considering which aspects of this we could use. In the European Commission's five-year plan to combat antibiotic resistance, research has an important place. Among the projects carried out so far, there is one on bacteriophage therapy carried out by the Queen Astrid Hospital in Brussels along with one French and one Swiss partner'. Scheres stresses that the 2–3 billion years of common evolution of bacteria and bacteriophages are extremely interesting. 'They're a goldmine. There are so many mechanisms to kill bacteria that we can investigate. No-one knows how to kill bacteria better than a bacteriophage'.

The Dutch company Micreos is carrying out research projects on controlling MRSA infections with phages. The company has developed a lotion for skin diseases that is already available. At a London conference in November 2014, Micreos presented its research findings on 'Staphefekt' as a new medicine against *S. aureus* infections, MSSA and MRSA. Five out of six patients had positive things to say about Staphefekt (The Washington Post 2014). Two reports were published, describing seven and two patients, respectively. The authors concluded that their positive results could provide a stimulus to carry out placebo-controlled clinical trials. Micreos' medicine works on the basis of the enzyme endolysin. Phages use endolysins to release themselves from the bacteria in which they are multiplying. Staphefekt contains specially manufactured endolysins that specifically target *Staphylococcus aureus*. Here endolysins appear to be much less affected by resistance development than antibiotics (Herpers et al. 2014). The company is now trying to develop similar products that are effective against other (multi)resistant bacteria. Since the introduction of Staphefekt Micreos developed food safety products based on bacteriophages against Salmonella (3M Science 2020), Listeria monocytogenes

(Reinhard et al. 2020) and the EHEC and HUS causing E. coli O157:H7[25] (Shebs et al. 2020), all three approved by the FDA.

## Media Attention

In autumn 2017, phage therapy somewhat suddenly received a great deal of attention in the non-specialist Dutch press. Several programmes aired on national television showed examples of patients who travelled all the way to the former Soviet republic of Georgia to undergo (apparently successful) phage therapy to treat chronic infections of wounds or the urinary tract. Doctors in the Netherlands had been unsuccessful in treating these infections with antibiotics owing to antimicrobial resistance. Dutch doctors are reluctant to use bacteriophages to treat infections caused by multiresistant microbes. They stress that very little is known about the safety or effectiveness of these medicines. The vast majority of the limited corpus of scientific articles on bacteriophages are in Russian or Georgian, and therefore difficult to access. Marc Bonten, Professor of Molecular Epidemiology at the UMC Utrecht, confirms the scepticism about bacteriophages that predominates in the Dutch medical world. 'A cocktail of specific bacteriophages may be an effective treatment against a certain number of subtypes of microbes that cause infections', he explains. 'But we don't know whether we have to put three or, for example, seven active phages in such a cocktail. Nor do we know when to check which strains are resistant to the phages. Or what the next cocktail of phages that you have to give the patient should be'.

## Obstacles for a Study

Bonten—who received oral requests and e-mails for bacteriophage therapy from patients every week—also announces that scientific research into the effectiveness of bacteriophage therapy is beginning. Early in 2018, Bonten's department began planning a clinical trial of bacteriophages, after the Netherlands health minister was questioned in parliament about Dutch reluctance to embrace phage therapy. At the time of writing the last lines of this book, early April 2021, it was still far from certain whether Bonten and his collaborators would receive permission for the clinical trials. 'Bacteriophages are not recognised medicines, so we cannot prescribe them without special permission'. Bonten hopes to be able to import the required bacteriophages from the pharmacy at the Queen Astrid Hospital in Brussels. 'They prepare phage-cocktails for patients there', he says. Even if he feels that bacteriophages may be of some use in treating infections caused by multiresistant microbes, Bonten stresses that they are not going to be a miracle cure for all the problems posed by antimicrobial resistance. The UMC Utrecht decided to organise a

---

[25] See Chap. 9 *The role of microbiology.*

conference on phage therapy late in February 2018, where some of the leading international specialists were invited to speak about the current state of phage therapy. At the Technical University of Delft, Stan Brouns is already carrying out a research project on the working mechanism of bacteriophages, and their possible role as an alternative to antibiotics. Brouns received funding in February 2019 to set up a phage bank in the Netherlands that opened its doors 2 months later. Brouns and his colleagues are looking for Dutch and foreign partners to introduce phage therapy as an alternative way to treat infections caused by (multi-)resistant microbes. A molecular biologist and one of the speakers at the Utrecht conference, Mr. Brouns also appeared in one of the TV programmes broadcast in autumn 2017. His appearance provoked responses from a number of patients looking for a cure for infections that were hard to treat.

These TV programmes led not only to parliamentary questions but also to a ministerial directive to the national health institute, the RIVM, to carry out a study of the current state of knowledge on the use of bacteriophages. In the report summarising their findings, published at the end of May 2018, the researchers wrote: 'Phages have a different mode of action compared to antibiotics. In theory, this should allow them to be used to treat infections that are resistant to antibiotics. However, the current scientific evidence is insufficient to determine the value of phage treatment, or to be able to use phages safely and for different types of infections. This is the outcome of a literature study carried out by the RIVM on the current scientific evidence for treatment of human infections with bacteriophages. A phage is very specifically targeted at one type of bacterium, while antibiotics are effective against multiple species of bacteria. This prohibits the use of phages for the treatment of acute infections: the causative bacterium has to be identified first, before (a) matching phage(s) can be found. Because of these practical concerns, antibiotics became more successful, and phages fell out of favour. Understanding of the precise mode of action of bacteriophages when treating infections—how they act in the human body, optimal dosage, length of treatment and risks of use—is still limited. Phages are not suitable for the treatment of acute infections because they are time-consuming and complex. In theory, phages should be useful for the treatment of chronic infections, such as superficial skin infections. More clinical research is needed to answer these questions. Aside from practical concerns, the current European legislative framework for pharmaceutical products is not suited to personalised biologicals such as phages. Efforts are being made at the European level to bring about a possible revision of the legislation on biologicals. Legislation on the use of biologicals is less strict in certain fields, e.g. agriculture and food production, than it is in human medicine. Phages are already being used in these fields' (RIVM 2018).

The RIVM sent a group of researchers to the Eliava Clinic in Tbilisi to see for themselves how phages are used on patients. They observed how phages and cocktails of phages made at the Eliava Clinic pharmacy were sold without prescription in pharmacies throughout Georgia. Phages are also available without prescription in Poland and Russia. 'The scientists at the Eliava Clinic agree that it is necessary to perform proper scientific studies on the application and use of bacteriophages', says Jaap van Dissel, head of the RIVM's infectious diseases department.[26] When I spoke to him at the end of May 2018, he stressed that antibiotics are also in common use in Georgia. 'In the university hospital we visited in Tbilisi, doctors used only antibiotics, not phages. And all of them told us that, for some decades now, phage therapy is no longer used to treat the infections of hospital patients in Georgia'.

## Proper Studies

All the media attention for bacteriophages led to a public petition demanding the admission of phage therapy in the Netherlands. The petition was presented to the Dutch Parliaments Health Committee at the beginning of October 2018. On that occasion specialist in internal diseases and intensive care doctor at the Erasmus Medical Centre in Rotterdam Ard van der Struijs announced the creation in his hospital of a center for phage therapy where the possibilities of using bacteriophages to cure patients with infections caused by (multi-)resistant bugs are going to be studied.

The center, that is the fruit of long discussions between phages promotor Van der Struijs, a number of his more sceptical colleagues and the leadership of the hospital was due to start his activities at the end of 2019 or at the beginning of 2020. At the beginning of 2021, it still didn't function and it was unclear if and when it would take off. Van der Struijs thinks that the general criticism on the lack of scientific proof for phage therapy is not fair. During a conversation in June 2019, he tells me that the library of the Eliava Institute in Tbilisi contains 'loads of proper scientific studies' which has been ignored for example by the visiting delegation of the RIVM 'simply because they are in Russian'. To counter this situation Van der Struijs is actually working, with the help of a Russian co-author, on an overview scientific article presenting the available studies on bacteriophages.

## Buying Licences

From 2010 to 2016, Mats Ulfendahl was General Secretary for Pharmacy and Health at the Swedish Research Council (Vetenskapsrådet). 'There is a high level of sensitivity to the problem of antibiotic resistance in Sweden: our knowledge is good, and the problem is small. This immediately makes it less credible if we talk about a "big problem". How can we make it clear, that the much greater problems with antibiotic resistance in most other countries are our problem as well?' Ulfendahl is glad that the European Action plan has been agreed, and particularly happy about the initiative for public–private partnerships. But he also has some criticisms. 'The

---

[26]As such he leads the Outbreak Management Team, the main scientific advisory board of the government, during the SARS-CoV-2 pandemic.

idea is perfectly good, but now it needs to be translated into concrete measures. As a scientist I'm always somewhat sceptical where the pharma industry is concerned, but in any case we need them for producing antibiotics. We wish to solve a clinical problem; the industry wants to make a profit. That's our point of departure. Some of the proposals they're making seem truly unimaginable: less strict studies, subsidies that ultimately bring them profits. But one thing is very clear: if the development of new antibiotics doesn't bring them enough profit, then they concentrate on other markets. So we don't have any choice'. Ulfendahl explains that the big pharma companies are increasingly outsourcing their research. 'AstraZeneca has closed its research departments in Sweden and Canada', he says. 'They constantly monitor everything that's going on, and buy licences to launch medicines developed by small biotech companies on the market.[27] But we can do that too. Why shouldn't the state buy these licences from university spin-off companies? And then grant pharmaceutical companies the right to market these medicines? Then there would still be a little bit left over for ourselves as well. The industry is cutting research costs and looking for discoveries financed by others. And they get part financing for clinical trials. We need them, that's for sure. But they need us as well. Good relationships with the public healthcare sector are indispensable for companies in order to carry out trials. Not just for developing antibiotics, but also for developing all other medicines. Of course they'd like to earn money, but I believe they also have a sense of responsibility. Even pharmaceutical manufacturers have children. And parents who are old and weak. Therefore in the last analysis, perhaps they're prepared to content themselves with less profit'.

Paul Huijts has fewer reservations about public–private partnerships than Ulfendahl. 'In the Netherlands', he said while still General Director at the Health Ministry, 'the state doesn't have billions of taxpayers' money lying around. It is far too expensive for the scientific sector to develop these medicines themselves. Scientific studies on humans are far too expensive. So we have to pool our resources. And then once again you wind up with the EU, which has an extensive research programme. As part of this programme, AstraZeneca and GlaxoSmithKline carried out a study that cost 224 million euros. Almost half of this, 109 million, was paid by the EU. In this market it is inevitable that we should opt for public-private partnerships. The EU provides a framework in which we can find a percentage of the resources we require'.

As part of the COMBACTE project—Combatting Bacterial Resistance in Europe—(Imi 2020), in February 2013 the University Medical Centre Utrecht

---

[27] At the end of January 2014 AstraZeneca signed an agreement with FOB Synthesis of Atlanta in the US. The company is developing two new carbapenem antibiotics FSI-1671 and FSI 1686. AstraZeneca want to combine these with their own medicines. In an e-mail to the author sent in January 2018, a spokesperson from AstraZeneca said that the company had sold their antibiotics franchise portfolio to Pfizer. In January 2019 FSI-1671 combined with sulbactam was still in the preclinical development (Isler et al. 2019). FSI-1686 is also still in preclinical development. Both potentially new carbapenems are now being developed by Achillion, since January 2020 part of Alexion Pharmaceuticals, and FOB Synthesis (Adis Insight 2020).

received 5.5 million euros to set up a network of European hospitals where new antibiotics could be tested quickly in properly conducted clinical trials. This is one way of getting medicines to the market more quickly and thus reducing the development costs. The European pharma industry is investing 104 million euros in COMBACTE, and the European Commission 83 million. COMBACTE is part of the wider European programme against antibiotic resistance, 'New Drugs for Bad Bugs' (ND4BB), and is intended to support and promote collaboration between industry and science. One of the initiatives being carried out under the umbrella of COMBACTE is a clinical trial of the effectiveness of GSK1322322, a new antibiotic from GlaxoSmithKline which is possibly effective against infections of the respiratory tracts, skin and soft tissues by methicillin-resistant *Staphylococcus aureus* (MRSA) or multiresistant *Streptococcus pneumoniae*. GSK1322322 is said to represent a new class of antibiotics with a new mode of action, which attack the enzyme peptide deformylase (PDF). PDF is an enzyme that is necessary for the maturation of bacterial proteins that are required for the growth and reproduction of bacteria (Naderer et al. 2013; Corey et al. 2014). At the end of January 2017, GlaxoSmithKline informed the author in an e-mail that it had discontinued the development of GSK1322322. In January 2018 Ad Antonisse, Director of Economic Affairs at AstraZeneca, told the author via e-mail that his company had sold its antibiotics franchise portfolio to Pfizer.

At the beginning of 2014, a new project was starting under the ND4BB programme. Called ENABLE (European Gram-Negative Antibacterial Engine), the project is a cooperative association of 32 universities and companies from 13 European countries. The 6-year-long programme is being managed by Uppsala University in Sweden and GlaxoSmithKline and funded by the Innovative Medicines Initiative (IMI). The IMI is financed by the European Commission and the European pharmaceutical industry. By 2019, at least one new antibiotic needs to have been developed to the point where it can be tested on humans. A total of 85 million euros was available to achieve this (Uppsala Universitet 2014) and the goal was reached (ENABLE 2020).

In March 2019, a group of researchers from different university hospitals and the local hospital in Hilversum published an overview article in which they were pretty optimistic about the efforts of the industry and public authorities to increase the investments in the development of novel antibiotics. They were also positive in the results of pre-clinical trials in the efficacy and safety of the potential new antibiotics. As they put it in the English abstract from their article published in Dutch in the *Nederlands Tijdschrift voor Geneeskunde* (Lemkes et al. 2019):

- 'The worldwide rapid increase in antibiotic resistance means that new therapeutic measures are urgently needed.
- Older antibiotics, such as colistin, fosfomycin, minocycline, mecillinam and temocillin, which had fallen from grace due to the development of more effective and less toxic drugs are now of renewed interest in the treatment of infections caused by multiresistant bacteria.

- Two new glycopeptides (oritavancin and dalbavancin) and a new oxazolidinone (tedizolid) are now registered for the treatment of acute skin and soft-tissue infections.
- In the treatment of infections caused by Gram-negative bacteria, cephalosporins are combined with beta-lactamase inhibitors which protect them from various beta-lactamases and also make them effective against extended spectrum beta-lactamase-producing bacteria. Examples of these are ceftolozane-tazobactam, ceftazidime-avibactam and meropenem-vaborbactam.
- Results of preclinical research on the effectiveness of new antibiotics are hopeful. There has been a great increase in investment in the development of new antimicrobials. Also, regulatory agencies have accelerated their assessment of these new—and urgently needed—drugs'.

## A Very Promising Molecule

Before the new public–private partnerships bear fruit, at least 10 years will have passed. In the interim, hardly a single antibiotic with a new working mechanism will come on the market. And very likely, none against Gram-negative bacteria. At the beginning of August 2010, The Wellcome Trust[28] issued a very promising press release about a possible new antibiotic (Wellcome Trust 2010). At the same time, they published an article in *Nature,* describing a new molecule they are developing (Bax et al. 2010). This new molecule—GSK 299423—is supposed to block an enzyme that is indispensable for the reproduction of bacteria.[29] The new medicine might possibly be effective against Gram-positive bacteria such as MRSA and, even more importantly, Gram-negative bacteria such as *E. coli*, Klebsiella, pseudomonas and Acinetobacter. The Wellcome Trust and the US government part-financed the development costs of the potential new antibiotic. At the end of January 2017, GlaxoSmithKline told the author in an e-mail that the company had also discontinued the development of GSK299423. In the same e-mail, GSK underscored the importance of its public–private partnership with US Biomedical Advanced Research and Development Authority (BARDA). GSK had developed the novel antibiotic with a grant of up to 200 million dollars of this organisation. 'Our most advanced antibiotic asset—a topoisomerase inhibitor, gepotidacin (GSK2140944)[30]—has been developed as part of this collaboration. This asset has

---

[28]Founded in 1936, the Wellcome Trust administers the estate of the pharmaceutical magnate Sir Henry Wellcome. Born in America, Wellcome founded his pharmaceutical business in England in 1880. The Wellcome Trust supports medical research and is the second largest foundation of its kind after the Bill & Melinda Gates Foundation, with available assets of ca. 14 billion pounds sterling.

[29]GSK 299423 is intended to block the functioning of the topoisomerase enzyme and with it the reproduction of the bacteria.

[30]The new compound gepotidacin (GSK2140944) blocks the enzyme topoisomerase, thus blocking reproduction of the bacteria:

a novel mechanism of action and the potential to address multiple indications, and is now moving towards phase III studies, following positive phase II results' (Jones et al. 2016; Flamm et al. 2017; O'Riordan et al. 2017; Taylor et al. 2018).

The American pharma company Tetraphase engaged in a phase 3 study of the new medicine eravacycline, a fluorocycline antibiotic (Grossmann et al. 2012; Zhanel et al. 2016). The medicine is supposed to show strong *in vitro* activity against carbapenem-resistant *Acinetobacter baumannii* (Abdallah et al. 2015). Chinese researchers report that in a study carried out recently, two-thirds of all *Acinetobacter baumannii* isolates were resistant to doripenem (Li et al. 2015). Eravacycline was approved in August 2018 by the FDA after it was proven clinically noninferior compared to the carbapenem antibiotics meropenem and ertapenem for the treatment of complicated intraabdominal Gram-Negative infections in adults (Alosaimy et al. 2020). The development of eravacycline was the beginning of the end of Tetraphase. The company was sold for very little money (Rex 2020).

Besides GSK, of all the big pharma companies AstraZeneca was for a long time perhaps the most active in the field of researching new antibiotics. At the end of August 2012, the company obtained permission from the European Commission to launch the new antibiotic ceftaroline fosamil on the market, after the medicine had previously been evaluated positively by the European Medicines Agency (AstraZeneca 2012; EMA 2012). The drug in question is a cephalosporin for intravenous administration developed by Forest Laboratories Inc. AstraZeneca has sold the licence all over the world with the exception of the USA, Canada and Japan.

AstraZeneca's Ad Antonisse explained to me the problems of developing new antibiotics on the basis of the ceftaroline case. 'We launched ceftaroline on the Dutch market in 2013. Two patients received the medicine. We sold a total of six packets. But they were able to save human lives'. The antibiotic is effective against MRSA infections, directly subcutaneous infections, and in part also against pneumonia. AstraZeneca has limited reserves of ceftaroline in stock. 'We've already thrown away 100,000 euros' worth of ceftaroline', says Antonisse, 'because it was past its sell-by date. But we're remaining active in the antibiotics sector'. That was true, as noted above, until January 2018.

Ceftaroline is primarily intended for adult patients who are suffering from acute skin infections or pneumonias that have been acquired outside healthcare facilities. The medicine is effective against Gram-positive bacteria such as *Staphylococcus aureus*, including its methicillin-resistant form MRSA. This means it could become an important medicine, because MRSA infections accounted in 2019 for an average of 15.5% of all infections by *Staphylococcus aureus* in the European Union (ECDC 2020b). In 2005, an estimated 95,000 people suffered from an MRSA bloodstream infection in the USA and 19,000 people died of it (Klevens et al. 2007). Ten years later the decrease since 2007 in the number of MRSA bloodstream infections slowed down and the mortality remained high. In 2017 almost 20,000 people died of a Staphylococcus aureus infection, MRSA and the variant susceptible to methicillin

MSSA (Kourtis et al. 2019). On the other hand, there are still several antibiotics that are effective against MRSA infections.[31]

In 2016, AstraZeneca[32] received marketing approval for ceftazidime/avibactam, a medicine for use against Gram-negative bacteria (EMA 2016). 'Avibactam is a new beta-lactamase inhibitor[33] that is used to supplement older antibiotics such as ceftazidime or imipenem', says Professor Inge Gyssens. 'So something is already happening in our research field. AstraZeneca is working on a larger observational study, the REACH study. As part of this, 4000 patients were investigated retrospectively. Half of them had community-acquired pneumonia, the other half skin or soft tissue infections.[34] An investigation of this kind, designed to find out more about the characteristic features of potential patients, has never been carried out by a company before this'. The initial findings of the study were presented at the ECCMID 2012 in London. For almost a third of all patients with community-acquired pneumonia, the initial empirically selected antibiotic treatment had to be changed (Blasi et al. 2013). In the case of skin or soft tissue infections, the initial antibiotic therapy had to be changed to a different antibiotic in about 40% of all cases (Garau et al. 2015). The researchers analysed data for both types of infections from 128 and 129 European hospitals, respectively, in 10 European countries. At the moment a follow-up study is in progress that is intended to deliver additional information on why the antibiotics were changed, and how.

## Back to the Old Antibiotics, Then?

At the 2012 symposium of the Dutch Working Party on Antibiotic Policy (SWAB), Gyssens gave a presentation with the provocative title 'Forgotten antibiotics'. Forgotten antibiotics? Are there such things? It was only an idea that Gyssens had had, which she'd mentioned in a conversation with her Danish colleague Niels Frimodt Møller of the University of Copenhagen. In fact, there are some old medicines whose existence has been forgotten, for example because better products came on the market afterwards. Using their international network, Gyssens and Frimodt Møller consulted hospital pharmacists, microbiologists and specialists for infectious diseases in 38 different countries, including the EU member states, the USA, Canada and Australia. This led to some quite astonishing discoveries, which were published in *Clinical Infectious* Diseases (Pulcini et al. 2012). Colistin, one of

---

[31]Professor Inge Gyssens mentions vancomycin, teicoplanin, linezolid, daptomycin and telavancin. Some antibiotics, such as cotrimoxazol, clindamycin and doxycyclin, also help fight livestock-associated MRSA.

[32]AstraZeneca was formed in 1999 from a merger between the Swedish firm Astra AB and the Zeneca Group PLC of the UK.

[33]Beta-lactamases are enzymes that make bacteria resistant to beta-lactam antibiotics. A beta-lactamase inhibitor restricts these enzymes and thus prevents resistant bacteria from forming. These inhibitors have their own antibacterial effect, although as a rule it is only very weak.

[34]Soft tissue infections are infections of the tissue directly under the skin.

the two medicines that are still effective against bacteria resistant to carbapenem antibiotics, was only available in 25 of the 38 countries.

'Only 14 of the 33 antibiotics we classed as most important are approved in the Netherlands. In Belgium the figure is 15. For example aztreonam, a monobactam, is a medicine that provides a good alternative in cases of sepsis if the patient has an allergic reaction to beta-lactam antibiotics. But it is only available in half of these 38 countries. Ertapenem is not available in Belgium. In the Netherlands and Germany it continues to be available. Ertapenem is a carbapenem antibiotic, and it's very expensive. Belgian patients sometimes buy it in the Netherlands, but then they have to pay for it themselves. Fusidic acid is not available in Germany and Belgium, but in the Netherlands it is.[35] Here's another example: there are signs that temocillin could be used for urinary tract infections caused by ESBL-producing *E. coli*. Temocillin is only available in Belgium and the United Kingdom. Not in the other 36 countries. And there are similar differences between approved antibiotics amongst all the 38 countries. We know much less still about the availability of antibiotics in developing countries and south-east Asia', says Gyssens. 'Perhaps we have a kind of reserve arsenal at our disposal here. Should we approve all of these medicines everywhere? There are still many questions to be cleared up. For example, are there still medicines in the veterinary or agricultural sectors that can also be used for humans?'[36]

## New Knowledge on Old Medicines

During a contribution to ECCMID 2012 in London, Gyssens' late colleague Johan Mouton, who was working in Nijmegen at the time, spoke about the irresponsible use of old antibiotics. He warned that antibiotics that were launched on the market 30 or more years ago do not fulfil the strict approval conditions that apply today. In general, moreover, little is said about new data that has come to light regarding these old medicines, even though new understanding, for example regarding the dosage of a medicine, is of crucial importance. For a long time now, for example, the old medicine colistin has hardly been used anymore because of its toxicity. But with the right dosage, the toxicity does not appear to be quite so pronounced (Mouton 2012).

At her home in the Berchem district of Antwerp, Inge Gyssens tells me more about her quest for old antibiotics and the possibilities that might be incorporated into treatment again. 'There are medicines that work very well which have never been used in the Scandinavian countries or the Netherlands, because there were no

---

[35]Fusidic acid is a bactericidal antibiotic that is mainly used to combat superficial infections of the skin, for example those caused by *Staphylococcus aureus*.

[36]In June 2012, scientists from the UK, Switzerland and the USA published a study in *Proceedings of the National Academy of Sciences* concerning apramycin, an antibiotic used in the veterinary sector that can possibly be used against bacteria that are resistant to aminoglycoside antibiotics (broad-spectrum antibiotics) (Matt et al. 2012). Before this, however, studies must first be carried out on humans.

resistance problems. Therefore, sometimes they're not even approved. Or they have been approved, but never came on the market'. The example of ertapenem, which has already been mentioned, speaks for itself. In the Netherlands it is available, and in Belgium it is not. It is a strong carbapenem that remains effective for a long period. 'It only needs to be administered once a day by injection. Other carbapenems need to be administered three or four times a day as infusions. Ertapenem is only used for severe infections that demand long treatment. Its advantage is that the patients can be sent home and only have to come once a day to receive their injection. In Belgium there seemed no need to approve it, since other carbapenems were available and there is no tradition of outpatient treatment. I know one case of a patient who wanted ertapenem and paid for it himself. This treatment cost him around 500 euros. Other patients who didn't receive ertapenem—because the costs were not met and they couldn't afford it themselves—spent three weeks in hospital. The per diem costs there are probably just as high as what that single patient paid for his ertapenem. But the health insurance provider was not convinced by this'.

Gyssens mentioned one more example: mecillinam, a medicine produced by the Danish pharma company LEO Pharma that is approved neither in the Netherlands nor Belgium and is only available in two countries. 'Niels Frimodt Møller has discovered that it is a very good medicine for treating ESBL infections in mice. The patent has expired, and the industry has absolutely no interest in carrying out further expensive trials of it on human beings'. Now there is European funding that is being made available for further research, coordinated until his death by Johan Mouton, into some of these old antibiotics (CORDIS 2017; Theuretzbacher 2017). Professor Gyssens describes another phenomenon as well. 'Sometimes we see a situation where some medicines can't be supplied either temporarily or long-term, but a more expensive medicine can be used as an alternative. This is an ideal situation for carrying out a type of "market research". I don't know whether there's anyone who thinks in such a devious way. I don't want to make insinuations about anybody either, but sometimes this is the way it looks'.

The possibilities offered by these forgotten antibiotics in the fight against multiresistant bacteria were intensively discussed at the end of October 2014, at the 3-day-long 'Reviving Old Antibiotics' conference in Vienna. Around 300 doctors and scientists, plus representatives of government and the pharma industry, took part in the meeting, organised by the European Society of Clinical Microbiology and Infectious Diseases (ESCMID). 'We had a very successful and fruitful conference', said Dr. Ursula Theuretzbacher, founder of the Centre for Anti-Infective Agents (CEFAIA) in Vienna (ESCMID 2014). 'We'd known for some time that old generations of antibiotics that were developed up to 55 years ago are effective against multiresistant germs in certain clinical situations. However, these old medicines were not developed any further. Without a solid strategy for "redeveloping" these old medicines and thoroughly testing them to modern standards, we run the risk that we will damage patients with them, or accelerate the development of resistance. We urgently need to bring our present-day state of knowledge to bear on the regulatory and therapeutic processes, in order to beneficially use these old antibiotics as an interim solution until we have developed completely new generations of antibiotics'.

The most important old antibiotics include colistin and colistimethate sodium, which belong to the polymyxin antibiotics. Colistimethate sodium is a solution that is converted into colistin in the body. For a long time, colistin was hardly used, particularly in the Western world, because it caused severe side-effects. For example, it sometimes caused permanent kidney damage. Thanks to a new manufacturing method, colistin now causes fewer side-effects than before. At the end of October 2014, the European Medicines Agency published new recommendations for the safe use of colistin for patients with severe infections caused by bacteria that were resistant to all other antibiotics. The recommendations included correct dosages, the way to administer the drug, and indications for the use of colistin (EMA 2014).

## Long-Term Goals

New antibiotics, old antibiotics—all that requires a lot of research, and a lot of time and money. And responsible handling of antibiotics can't be implemented overnight either. Perhaps it is a realistic goal in the Scandinavian countries and the Netherlands, but in many other (European) countries the use of antibiotics still remains sky-high. In November 2012, to mark 'European Antibiotic Awareness Day', for the first time the ECDC published figures on antibiotic use in the community for 27 EU member states. In 2010, Greece used roughly three and a half times as many antibiotics as Estonia, Lithuania and the Netherlands.[37] Belgium, France and Italy used approximately two and a half times as many (ECDC 2013). The figures in the sixth annual ECDC Report, published in November 2017, are basically more or less the same as those in the first report. The use of antibiotics in the community was in 2016 the lowest in the Netherlands. In Greece, it is almost 3.5 times as much, and still remains the highest of all the EU/EEA countries. Romania, France and Cyprus use approximately three times as many antibiotics as the Dutch. Italy and Belgium use 2.5 times as many, and the UK twice as many. The Dutch also use the fewest antibiotics in the hospital sector. Denmark, Latvia and France use twice as many; Greece, Italy, Lithuania and the UK 2.5 times as many; and Malta three times as many (ECDC 2017). The 2020 ECDC report, which contains data on 2019, also shows few changes compared to previous years. The big users remained big users, both in the community and in the hospital sector. The big users Greece, Cyprus, Romania and France and Spain continue to use (far) more than the EU average. The countries—the Netherlands, Austria, Germany, Sweden, Norway—who used relatively few antibiotics continued to do so (ECDC 2020a).

---

[37] As a whole Lithuania uses relatively few antibiotics, but it has the highest use of carbapenems amongst the 18 countries that sent data to the ECDC for the report on the antibiotic consumption data over 2010. Three times as many carbapenems are prescribed in Lithuania as in the Netherlands.

'In 2019', says the ECDC 2020 report on antimicrobial consumption, 'the average total (community and hospital sector combined) consumption of antibacterials for systemic use in the EU/EEA was 19.4 defined daily doses (DDD) per 1000 inhabitants per day (country range: 9.5–34.1). During the period 2010–2019, a statistically significant decrease was observed for the EU/EEA overall. Statistically significant decreasing trends were observed for 13 countries. Statistically significant increasing trends were observed for four countries'.

In the *Proceedings of the National Academy of Science* (PNAS) of 10 April 2018, an international group of researchers noted that between 2000 and 2015 there had been a dramatic global increase in the consumption of antibiotics. The report, with data on 76 countries over 16 years, found 'that the antibiotic consumption rate in low- and middle-income countries (LMICs) has been converging to (and in some countries surpassing) levels typically observed in high-income countries. However, inequities in drug access persist, as many LMICs continue to be burdened with high rates of infectious disease-related mortality and low rates of antibiotic consumption. Our findings emphasise the need for global surveillance of antibiotic consumption to support policies to reduce antibiotic consumption and resistance while providing access to these lifesaving drugs'. The figures the researchers have uncovered are striking: from 2000 to 2015 inclusive, the global antibiotic consumption expressed in defined daily doses increased from 21.1 to 34.8 billion DDDs, a 65% rise. The antibiotic consumption rate increased by 39%, from 11.3 to 15.7 DDDs per 1000 inhabitants per day. The rise in consumption is driven by low- and middle-income countries, where the increase in antibiotic consumption was correlated to a rise in per capita GDP. 'Of particular concern was the rapid increase in the use of last-resort compounds, both in HICs and LMICs, such as glycylcyclines, oxazolidinones, carbapenems, and polymyxins. Projections of global antibiotic consumption in 2030, assuming no policy changes, were up to 200% higher than the 42 billion DDDs estimated in 2015. Although antibiotic consumption rates in most LMICs remain lower than in HICs despite higher bacterial disease burden, consumption in LMICs is rapidly converging to rates similar to HICs. Reducing global consumption is critical for reducing the threat of antibiotic resistance, but reduction efforts must balance access limitations in LMICs and take account of local and global resistance patterns' (Klein et al. 2018). In another study on the same data, a research group led by Elli Klein focused on the consumption of antibiotics that are on WHO's Watch-list. The global consumption of these Watch-list antibiotics increased between 2000 and 2015 with more than 90% from 3.3 to 6.3 defined daily doses (DDD) per 1000 inhabitants. The overall use of all available antibiotics increased by 26% from 8.4 to 10.6 DDD per 1000 inhabitants. In low-income and middle-income countries, the increase in the use of Watch-list antibiotics was 165% from 2.0 to 5.3 DDD per 1000 inhabitants. The WHO has set as a target for 2023 that 60% of the total antibiotic consumption will consist of antibiotics that are not on the Watch-list but in the Access category. In 2000, 50 out of 66 countries achieved already this goal. In 2015, their number had dropped to 42 out of 76 countries studied (Klein et al. 2021).

## Overconsumption and Underconsumption

In addition to the global rise in the consumption of antibiotics, there are wide differences between the antibiotics consumption of different countries. Data published by the WHO in November 2018 reveal these differences in antibiotics consumption in human healthcare. The discrepancies in use range from 4 DDD/1000 inhabitants per day to more than 64 DDD. These data suggest under-consumption of antibiotics in some countries and overconsumption in others. In the European WHO region, the median consumption is 17.9 DDD/1000 inhabitants per day. But in Europe, there is also an almost fourfold difference between the highest- and lowest-consuming countries. The WHO stresses the need for better data, as the quality and completeness of the data used vary widely (WHO 2018b).

In India and China, on the African continent, in large parts of Latin America, in Eastern Europe and even in the USA, responsible use of antibiotics is still further from being everyday reality than in Europe. The completely different causes that are responsible for this make a global approach to tackling this problem almost impossible. For example, India, with its extremely rich upper class and equally poor general population, has excessive use of antibiotics in the first case, and inadequate access to antibiotics in the latter. But it also has a lack of toilet facilities, sewerage and wastewater purification systems.[38] In Africa, the key issues are the inadequate availability of antibiotics for extremely poor social strata, and the lack of sanitary facilities. In the USA, it is much more a question of unjustified use of antibiotics for humans and animals. Scientific data published in November 2012 show that large quantities of MRSA were present in the inflows of clarification plants in various US states (Rosenberg Goldstein et al. 2012). A study in the French town of Besançon showed that wastewater from hospitals contains more ESBL than normal wastewater (Brëchet et al. 2014). Scientists at the University of Warwick in the UK also demonstrate that wastewater contains large amounts of ESBL (Amos et al. 2014).

Large concentrations of ampicillin-resistant *E. faecium* bacteria, which are often present in hospitals, are found in the water of clarification plants (Sadowy and Luczkiewicz 2014; Taucer-Kapteijn et al. 2016). According to a recent German study, this does not only apply to *Enterecocci spp.* but also to several other bacteria like *Escherichia coli, Pseudomonas aeruginosa, Klebsiella pneumoniae* and *Acinetobacter baumannii* (Alexander et al. 2020). These bacteria are also found frequently amongst the general population. The increased prevalence of these bacteria in the drainage outlets of clarification plants may have something to do with the process cycles of these facilities. Clarification plants are in fact a kind of bioreactor where transfer of resistance genes is possible. But the livestock industry certainly plays a significant role as well, because the slurry from poultry, calves and

---

[38]On 2 October 2014, the birthday of Mahatma Gandhi and Indian Independence Day, the new Indian Prime Minister Narendra Modi launched the *Swachh Bharat* ('Clean India') campaign. Through this initiative, he hopes to have 120 million toilets built in 5 years' time for the 600 million Indians who at present do not have one. According to an Indian factchecker-site, in 3 years 50 million household toilets have been constructed (FactChecker 2017).

pigs is contaminated with ESBL-positive *E. coli* in almost three-quarters of cases. Remarkably high concentrations of ESBL-positive *E. coli* are frequently found in ditches and canals near farms. This is caused by the flushing of slurry into the ditches, but also by the water that flows into the ditches when the animal sheds are cleaned. The ESBL bacteria are further spread by using the water from the ditches to water vegetables, just as they are by using dung contaminated with ESBL-positive bacteria on the fields. Roughly a half of all the water used for irrigation contains ESBL bacteria. At the end of this cycle, they also wind up in bathing and recreational water, and therefore in human beings (Blaak et al. 2015). The same applies to other resistant bacteria (Piccirilli et al. 2019).

However, the contribution of ESBLs originating from livestock to the spread of ESBL producing bacteria in humans, through meat eating, swimming and livestock farming, seems low, according to a Dutch interdisciplinary study. 'Based on swimming frequency, water absorption and water contamination, the exposure of swimmers is estimated', write the authors. 'The same has been done for the exposure through consumption of pork, chicken and beef. To this end, data on the degree of contamination of meat and meat products are combined with information about the frequency of consumption. The analyzes show that both swimmers and consumers are exposed to low concentrations of ESBLs. The exposure through consumption of meat, and in particular raw meat products, is higher than the exposure to ESBLs via swimming. At present, there are no epidemiological studies in the Netherlands that show that exposure through meat or swimming leads to an increased risk of carrier status in the general population or infections in patients. Residents living in livestock-dense areas are exposed to ESBLs through the environment, for example by ESBLs in the air. Research among these residents showed that this exposure does not result in an increased chance of carrier status' (ESBLAT 2018).

In the Netherlands, the problems with antibiotics use are primarily concentrated in the veterinary sector, although a significant decrease in usage has been achieved since 2009. In Belgium, too many antibiotics are used in both the human and veterinary medicine sectors. In Greece and Spain, the biggest problem is the availability of antibiotics without prescription. Irresponsible use of antibiotics—and therefore antibiotic resistance—is a many-headed monster. And every one of these heads must be fought in a different way. How intractable this problem is can perhaps best be illustrated by looking at the eternal struggle to improve hygiene in hospitals.

## Washing Hands

Hygiene—above all hand hygiene—is the mother and father of all approaches to improving infection prevention in hospitals. Alex Friedrich has a nice metaphor that underscores the importance of good hygiene: 'Antibiotics are the motor of resistance; lack of hygiene is the photocopier', he says. In his statement, Friedrich is not so much referring to the lack of water pipes and sewerage as to the inadequate hand hygiene of doctors and nursing staff. Education and training on the utility and necessity of hand hygiene have proven beneficial properties. The health scientist Agnes van den Hoogen described this in her doctoral dissertation for the UMC Utrecht. Van den Hoogen carried out her studies at neonatal intensive care units in the university medical centre. She gave training sessions on good hand hygiene for all staff and combined them with information on the number of healthcare-associated infections in the department. She also put up posters at prominent, easily visible locations around the department, to sensitise staff to the importance of good hand hygiene. In addition to this, she uploaded a film on this subject onto the desktop of all the computers in the department. Van den Hoogen's approach led to a clear improvement in hand hygiene, from 23% before the study to 50% afterwards. 'But', she notes, '50 per cent is much too little, that needs to be further improved' (Van den Hoogen 2009). In spring 2012, the behavioural scientist Vicki Erasmus obtained her doctorate from the Erasmus University Medical Centre with a study on compliance with hygiene regulations. Doctors and nurses only wash their hands in 20% of the cases where it is prescribed. Erasmus researched this using an observational study in intensive care units and surgical wards, in a representative random sample of 24 Dutch hospitals. Compliance with hygiene regulations was worst in teaching hospitals (Erasmus 2012).

## Sufficient Nurses

A good structure for infection prevention and hygiene begins by providing a sufficient number of nurses, says Alex Friedrich. 'In Dutch intensive care units there is a maximum of 1.5 to 2 patients per nurse. In Germany there are around 3.5. In other words, twice as many! How are nursing staff supposed to observe the rules for hand hygiene, when there aren't enough hands at each individual bed? This combination of "overcrowding" and "understaffing" plays an important role in many institutions'.

The existing problems with hygiene are now being compounded by new problems created by modern lifestyles. Smartphones and mobile computers used by doctors and nurses while caring for patients are covered with microbes but are rarely disinfected. And hand hygiene after the use of such equipment is poor (Manning et al. 2013; Morubagal et al. 2017).

## Prevention at Low Cost

As long as in the Netherlands, and the rest of the world, hygiene regulations are not well enough observed in medical institutions, as long as antibiotics are often not used responsibly, as long as antibiotics are used excessively in the livestock industry, and as long as no new antibiotics with a really novel working mechanism appear, fighting antibiotic resistance will continue to be tilting at windmills. However, a relatively small effort, with limited financial costs, would be able to make a huge difference. In November 2018, the Organisation for Economic Cooperation and

Development (OECD) published the report *Stemming the superbug tide: just a few dollars more* (OECD 2018). The researchers who wrote the report analysed all kinds of available data on antibiotic resistance in order 'to model future patterns of resistance and identify "best practice" public health measures to tackle the problems'. According to the report, based on current trends an estimated 2.4 million people would die in OECD countries between 2015–50 because of infections caused by multiresistant bacteria. 'Southern Europe risked being particularly affected, and Greece, Italy and Portugal were likely to have the highest mortality rates due to antimicrobial resistance'. But preventative measures could change this bleak scenario dramatically. 'Three quarters of all deaths from antibiotic-resistant bacterial infections could be prevented if countries spent 2 US dollars (€1.75) per person per year on measures to prevent the predicted increase in antimicrobial resistance'. If only....

## References ·

3M Science. (2020). *Testing of Salmonella bacteriophage preparation for presence of free Salmonella DNA*. Accessed January 1, 2021, from https://bit.ly/3o19DhI

Abdallah, M., Olafisoye, O., Cortes, C., et al. (2015). Activity of Eravacycline against enterobacteriaceae and Acinetobacter baumannii, including multidrug-resistant isolates, from New York City. *Antimicrobial Agents and Chemotherapy, 59*(3), 1802–1805. Accessed from https://bit.ly/3rNFq88

Access to Medicine. (2017). *Access to Vaccines Index 2017*. Accessed December 30, 2020, from https://bit.ly/3oaM0n0

Access to Medicine. (2018). *Shortages, stockouts and scarcity: The issues facing the security of antibiotic supply and the role for pharmaceutical companies*. Accessed December 30, 2020, from https://bit.ly/34SMWVh

Access to Medicine. (2020a). *Biannual reports on access to medicine*. Accessed December 30, 2020, from https://bit.ly/2X5arq1

Access to Medicine. (2020b). *Biannual AMR Benchmark*. Accessed December 30, 2020, from https://bit.ly/3b35MwR

Adis Insight. (2020). *Research programme: Antibacterials - Achillion/FOB Synthesis. Alternative Names: FSI-1297; FSI-1671; FSI-1686*. Accessed January 1, 2020, from https://bit.ly/39w7Z1N

Alexander, J., Hembach, N., & Schwartz, T. (2020). Evaluation of antibiotic resistance dissemination by wastewater treatment plant effluents with different catchment areas in Germany. *Scientific Reports, 10*, 8952. https://doi.org/10.1038/s41598-020-65635-4.

Alosaimy, S., Abdul-Mutakabbir, J. C., Kebriaei, R., et al. (2020). Evaluation of eravacycline: a novel fluorocycline. *Pharmacotherapy, 40*(3), 221–238. https://doi.org/10.1002/phar.2366.

Amos, G. C. A., Hawkey, P. M., Gaze, W. H., et al. (2014). Waste water effluent contributes to the dissemination of CTX-M-15 in the natural environment. *The Journal of Antimicrobial Chemotherapy, 69*(7), 1785–1791. https://doi.org/10.1093/jac/dku079.

AMR Action Fund. (2020). *Bridging the gap between science and patients. 2 to 4 novel antibiotics by 2030*. Accessed January 10, 2020, from https://amractionfund.com/

AMR Industry Alliance. (2018). *Tracking progress to address AMR*. Accessed December 30, 2020, from https://bit.ly/34VQYw9

AstraZeneca. (2012). *European Commission approves ZINFORO™ (ceftaroline fosamil) for adult patients with serious skin infections or community acquired pneumonia*. Accessed January 2, 2021, from https://bit.ly/3od0faU

Barber, S. L., Borowitz, M., Bekedam, H., et al. (2014). The hospital of the future in China: China's reform of public hospitals and trends from industrialized countries. *Health Policy and Planning, 29*(3), 367–378. https://doi.org/10.1093/heapol/czt023.

Bax, B. D., Chan, P. F., Eggleston, D. R., et al. (2010). Type IIA topoisomerase inhibition by a new class of antibacterial agents. *Nature, 466*, 935–940. https://doi.org/10.1038/nature09197.

Bergström, R. (2011). *EFPIA Director Genral's lectur: Is society ready for the new science?* Accessed January 1, 2021, from https://bit.ly/351cNdV

Blaak, H., van Hoek, A. H., Hamidjaja, R. A., et al. (2015). Distribution, numbers, and diversity of ESBL-producing E. coli in the poultry farm environment. *PLoS One, 10*(8), e0135402. https://doi.org/10.1371/journal.pone.0135402.

Blasi, F., Garau, J., Medina, J., et al. (2013). Current management of patients hospitalized with community-acquired pneumonia across Europe: Outcomes from REACH. *Respiratory Research, 14*(1), 44. https://doi.org/10.1186/1465-9921-14-44.

Bréchet, C., Plantin, J., Sauget, M., et al. (2014). Wastewater treatment plants release large amounts of extended-spectrum β-lactamase-producing Escherichia coli into the environment. *Clinical Infectious Diseases, 58*(12), 1658–1665. https://doi.org/10.1093/cid/ciu190.

Carlet, J. (2014). *World alliance against antibiotic resistance: The WAAAR declaration against antibiotic resistance.* Accessed from https://www.efort.org/waaar/

Carlet, J., Rambaud, C., & Pulcini, C. (2012). WAAR (World Alliance against Antibiotic Resistance): Safeguarding antibiotics. *Antimicrobial Resistance and Infection Control 1*, 25. Accessed from https://bit.ly/38r7lmL

Cars, O., Hedin, A., & Heddini, A. (2011). The global need for effective antibiotics—Moving towards concerted action. *Drug Resistance Updates, 14*(68–69). All conference materials are accessible through this link. Accessed December 27, 2020, from https://bit.ly/3mT5riO

Cassini, A., Högberg, L. D., Plachouras, D., et al. (2019). Attributable deaths and disability-adjusted life-years caused by infections with antibiotic-resistant bacteria in the EU and the European Economic Area in 2015: A population-level modelling analysis. *Lancet Infectious Disease, 19*(1), 56–66. https://doi.org/10.1016/S1473-3099(18)30605-4.

CDDEP. (2012). *The Global Antibiotic Resistance Partnership. Joint Statement on Antibiotic Resistance with the U.S. Centers for Disease Control and Prevention (CDC) and 25 National Health Organizations.* Accessed December 27, 2020, from https://bit.ly/3pvAlzx

CDDEP. (2020). *The Global Antibiotic Resistance Partnership. GARP Network.* Accessed December 19, 2020, from https://bit.ly/39gcahY

CenterWatch. (2014). *Antibacterial drugs market to top $45B globally in 2019.* Accessed December 27, 2020, from https://bit.ly/2MFOqMq

Chan, M. (2012). *Antimicrobial resistance in the European Union and the world.* Accessed December 27, 2020, from https://bit.ly/3nNDQRg

CORDIS. (2017). *Preserving old antibiotics for the future: Assessment of clinical efficacy by a pharmacokinetic/pharmacodynamic approach to optimize effectiveness and reduce resistance for off-patent antibiotics.* Accessed January 2, 2021, from https://bit.ly/3s73YZX

Corey, R., Naderer, O. J., O'Riordan, W. D., et al. (2014). Safety, tolerability, and efficacy of GSK1322322 in the treatment of acute bacterial skin and skin structure infections. *Antimicrobial Agents and Chemotherapy, 58*(11), 6518–6527. https://doi.org/10.1128/AAC.03360-14.

Council of Europe. (2017). *Two Danish Journalists prosecuted for exposing a public health hazard.* Accessed December 26, 2020, from https://bit.ly/38r7xlZ

Davos Declaration. (2016). *Declaration by the pharmaceutical, biotechnology and diagnostics industries on combating antimicrobial resistance January 2016.* Accessed December 30, 2020, from https://bit.ly/3aP9QAW

De Kraker, M. E. A., Stewardson, A. J., & Harbarth, S. (2016). Will 10 million people die a year due to antimicrobial resistance by 2050? *PLoS Medicine, 13*(11), e1002184. https://doi.org/10.1371/journal.pmed.1002184.

Deckers, D. (2014). *Speech on the conference joining forces for future health in The Hague, 25 and 26 June 2014.* Accessed December 27, 2020, from https://bit.ly/35srV46

Dijksma S (2014). *Speech by Minister for Agriculture Sharon Dijksma at the Ministerial Conference on Antibiotic Resistance.* Accessed December 27, 2020, from https://bit.ly/3nSuiEH

DISARM Act. (2019). *Developing an innovative strategy for antimicrobial resistant microorganisms Act of 2019 or the DISARM Act of 2019.* Accessed January 10, 2021, from https://www.congress.gov/bill/116th-congress/senate-bill/1712

DNDi. (2016). *Drugs for neglected diseases initiative.* Accessed December 30, 2020, from https://bit.ly/3mXXI2R

EC (European Commission). (2011). *Directorate-general for Health & Consumers. Communication from the Commission to the European Parliament and the Council. Action plan against the rising threats from Antimicrobial Resistance.* Accessed December 26, 2020, from https://bit.ly/37O7Fvj

EC (European Commission). (2017a). *New EU Action Plan on Antimicrobial Resistance – Questions and answers.* Accessed January 1, 2021, from https://bit.ly/3i0689i

EC (European Commission). (2017b). *A European One Health Action Plan against Antimicrobial Resistance (AMR).* Accessed January 1, 2021, from https://bit.ly/351rBt4

ECDC (European Centre for Disease Prevention and Control). (2013). *Surveillance of antimicrobial consumption in Europe, 2010.* Accessed January 2, 2021, from https://bit.ly/3b1qz41

ECDC (European Centre for Disease Prevention and Control). (2017). *Summary of the latest data on antibiotic consumption in the European Union ESAC-Net surveillance data November 2017.* Accessed January 2, 2021, from https://bit.ly/3rNhO3z

ECDC (European Centre for Disease Prevention and Control). (2020a). *Antimicrobial consumption in the EU/EEA Annual Epidemiological Report for 2019.* Accessed January 2, 2021, from https://bit.ly/3pIQf9L

ECDC (European Centre for Disease Prevention and Control). (2020b). *Antimicrobial resistance in the EU/EEA (EARS-Net) Annual Epidemiological Report for 2019.* Accessed January 2, 2021, from https://bit.ly/3o9ZLlM

ECDC/EMEA. (2009). *ECDC/EMEA JOINT TECHNICAL REPORT: The bacterial challenge: Time to react A call to narrow the gap between multidrug-resistant bacteria in the EU and the development of new antibacterial agents.* Accessed December 27, 2020, from https://bit.ly/37NQhqK

EMA (European Medicines Agency). (2012). *Assessment Report Zinforo (ceftaroline fosamil).* Accessed January 2, 2021, from https://bit.ly/2JCelUa

EMA (European Medicines Agency). (2014). *European Medicines Agency completes review of polymyxin-based medicines recommendations issued for safe use in patients with serious infections resistant to standard antibiotics.* Accessed January 2, 2021, from https://bit.ly/3pADtdo

EMA (European Medicines Agency). (2016). *Zavicefta (ceftazidime/avibactam).* Accessed January 2, 2021, from https://bit.ly/2LBTaCc

ENABLE. (2020). *European Gram Negative Antibacterial Engine. What have we achieved?* Accessed January 1, 2021, from https://bit.ly/3pGWxXy See also the press releases form January and November 2020 https://bit.ly/3pMfpo5

Encyclopeadia Brittanica. (2020). *Soviet invasion of Afghanistan 1979.* Last updated 11 May 2020. Accessed January 1, 2021, fromhttps://bit.ly/38uZ4y9

Erasmus, V. (2012). *Compliance to hand hygiene guidelines in hospital care. A stepwise behavioural approach.* Doctorate thesis. Accessed January 3, 2021, from https://repub.eur.nl/pub/32161/

ESBLAT. (2018). *Summary ESBL-Attribution-analysis (ESBLAT). Searching for the sources of antimicrobial resistance in humans.* Accessed January 3, 2021, from https://bit.ly/3rQ9hwz

ESCMID. (2014). *Conference outlines a global plan to use old antibiotics to tackle multi-drug resistant 'Superbugs' and confront the imminent threat of a 'post-antibiotic age' which could see millions die from once commonplace, treatable infections.* Accessed January 2, 2021, from https://bit.ly/3o96xbA

FactChecker. (2017). *3 Years of Swachh Bharat: 50 Million more toilets; unclear how many are used.* Accessed January 2, 2021, from https://bit.ly/3pGAmk7

Flamm, R. K., Farrell, D. J., Rhomberg, P. R., et al. (2017). Gepotidacin (GSK2140944) *in vitro* activity against gram-positive and gram-negative bacteria. *Antimicrobial Agents and Chemotherapy, 61*(7), e00468–e00417. https://doi.org/10.1128/AAC.00468-17.

Fruciano, D. E., & Bourne, S. (2007). Phage as an antimicrobial agent: d'Herelle's heretical theories and their role in the decline of phage prophylaxis in the West. *Canadian Journal of Infectious Diseases and Medical Microbiology, 18*(1), 19–26. https://doi.org/10.1155/2007/976850.

G7 Health Ministers. (2015). *Declaration of the G7 Health Ministers 8-9 October 2015 in Berlin. Think ahead, act together.* Accessed December 26, 2020, from https://bit.ly/2WLBgiN

Garau, J., Blasi, F., Medina, J., et al. (2015). Early response to antibiotic treatment in European patients hospitalized with complicated skin and soft tissue infections: Analysis of the REACH study. *BMC Infectious Diseases, 15*, 78. https://doi.org/10.1186/s12879-015-0822-2.

Ghafur, A., Mathai, D., Muruganathan, A. et al. (2013). The Chennai declaration: A roadmap to tackle the challenge of antimicrobial resistance. *The Indian Journal of Cancer, 50*(1): 71–73. https://doi.org/10.4103/0019-509X.104065. Accessed from https://bit.ly/3gZuOy4

Goossens, H. (2013). The Chennai declaration on antimicrobial resistance in India. *The Lancet Infectious Diseases, 13*(2): 105–106. Accessed from https://bit.ly/3s6Z4vX

Government of the Netherlands. (2012). *The responsible use of medicines, setting policies for better and cost-effective healthcare.* Accessed December 26, 2020, links to speech of the Dutch Health Minister and to the conference report https://bit.ly/37NcXra

Grand View. (2016). *Antibiotics market size to reach $57.0 billion by 2024. Grand View Research, Inc.* Accessed December 27, 2020, from https://bit.ly/3mTlVYf

Grossmann, T. H., Starosta, A. L., Fyfe, C., et al. (2012). Target- and resistance-based mechanistic studies with TP-434, a novel fluorocycline antibiotic. *Antimicrobial Agents and Chemotherapy, 56*(5), 2559–2564. https://doi.org/10.1128/AAC.06187-11.

Gyssens, I. C. (2008). All EU hands to the EU pumps: The Science Academies of Europe (EASAC) recommend strong support of research to tackle antibacterial resistance. *Clinical Microbiology and Infection, 14*(10), 889–891. https://doi.org/10.1111/j.1469-0691.2008.02067.x.

Hellamand, M., & Rafiqi, F. (2020). Evidence shows the antibiotics market is failing, but here is how it can be revived. *The Pharmaceutical Journal, 305*(7940). https://doi.org/10.1211/PJ.2020.20208270. Accessed from https://bit.ly/3500qi5

Herpers, B. L, Badoux, P., Totté, J. E. E., et al. (2014). *Specific lysis of Staphylococcus aureus by the bacteriophage endolysin Staphefekt SA. 100: In vitro studies and human case series.* Oral presentation on 5 Nov 2014 during the EuroSciCon conference Antibiotic alternatives for the new millennium 5th–7th Nov 2014, London, UK. Accessed January 1, 2021, from https://bit.ly/3n4tFqp

IDSA - Infectious Diseases Society of America. (2008). Position paper: Recommended design features of future clinical trials of antibacterial agents for community-acquired pneumonia. *Clinical Infectious Diseases, 47*(3), 249–265. https://doi.org/10.1086/591411.

IFPMA (International Federation of Pharmaceutical Manufacturers & Associations). (2016). *Industry roadmap for progress on combating antimicrobial resistance – September 2016.* Accessed December 30, 2020, from https://bit.ly/38LBfBc

Imi. (2020). *Innovative medicines initiative. COMBACTE-NET. Combatting bacterial resistance in Europe.* Accessed January 1, 2021, from https://bit.ly/2LywAuj

Investigative Report Denmark. (2014). *Danish journalists sentenced to fine for releasing names of infected farms – They will try to appeal the case.* Accessed December 26, 2020, from https://bit.ly/3poqqLV

Investigative Reporting Denmark. (2010). *Results of coverage of swine-MRSA in Denmark.* Accessed January 9, 2021, from https://bit.ly/2LEQmnR

Isler, B., Doi, Y., Bonomo, R. A., et al. (2019). New treatment options against carbapenem-resistant *Acinetobacter baumannii* infections. *Antimicrobial Agents and Chemotherapy, 63*(1), e01110–e01118. https://doi.org/10.1128/AAC.01110-18.

Joining Forces for Future Health. (2014, 25–26 June). *Outcome statement*. The Hague ministerial meeting "Joining Forces for Future Health". Accessed December 27, 2020, from https://bit.ly/38T2JF9

Jones, R. N., Fedler, K. A., Scangarella-Oman, N. E., et al. (2016). Multicenter investigation of Gepotidacin (GSK2140944) Agar Dilution quality control determinations for *Neisseria gonorrhoeae* ATCC 49226. *Antimicrobial Agents and Chemotherapy, 60*(7), 4404–4406. https://bit.ly/38tdb6W.

Klein, E. Y., Van Boeckel, T. P., Martinez, E. M., et al. (2018). Global increase and geographic convergence in antibiotic consumption between 2000 and 2015. *PNAS, 115*(15), E3463–E3470. https://doi.org/10.1073/pnas.1717295115.

Klein, E. Y., Milkowska-Shibata, M., Tseng, K. K., et al. (2021). Assessment of WHO antibiotic consumption and access targets in 76 countries, 2000-15: An analysis of pharmaceutical sales data. *The Lancet Infectious Diseases, 21*(1), 107–115. https://doi.org/10.1016/S1473-3099(20)30332-7.

Klevens, R. M., Morrsisson, M. A., Nadle, J., et al. (2007). Invasive methicillin-resistant Staphylococcus aureus infections in the United States. *JAMA, 298*(15), 1763–1771. https://bit.ly/2JCldAW.

Koenders, B. (2016). *Nederlands EU-voorzitterschap 2016*. Accessed December 27, 2020, from https://bit.ly/37Ti2hq

Kourtis, A. P., Hatfield, K., Baggs, J., et al. (2019). Vital signs: Epidemiology and recent trends in methicillin-resistant and methicillin-susceptible Staphylococcus aureus bloodstream infections – United States. *MMWR (Morbidity and Mortality Weekly), 68*(9), 214–219. Accessed from https://bit.ly/2KV67XV

Lemkes, B. A., Richel, O., Bonten, M. J., et al. (2019). New antibiotics: An overview. *Nederlands Tijdschrift voor Geneeskunde, 163*, D3107. Accessed from https://bit.ly/39gJipN

Lepore, C., & Kim, W. (2021). *Opportunities in 2021 to fix the broken antibiotics market*. The Pew Charitable Trusts. Accessed January 10, 2021, from https://bit.ly/2XrgAwV

Li, Y., Lv, Y., Xue, F., et al. (2015). Antimicrobial resistance surveillance of doripenem in China. *The Journal of Antibiotics, 68*, 496–500. https://doi.org/10.1038/ja.2015.25.

Manning, M. L., Davis, J., Sparnon, E., et al. (2013). iPads, droids, and bugs: Infection prevention for mobile handheld devices at the point of care. *American Journal of Infection Control, 41*(11), 1073–1076. https://doi.org/10.1016/j.ajic.2013.03.304.

Matt, T., Ng, C. L., Lang, K., et al. (2012). Dissociation of antibacterial activity and aminoglycoside ototoxicity in the 4-monosubstituted 2-deoxystreptamine apramycin. *PNAS, 109*(27), 10984–10989. https://doi.org/10.1073/pnas.1204073109.

Morubagal, R. R., Shivappa, S. G., Mahale, R. P., et al. (2017). Study of bacterial flora associated with mobile phones of healthcare workers and non-healthcare workers. *Iranian Journal of Microbiology, 9*(3), 143–151. Accessed from https://bit.ly/38rsrBu.

Mossialos, E., Morel, C. M., Edwards, S., et al. (2010). *Policies and incentives for promoting innovation in antibiotic research*. Accessed December 27, 2020, from https://bit.ly/3mSvxm7

Mouton, J. W. (2012). *Optimising use of old antibiotics: The PK/PD perspective*. Oral presentation at the ECCMID 2012 in London, 31 March–April, ExCel Centre, London UK. Accessed January 2, 2021, from https://bit.ly/2JDOxqR

Naderer, O. J., Jones, L. S., Zhu, J., et al. (2013). Safety, tolerability, and pharmacokinetics of oral and intravenous administration of GSK1322322, a peptide deformylase inhibitor. *The Journal of Clinical Pharmacology, 53*(11), 1168–1176. https://doi.org/10.1002/jcph.150.

O'Neill, J. (2014). *The review on antimicrobial resistance. antimicrobial resistance: Tackling a crisis for the health and wealth of nations*. Accessed December 27, 2020, from https://bit.ly/3aPsOCv

O'Neill, J. (2016). *The review on antimicrobial resistance. Tackling drug resistant-infections globally: Final report and recommendations*. Accessed December 27, 2020, from https://bit.ly/38AXI3P

O'Riordan, W., Tiffany, C., Scangarella-Oman, N., et al. (2017). Efficacy, safety, and tolerability of Gepotidacin (GSK2140944) in the treatment of patients with suspected or confirmed gram-positive acute bacterial skin and skin structure infections. *Antimicrobial Agents and Chemotherapy, 61*(6), e02095–e02016. https://doi.org/10.1128/AAC.02095-16.

OECD. (2018). *Stemming the superbug tide. Just a few dollars more. Policy brief.* Accessed January 3, 2020, from https://bit.ly/3n9V4qW

Piccirilli, A., Pompilio, A., Rossi, L., et al. (2019). Identification of CTX-M-15 and CTX-M-27 in antibiotic-resistant gram-negative bacteria isolated from three rivers running in Central Italy. *Microbial Drug Resistance, 25*(7), 1041–1049. https://doi.org/10.1089/mdr.2019.0016.

PSCI. (2020). *Pharmaceutical supply chain initiative.* Accessed December 30, 2020, from https://pscinitiative.org/about

Pulcini, C., Bush, K., Craig, W. A., et al. (2012). Forgotten antibiotics: An inventory in Europe, the United States, Canada, and Australia. *Clinical Infectious Diseases, 54*(2), 268–274. https://doi.org/10.1093/cid/cir838.

Reinhard, R. G., Kalinowski, R. M., Bodnaruk, P. W., et al. (2020). Fate of Listeria on various food contact and noncontact surfaces when treated with bacteriophage. *Journal of Food Safety, 40*(3), e12775. Accessed from https://bit.ly/3rSpOAv.

Rex, J. H., (2020). *Tetraphase sold for 14m… and 600m goes up in smoke!* Antimicrobial Resistance Solutions. Accessed April 9, 2021, from https://bit.ly/3ta5Mle

RIVM. (2018). *Bacteriophages: Insufficient understanding of phage treatment of human infections.* Accessed from https://bit.ly/3aYnv8J

Rosdahl, V. T., & Pedersen, K. B. (eds.) (1998). *The Copenhagen recommendations report from the invitational EU conference on the microbial threat.* Copenhagen, Denmark 9–10 September 1998. Accessed December 26, 2020, from https://bit.ly/38zw4nD

Rosenberg Goldstein, R. E., Micallef, S. A., Gibbs, S. G., et al. (2012). Methicillin-resistant *Staphylococcus aureus* (MRSA) detected at four U.S. Wastewater Treatment Plants. *Environmental Health Perspectives, 120*(11). https://doi.org/10.1289/ehp.1205436

Sadowy, E., & Luczkiewicz, A. (2014). Drug-resistant and hospital-associated *Enterococcus faecium* from wastewater, riverine estuary and anthropogenically impacted marine catchment basin. *BMC Microbiology, 14*(66). https://doi.org/10.1186/1471-2180-14-66

Schippers, E. I. (2012). *Letter to Parliament and report on the trip to China of the Minsiter of Health.* In Dutch. Accessed December 19, 2020, from https://bit.ly/3q2R25n

Schippers, E. I. (2013a). *Letter to parliament on the life sciences and health mission to Russia from 5-9 November 2013.* In Dutch. Accessed December 19, 2020, from https://bit.ly/39iMFwm

Schippers, E. I. (2013b). *Report on the life sciences and health mission to China from 8-13 September.* In Dutch. Accessed December 19, 2020, from https://bit.ly/2LA81x4

Schippers, E. I. (2014a). B*rief regering; Verslag een werkbezoek aan India van 29 tot en met 31 januari 2014.* Letter to Parliament on the trip of the Health Minister to India from 29-31 January 2014. In Dutch. Accessed December 26, 2020, from https://bit.ly/3hWBcXa

Schippers, E. I. (2014b). *Minister Schippers opens conference on antibiotic resistance.* Accessed December 27, 2020, from https://bit.ly/38tK8jJ

Schippers, E. I. (2016). *Statement by Dutch Minister of Health, Welfare and Sport, at the meeting of the committee on the Environment, Public Health and Food Safety, in Brussels 14 January 2016.* Accessed December 27, 2020, from https://bit.ly/3hns11D

Shebs, E. L., Lukov, M. J., Giotto, F. M., et al. (2020). Efficacy of bacteriophage and organic acids in decreasing STEC O157:H7 populations in beef kept under vacuum and aerobic conditions: A simulated high event period scenario. *Meat Science, 162*(108023). Accessed from https://bit.ly/3rLXe3l

Skipr. (2013). *Wereldwijde aanpak antibioticaresistentie.* In Dutch. Accessed December 20, 2020, from https://bit.ly/3oyAbag

Spellberg, B., Fleming, T. R., & Gilbert, D. N. (2008). Executive summary: Workshop on issues in the design and conduct of clinical trials of antibacterial drugs in the treatment of community-acquired pneumonia. *Clinical Infectious Diseases, 47*(3), 105–107. https://doi.org/10.1086/591389.

Statens Serum Institut. (2016). *Danmap 2015*. Accessed December 26, 2020, from https://www.danmap.org/reports/2015

Statens Serum Institut. (2020). *Danmap 2019*. Accessed December 26, 2020, from https://www.danmap.org/reports/2019

StopTB. (2020). *StopTB Partnership*. Accessed December 30, 2020, from https://bit.ly/3n1IdHk

Sulakvelidze, A., Alavidze, Z., & Morris, J. G., Jr. (2001). Bacteriophage therapy. *Antimicrobial Agents and Chemotherapy, 45*(3), 649–659. https://doi.org/10.1128/AAC.45.3.649-659.2001.

SumOfUs. (2015). *Bad Medicine. How the pharmaceutical industry is contributing to the global rise of antibiotic-resistant superbugs*. Accessed December 19, 2020, from https://bit.ly/37wTgDF

Swedish EU-Presidency. (2009). *Innovative incentives for effective antibacterials*. Accessed December 26, 2020, from https://bit.ly/2Jkj5xy

TATFAR. (2011). *Transatlantic Taskforce on Antimicrobial Resistance. Recommendations for future collaboration between the U.S. and EU*. Accessed January 1, 2021, from https://bit.ly/3hAkRaD

Taucer-Kapteijn, M., Hoogenboezem, W., Heiliegers, L., et al. (2016). Screening municipal wastewater effluent and surface water used for drinking water production for the presence of ampicillin and vancomycin resistant enterococci. *International Journal of Hygiene and Environmental Health, 219*(4-5), 437–442. https://doi.org/10.1016/j.ijheh.2016.04.007.

Taylor, S. N., Morris, D. H., Avery, A. K., et al. (2018). Gepotidacin for the treatment of uncomplicated urogenital gonorrhea: A phase 2, randomized, dose-ranging, single-oral dose evaluation. *Clinical Infectious Diseases, 67*(4), 504–512. https://doi.org/10.1093/cid/ciy145.

The Danish Council of Ethics. (2014). *The Danish Council of Ethics' statement on the use of antibiotics*. Accessed December 26, 2020, from https://bit.ly/3aN4ztx

The Federal Government. (2016). *Final Report on the G7 Summit*. See page 26 of the full report. Accessed December 26, 2020, from https://bit.ly/399C1rC

The Guardian. (2016). *GSK's Andrew Witty: The man who sold the world cheaper medicines*. Accessed January 1, 2021, from https://bit.ly/3aZAZBd

The Times of India. (2011). *Plan to ban OTC sale of antibiotics put off*. Accessed December 19, 2020, from https://bit.ly/2WIl2XX

The Times of India. (2012). *Curb on over-the-counter sale of 92 antibiotics soon*. Accessed December 19, 2020, from https://bit.ly/2WrXoid

The Times of India. (2014). *Over-the-counter sale of 46 drugs to be restricted from March 1*. Accessed December 19, 2020, from https://bit.ly/37w4NmT

The Wall Street Journal. (2014). *Drug makers Tiptoe back into antibiotic R&D. As superbugs spread, regulators begin to remove roadblocks for new treatments*. Accessed January 1, 2021, from https://on.wsj.com/2X1RFA0

The Washington Post. (2014). *Beyond antibiotics: A new weapon against superbugs shows promise share on Facebook share on Twitter share on Google Plus share via email more options*. Accessed January 1, 2021, from https://bit.ly/350sP82

Theuretzbacher, U. (2017). *AIDA. Preserving old antibiotics for the future*. Accessed January 2, 2021, from https://theuretzbacher.wordpress.com/aida/

UN. (2016). *Draft political declaration of the high-level meeting of the General Assembly on antimicrobial resistance*. Accessed December 30, 2020, from https://bit.ly/34XxLKB

UN News. (2016). *At UN, global leaders commit to act on antimicrobial resistance*. Accessed December 30, 2020, from https://bit.ly/38Rwkyz

Uppsala Universitet. (2014). *€85 million European programme targets novel antibiotics*. Accessed January 1, 2021, from https://bit.ly/3oceqNg

USCC. (2014). *Annual Report to Congress of the US-China Economic and Security Commission (USCC)*. See section 3 pp 127–182. Accessed December 19, 2020, from https://bit.ly/389kZLb

Van den Hoogen, A. (2009). *Infections in neonatal intensive care prevalence, prevention and antibiotic use*. Doctorate thesis. Accessed January 3, 2021, from https://bit.ly/352l4yo

Vlieghe, E. (2012). The first global forum on bacterial infections calls for urgent action to contain antibiotic resistance. *Expert Review of Anti Infective Therapy, 10*(2). https://doi.org/10.1586/eri. 11.162.

Wellcome Trust. (2010). *Image of new antibiotic in action opens up new opportunities to combat antibacterial resistance.* Accessed January 2, 2021, from https://bit.ly/355n8FA

WHO. (2011). *Millennium Development Goal 6.* Accessed December 27, 2020, from https://bit.ly/ 357ias9

WHO. (2013). *The use of Bedaquiline in the treatment of multidrug-resistant tuberculosis Interim policy guidance.* Accessed December 30, 2020, from https://bit.ly/2WUizJZ

WHO. (2015). *Global action plan on antimicrobial resistance.* Accessed December 27, 2020, from https://bit.ly/38aRLLG

WHO. (2018a). *Cancer. Key facts.* Accessed December 27, 2020, from https://bit.ly/389R4mc

WHO. (2018b). *WHO report on surveillance of antibiotic consumption 2016 - 2018 early implementation.* Accessed January 2, 2021, from https://bit.ly/3ogzxhO

WHO. (2020). *WHO model lists of essential medicines.* Accessed December 30, 2020, from https:// bit.ly/34ZsrXk

WHO Europe. (2014). *The role of pharmacist in encouraging prudent use of antibiotic medicines and averting antimicrobial resistance – A review of current policies and experiences in Europe (2014).* Accessed December 19, 2020, from https://bit.ly/2J551rL

Willemsen, I. E. (2010). *Improving antimicrobial use and control of resistant micro-organisms in the hospital.* Dissertation. Accessed January 1, 2021, from https://bit.ly/34WTaDB

World Bank. (2020). *New World Bank country classifications by income level: 2020-2021.* Accessed December 19, 2020, from https://bit.ly/38o9pdS

Zhanel, G. G., Cheung, D., Adam, H., et al. (2016). Review of Eravacycline, a novel fluorocycline antibacterial agent. *Drugs, 76*(5), 567–588. https://doi.org/10.1007/s40265-016-0545-8.

Printed in the United States
by Baker & Taylor Publisher Services